Care of the
Critically Ill Patient

SERIES EDITOR

Fred F. Ferri, M.D., F.A.C.P.

Clinical Assistant Professor
Department of Medicine
Brown University

Chief, Division of Internal Medicine
St. Joseph's Hospital
Providence, Rhode Island

OTHER VOLUMES IN THE
"PRACTICAL GUIDE TO THE CARE OF" SERIES

Ambulatory Patient

Geriatric Patient

Gynecologic/Obstetric Patient

Medical Patient

Pediatric Patient

Psychiatric Patient

Surgical Patient

Practical Guide to the
Care of the
Critically Ill Patient

Joseph Varon, M.D.

Assistant Professor of Anesthesiology,
Critical Care, and Medicine
Assistant Director, Surgical Intensive Care Unit
The University of Texas
M.D. Anderson Cancer Center
Houston, Texas

with 40 *illustrations*

Mosby

St. Louis Baltimore Berlin Boston Carlsbad Chicago London Madrid

Naples New York Philadelphia Sydney Tokyo Toronto

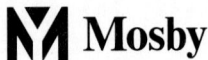

Mosby
Dedicated to Publishing Excellence

Executive Editor: Susan M. Gay
Developmental Editor: Sandra Clark Brown
Project Manager: John Rogers
Sr. Production Editor: Kathleen L. Teal
Manufacturing Supervisor: Kathy Grone
Design Coordinator: Renee Duenow
Cover Design: Malka Levy

Printed in the United States of America
Composition by the Clarinda Company
Printing/binding by R.R. Donnelley

Mosby–Year Book, Inc.
11830 Westline Industrial Drive
St. Louis, MO 63146

International Standard Book Number 0-8016-8106-5

94 95 96 97 98   9 8 7 6 5 4 3 2 1

Contributors

Stephen Brennan, M.D.
Assistant Professor of Medicine
Department of Medicine
Baylor College of Medicine
Houston, Texas

Robert J. Carpenter, Jr., M.D.
Associate Professor
Department of Obstetrics and
   Gynecology
Associate Professor
Department of Molecular and
   Human Genetics
Baylor College of Medicine
Houston, Texas

Arthur H. Combs, M.D.
Associate Professor of Medicine
Director, Medical Intensive Care
   Unit
Division of Pulmonary and
   Critical Care Medicine
Medical College of Pennsylvania
Philadelphia, Pennsylvania

Cynthia Curioso, M.D.
Resident
Department of Medicine
Providence Hospital
Washington, DC

Victor Fainstein, M.D.
Infectious Diseases Associates of
   Houston
Clinical Associate Professor
Baylor College of Medicine
Houston, Texas

Robert E. Fromm, Jr., M.D.,
   M.P.H.
Associate Professor of Medicine
Division of Cardiology
Baylor College of Medicine
Houston, Texas

Alex A. Lechin, M.D.
Pulmonary and Critical Care
   Fellow
Department of Internal Medicine
Section of Pulmonary and Critical
   Care
Baylor College of Medicine
Houston, Texas

J. Gabriel Martinez, M.D.
Resident
Department of Medicine
Providence Hospital
Washington, DC

Mauricio Reinoso, M.D.

Assistant Professor of Medicine
Baylor College of Medicine
Medical Director, Diagnostic
  Services
Pulmonary and Critical Care
  Section
Veteran Affairs Medical Center
  Houston
Houston, Texas

Pamela R. Roberts, M.D.

Assistant Professor of
  Anesthesia/Critical Care
  Medicine
Bowman Gray School of
  Medicine
Wake Forest University
Winston-Salem, North Carolina

Luviza Santos, M.D.

Resident
Department of Medicine
Providence Hospital
Washington, DC

George L. Sternbach, M.D.

Clinical Associate Professor
Department of Surgery
Stanford University Medical
  School
Stanford, California;
Emergency Physician
Seton Medical Center
Daly City, California

Joseph Varon, M.D.

Assistant Professor of
  Anesthesiology, Critical Care,
  and Medicine
Assistant Director, Surgical
  Intensive Care Unit
The University of Texas
M.D. Anderson Cancer Center
Houston, Texas

To my parents for pointing me in the right direction.

To my children, Adylle, Jacques and *Daryelle* for all the time taken away from them over the years.

To my wife Sara for all her love, support, and encouragement.

To the students and practitioners of Critical Care, who have provided me with a constant source of stimulation.

Preface

Intensive Care Medicine (Critical Care Medicine) is a relatively new subspecialty. However, over the past decade we have seen an enormous growth in the number of intensive care units (ICU) in the United States. In these units, thousands of medical students, residents, fellows and attending physicians (irrespective of their ultimate specialty), spend several months or years of their professional lives, taking care of critically ill or severely injured patients. These clinicians must have special training, experience, and competence in managing complex problems in their patients. They must interpret the data obtained by many kinds of monitoring devices, and they must integrate this information with their knowledge of the pathophysiology of disease.

This book was written for everyone engaged in Intensive Care Medicine. However, the primary beneficiaries of this book are more likely to be medical students, house officers, and other critical care physicians who consult their libraries as the clinical situation warrants. In addition, internists and surgeons involved with critical care medicine will find this book to be a valuable source of up-to-date information with respect to their own specialty and, perhaps more importantly, with respect to all other aspects of critical care.

We have attempted to depict both, basics and generally accepted standards of Intensive Care Medicine, as well as our personal points of view in each chapter. It contains numerous practical points regarding important procedures. Because the daily ICU routine is so important, a full chapter on this topic has been provided.

As a practical guide, this book follows an outline format providing the most important points in each subject. The chapters are divided by organ-system (i.e., neurologic disorders, cardiovascular disorders), as well as special topics (i.e., environmental disorders, trauma, toxicology). Some subjects, such as respiratory failure, are discussed in more than one section, but the management is essentially similar. In addition, each chapter reviews every topic systematically and uses reference citations *only* to complement the subject. However, Intensive Care Medicine is not a static field and there are changes occurring every day. Therefore, this book is not meant to be used to define standard of care but rather to be a general guide to current therapy.

Joseph Varon, M.D.

Acknowledgments

I am deeply indebted to Robert E. Fromm, Jr, M.D., M.P.H. and George L. Sternbach, M.D. for their energetic support in the realization of this project.

Contents

6   Endocrinologic Disorders, 95
Pamela R. Roberts

7   Environmental Disorders, 125
George L. Sternbach, Joseph Varon

8   Gastrointestinal Disorders, 149
Alex E. Lechin, Joseph Varon

9   Hematologic Disorders, 161
Alex E. Lechin

19 Trauma, 363
George L. Sternbach, Joseph Varon

20 Other Emergencies, 379
Joseph Varon

Key Telephone Numbers

This chapter is a listing of the phone numbers of departments and individuals in the hospital who might be needed for immediate consultation.

Department

Department	
Admitting	_____
Anesthesia	_____
CCU	_____
ECG	_____
EEG	_____
ER	_____
ICU	_____
Information	_____
IV Team	_____
Laboratory	_____
Chemistry	_____
Hematology	_____
Microbiology	_____
Other	_____
Medical Records	_____
Nuclear Medicine	_____
Paging	_____
Pathology	_____
Pharmacy	_____
Physical Therapy	_____
Pulmonary Function	_____
Radiology	_____
Recovery Room	_____
Respiratory Therapy	_____
Security	_____
Social Service	_____
Ultrasonography	_____
Other	_____

Nursing Stations

_____   _____
_____   _____
_____   _____
_____   _____
_____

House Staff

_____   _____
_____   _____
_____   _____
_____   _____
_____   _____
_____   _____
_____   _____
_____   _____
_____   _____
_____   _____
_____

Attending Staff

_____   _____
_____   _____
_____   _____
_____   _____
_____   _____
_____   _____
_____   _____
_____   _____
_____   _____
_____   _____
_____   _____
_____   _____
_____   _____
_____

Medical Record
Abbreviations

a arterial
(a-A)CO₂ arterial to alveolar gradient for partial pressure of carbon dioxide
(A-a)DO₂ alveolar to arterial gradient for partial pressure of oxygen
Aa alveolar/arterial
A₂ aortic second sound
āā of each
AB apical beat
ABC airway, breathing, and circulation
abd abdomen
ABG arterial blood gas
abn abnormal
ABVD doxorubicin (Adriamycin), bleomycin, vinblastine, dacarbazine (DTIC)
ac before meals
A/C assist control
ACE angiotensin converting enzyme, adrenocortical extract
acet acetone
aCL anticardiolipin (antibody)
ACLS advanced cardiac life support
ACT activated clotting time
ACTH adrenocorticotropic hormone
ADA American Diabetic Association, American Dietetic Association
ADH antidiuretic hormone
ADL activities of daily living
ad lib as desired, freely
adm admission
AF atrial fibrillation
AFB acid-fast bacilli
a fib atrial fibrillation
A/G albumin/globulin ratio
AG anion gap
AIDS acquired immune deficiency syndrome

AJ ankle jerk
AKA above-knee amputation
AL arterial line
alb albumin
alk phos alkaline phosphatase
ALL acute lymphoblastic leukemia
ALS amyotrophic lateral sclerosis
ALT alanine aminotransferase
AM morning
AMA against medical advice
AMI acute myocardial infarction
AML acute myelogenous leukemia
amp ampule
AMP adenosine monophosphate
amt amount
amy amylase
ANA antinuclear antibodies
ANCA antineutrophil cytoplasmic antibody
ANLL acute nonlymphocytic leukemia
AODM adult-onset diabetes mellitus
AOP aortic pressure
A&P auscultation and percussion
AP anteroposterior
APAG antipseudomonal aminoglycosidic penicillin
appt appointment
APSAC anisoylated plasminogen/streptokinase activator complex
APTT activated partial thromboplastin time
APUD amine precursor uptake decarboxylase
aq water
AR aortic regurgitation
ARC AIDS-related complex
ARDS acute respiratory distress syndrome, adult respiratory distress syndrome

ARF acute renal failure
ART assessment, review, and treatment
AS atriosystolic, aortic stenosis
asa aspirin
A.S.A. American Society of Anesthesiologists
ASH asymmetric septal hypertrophy
ASHD arteriosclerotic heart disease
ASLO anti–streptolysin O
AST aspartate aminotransferase
ATC around the clock
ATG antithymocyte globulin
ATN acute tubular necrosis
AV arteriovenous, atrioventricular
AVM arteriovenous malformation
AVP arginine vasopressin
AZT zidovudine
B black
ba barium
BACOD bleomycin, doxorubicin (Adriamycin), cyclophosphamide vincristine (Oncovin), dexamethasone
BACOP bleomycin, doxorubicin (Adriamycin), cyclophosphamide, vincristine (Oncovin), prednisone
BAL British anti-Lewisite (dimercaprol)
BBB bundle-branch block
BC blood culture
BCG bacillus Calmette-Guérin
BCNU carmustine
BCP birth control pill
BE barium enema
BEE basal energy expenditure
bid two times a day
bilat bilateral
bili bilirubin
BKA below-knee amputation
Bl s blood sugar
BM bowel movement
BMR basal metabolic rate
BP blood pressure
BPH benign prostatic hypertrophy
bpm beats per minute
BR bed rest
BRP bathroom privileges
BS or bs breath sounds, blood sugar, bowel sounds
BSA body surface area
BSO bilateral salpingo-oophorectomy
BTL bilateral tubal ligation
BUN blood urea nitrogen
BW body weight

Bx biopsy
c̄ with
C centigrade
C3 to C6 protein components of complement system
Ca cancer
Ca^{+2} calcium
(Ca-Cv̄) O$_2$ arterial to mixed venous difference in blood oxygen concentration
C/A Clinitest and acetone
CAB coronary artery bypass
CABG coronary artery bypass graft
CAD coronary artery disease
CAF cyclophosphamide, doxorubicin (Adriamycin), 5-fluorouracil
cal calorie
CaO$_2$ arterial oxygen content
cap capsule
CAT computerized axial tomography
cath catheterization
CAV cyclophosphamide, doxorubicin (Adriamycin), vincristine
CBC complete blood cell count
CBD common bile duct
cc cubic centimeter
CC chief complaint
CCr creatine clearance
CCU coronary care unit
CD4 helper-inducer T cells
CD8 suppressor-cytotoxic T cell
Cdyn dynamic compliance of the lung
CEA carcinoembryonic antigen
CF complement fixation, conversion factor
CGL chronic granulocytic (myelogenous) leukemia
CHD congenital heart disease
CHF congestive heart failure
CHO **cho** carbohydrate
CHOP cyclophosphamide, doxorubicin, vincristine (Oncovin), prednisone
CI cardiac index
CIE counterimmunoelectrophoresis
CK creatine kinase
CK-MB creatine kinase, myocardial band
cl clear
Cl$^-$ chloride
CLL chronic lymphocytic leukemia
cm centimeter
CM costal margin
CMF cyclophosphamide, methotrexate, 5-fluorouracil
CML chronic myelogenous leukemia

CMV cytomegalovirus, controlled mechanical ventilation
CNS central nervous system
CO cardiac output, carbon monoxide
c/o complains of
CO₂ carbon dioxide
CoA coenzyme A
COMLA cyclophosphamide, vincristine (Oncovin), methotrexate, leucovorin, cytosine arabinoside
conc concentrate
COPD chronic obstructive pulmonary disease
CPAP continuous positive airway pressure
CPK creatine phosphokinase
CPR cardiopulmonary resuscitation
Cr creatinine
CR cardiorespiratory
CRH corticotropin releasing hormone
C/S culture and sensitivity
CSF cerebrospinal fluid
C/sec cesarean section
Cst static compliance of the lung
CT computed tomography
Cu copper
CV cardiovascular
cva costovertebral angle
CVA cerebrovascular accident
CⱯO₂ mixed venous oxygen content
CVP central venous pressure
CXR chest X-ray
cysto cystoscopy
D&C dilation and curettage
D/C discontinue
D&S dilation and suction
DAT diet as tolerated
DBIL direct bilirubin
DCF 2′ deoxycoformycin
DDAVP desmopressin
ddI dideoxyinosine
DFA direct fluorescent antibody
DGI disseminated gonococcal infection
DHPG ganciclovir
Dial dialysis
DIC disseminated intravascular coagulation
dil dilute
DIP distal interphalangeal, desquamative interstitial pneumonitis
DKA diabetic ketoacidosis
DL_CO diffusing capacity of lung for carbon monoxide
dl deciliter

DLE drug-related lupus erythematosus
DM diabetes mellitus
DNA deoxyribonucleic acid
DOA dead on arrival
DO₂ oxygen delivery
DO₂(I) oxygen delivery index
DP dorsalis pedis
DPT diphtheria, pertussis, tetanus
DR delivery room
ds double strand
DSD dry sterile dressing
DTIC dacarbazine
DTR deep tendon reflex
DTs delirium tremens
DU duodenal ulcer
DUB dysfunctional uterine bleeding
DVT deep venous thrombosis
D₅W dextrose (5%) in water
Dx diagnosis
EBL estimated blood loss
EBV Epstein-Barr virus
ECF extended care facility, extracellular fluid
ECG electrocardiogram
ECM erythema chronicum migrans
ED emergency department
EDTA ethylene diamine tetraacetate
EEG electroencephalogram
EENT eyes, ears, nose, and throat
EF ejection fraction
EIA electroimmunoassay
EKG electrocardiogram
elect electrolyte
ELISA enzyme-linked immunoassay
elix elixir
EMD electromechanical dissociation
EMG electromyogram
ENT ear, nose, and throat
EOM extraocular movements
EPO erythropoietin
EPS extrapyramidal symptoms
ER emergency room, estrogen receptor
ERCP endoscopic retrograde cholangiopancreatography
ERS evacuation retained secundines
ERV expiratory reserve volume
ESR erythrocyte sedimentation rate
ESRD end-stage renal disease
EST, ECT electroshock therapy, electroconvulsive therapy
et al and others
EUA examination under anesthesia
ext extract, extremities
f respiratory rate
F Fahrenheit

FABM3 acute promyelocytic leukemia
FBS fasting blood sugar
FDP fibrin degradation products
Fe iron
FE fractional excretion
FEV forced expiratory volume
FF force fluids
FFP fresh frozen plasma
FH family history
FHM fetal heart monitor
FHR fetal heart rate
FIo$_2$ fraction of inspired oxygen
fl fluid, femtoliter
fL femtoliter
FMF familial Mediterranean fever
FNA fine needle aspiration
FRC functional residual capacity
FS frozen section
FSH follicle stimulating hormone
FTA-ABS fluorescent treponemal antibody absorbed
FTI free thyroxine index
5-FU 5-fluorouracil
FUO fever of undetermined origin
FVC forced vital capacity
fx fracture
g gram
Ga gallium
GA general anesthesia
GB gallbladder
Gc gonococcus
GERD gastroesophageal reflux disease
GFR glomerular filtration rate
GGT γ-glutamyltransferase
GGTP γ-glutamyltranspeptidase
GI gastrointestinal
GIP gastric inhibitory polypeptide
GITS gastrointestinal therapeutic system
glu glucose
GN glomerulonephritis
G$_6$PD glucose-6-phosphate dehydrogenase
gr grain
GSW gun shot wound
gtt drop
GTT glucose tolerance test
GU genitourinary
GVHD graft versus host disease
G/W enema glycerine and water enema
Gyn gynecology
H$_2$ histamine$_2$
H/A headache

HA hyperalimentation
HAV hepatitis A virus
Hb hemoglobin
HB$_c$Ag hepatitis B core antigen
HB$_s$Ag hepatitis B surface antigen
HBIG hepatitis B immune globulin
HBP high blood pressure
HBV hepatitis B virus
HCO$_3$$^-$ bicarbonate
hct hematocrit
HCV hepatitis C virus
HD hospital discharge
HDL high-density lipoprotein
HDV hepatitis D virus
HEENT head, eyes, ears, nose, and throat
Hg hemoglobin
H/H hemoglobin/hematocrit
5-HIAA 5-hydroxyindoleacetic acid
HIV human immunodeficiency virus
H&L heart and lungs
HLA human leukocyte antigen
HMG-CoA 3-hydroxy-3-methylglutaryl coenzyme A
HNP herniated nucleus pulposus
H$_2$O water
H$_2$O$_2$ hydrogen peroxide
HOCM hypertrophic obstructive cardiomyopathy
HORF high-output renal failure
H&P history and physical exam
HPI history of present illness
HR heart rate
HRS hepatorenal syndrome
hs hour of sleep (at bedtime)
HSV herpes simplex virus
ht height
HTN hypertension
hx history
I&D incision and drainage
IABP intraortic balloon pump
IBC iron-binding capacity
IBD inflammatory bowel disease
IBS irritable bowel syndrome
IC inspiratory capacity
ICF intracellular fluid
ICP intracranial pressure
ICU intensive care unit
ID intradermal
IDDM insulin-dependent diabetes mellitus
IFA immunofluorescent assay
Ig immunoglobulin
IHSS idiopathic hypertrophic subaortic stenosis
ILD interstitial lung disease

IM intramuscular
Imp impression
IMV intermittent mandatory ventilation
inf infusion
inh inhalation
inj injection
I&O intake and output
IOP intraocular pressure
IPG impedance plethysmography
iPLP parathyroid hormone–like protein by radioimmunoassay
IPPB intermittent positive pressure breathing
iPTH parathyroid hormone by radioimmunoassay
IQ Intelligence quotient
ISG immune serum globulin
ITP idiopathic thrombocytopenic purpura
IUD intrauterine device
IV intravenous
IVC inferior vena cava
IVP intravenous pyelogram
J joule
JG juxtaglomerular
JVD jugular venous distention
JVP jugular vein pulse
kat katal (mole/sec)
K⁺ potassium
KJ knee jerk
kg kilogram
17-KS 17-ketosteroid
KUB kidney, ureter, and bladder
l left
L liters, vascular volume
LA left atrium
lab laboratory
lac laceration
LAD left axis deviation
LAHB left anterior hemiblock
lap laparotomy
LAP leukocyte alkaline phosphatase
LAV lymphadenopathy-associated virus (same as HIV)
lb pound
LBBB left bundle-branch block
LBP low back pain
LDH lactate dehydrogenase
LDL low density lipoprotein
LES lower esophageal sphincter
LFT liver function test
LGV lymphogranuloma venereum
LH luteinizing hormone
LHRH luteinizing hormone–releasing hormone

Li lithium
Lip lipid
liq liquid
LLL left lower lobe
LLQ left lower quadrant
LMD local medical doctor
LMP last menstrual period
LNMP last normal menstrual period
LOC level of consciousness
LP lumbar puncture
LPHB left posterior hemiblock
LSB left sternal border
LSK liver, spleen, and kidney
LUL left upper lobe
LUSB left upper sternal border
LUQ left upper quadrant
LVEDP left ventricular end diastolic pressure
LVH left ventricular hypertrophy
LVSWI left ventricular stroke work index
L & W living and well
m murmur
M midnight, monoclonal
M1 to M7 categories of ANLL
MACE methotrexate, doxorubicin (Adriamycin), cyclophosphamide, epipodophyllotoxin
MAI *Mycobacterium avium intracellulare*
MAO monoamine oxidase
MAP mean arterial pressure
MAT multi-focal atrial tachycardia
max maximum
MB isoenzyme of cardiac origin
MBC minimum bactericidal concentration
MCA middle cerebral artery
MCL midclavicular line
MCP metacarpophalangeal
MCTD mixed connective tissue disease
MCV mean cell volume
med medication
MED medical
MEN multiple endocrine neoplasia
mEq milliequivalent
MERSA methicillin-resistant *Staphylococcus aureus*
mets metastases
MF maturation factor
mg milligram
Mg²⁺ magnesium
MH malignant hyperthermia
MHTAP microhemagglutination assay for antibody to *Treponema pallidum*

MI   myocardial infarction
MIBG   meta-iodobenzyl guanidine
MIC   minimum inhibitory concentration
min   minute
mixt   mixture
μkat   microkatal (micromole/sec)
ml   milliliter
ML   malignant lymphoma
μmol   micromole
mm   millimeter
mM, mmol   millimole
mod   moderate
MOM   milk of magnesia
MOPP   mechlorethamine, vincristine (Oncovin), procarbazine, prednisone
mOsm   milliosmol
MP   metacarpophalangeal
MPGN   membrane proliferative glomerulonephritis
MPTP   analog of meperidine (used by drug addicts)
MR   mitral regurgitation
MRI   magnetic resonance imaging
MS   mitral stenosis, mental status
MSU   monosodium urate
MTC   medullary thyroid carcinoma
MTP   metatarsophalangeal
MUGA   multiple gated (image) acquisition (analysis)
MVA   motor vehicle accident
MVP   mitral valve prolapse; mitomycin, vinblastine, cisplatin (Platinol)
MVV   maximum voluntary ventilation
N   normal
NA   not applicable
Na$^+$ sodium
NaHCO$_3$ sodium bicarbonate
NAPA   N-acetyl-procainamide, N-acetyl-paraaminophenol
NAS   no added sodium
NB   newborn
NCP   nursing care plan
neg   negative
NETT   nasal endotracheal tube
Neuro   neurology
ng   nanogram
NG   nasogastric
NGU   nongonococcal urethritis
NH$_3$ ammonia
NHL   non-Hodgkin's lymphoma
NIDDM   non–insulin-dependent diabetes mellitus

NKA   no known allergy
nkat   nanokatal (nanomole/sec)
NKDA   no known drug allergies
NM   neuromuscular
no   number
noc   night, nocturnal
NPH   normal pressure hydrocephalus, neutral protamine Hagedorn (insulin)
NPO   nothing by mouth
NS   normal saline
NSAID   nonsteroidal antiinflammatory drug
NSILA   nonsuppressible insulin-like activity
NSR   normal sinus rhythm
NTG   nitroglycerin
NYHA   New York Heart Association
OA   oral airway
OAF   osteoclast activity factor
OB   obstetrics
OD   overdose; right eye
OETT   oral endotracheal tube
17-OHCS   17-hydroxycorticosteroid
25-OHD   1, 25-dihydroxyvitamin D
oint   ointment
OOB   out of bed
OPD   outpatient department
opt   optimum
ophth   ophthalmology
OR   operating room
Oral   oral surgery
Ortho or ortho   orthopedics
OS   left eye
osm   osmolality
OT   occupational therapy
OU   each eye
oz   ounce
p   pulse
p̄   after
P wave   part of the electrocardiographic cycle representing atrial depolarization (stimulation)
P$_2$ pulmonic second sound
Paco$_2$ partial pressure of CO_2 in arterial blood
Pao$_2$ partial pressure of O_2 in arterial blood
P$_A$o$_2$ partial pressure of oxygen in the alveolar gas
P&A   percussion and auscultation
PA   posteroanterior, pulmonary artery
PADP   pulmonary artery diastolic pressure

P_{ALV} alveolar pressure

PA$\overline{OP}$ pulmonary artery occlusion pressure (wedge)

Pap   Papanicolaou

PAP   pulmonary artery pressure

para   number of pregnancies

PAS   paraaminosalicylic acid

PASP   pulmonary artery systolic pressure

PAT   paroxysmal atrial tachycardia

PAWP   pulmonary artery wedge pressure

pc   after meals

P_{CO_2} carbon dioxide tension

PCP   *Pneumocystis carinii* pneumonia, phencyclidine

PCWP   pulmonary capillary wedge pressure

PE   physical exam, pulmonary embolism

PEA   pulseless electrical activity

ped   pediatric

PEEP   positive end-expiratory pressure

PEEP$_i$ intrinsic PEEP, autoPEEP

PEFR   peak expiratory flow rate

per   by

PERRLA   pupils equal, round, reactive to light and accommodation

PFT   pulmonary function test

pg   picogram

PGE   prostaglandin E

PH   past history

phos   phosphorus

PHP   pseudohypoparathyroidism

PHR   peak heart rate

PI   present illness

PID   pelvic inflammatory disease

PIP   proximal interphalangeal

PKU   phenylketonuria

PLA   plasminogen activator

PLP   parathyroid hormone–like protein

PM   afternoon

PMI   point of maximum impulse

PMN   polymorphonuclear leukocyte

PMP   previous menstrual period

PM & R   physical medicine and rehabilitation

PMR   polymyalgia rheumatica

PND   paroxysmal nocturnal dyspnea

PNH   paroxysmal nocturnal hemoglobinuria

PO   by mouth

PO_4^{-3} phosphate

postop   postoperative

P_{O_2} oxygen tension

PP   postpartum

PPD   purified protein derivative

PPNG   penicillinase-producing *Neisseria gonorrhoeae*

PR   per rectum, pulmonic regurgitation, progesterone receptor

PR interval   part of electrocardiographic cycle from onset of atrial depolarization to onset of ventricular depolarization

Pra   right atrial pressure

preop   preoperative

prep   preparation

PROM   premature rupture of membranes

prn   as needed

PRSP   penicillinase-resistant synthetic pencillin

PS   pulmonic stenosis

(PS)   pressure support

PSGN   post-streptococcal glomerulonephritis

psi   pounds per square inch

PSVT   paroxysmal supraventricular tachycardia

Psych or psych   psychiatry

pt   patient

PT   prothrombin time, physical therapy, posterior tibia

PTA   prior to admission

PTC   percutaneous transhepatic cholangiography

PTCA   percutaneous transluminal coronary angioplasty

Pth   pathology

PTH   parathormone

PTRA   percutaneous transluminal renal angioplasty

PTT   partial thromboplastin time

PTU   propylthiouracil

PUD   peptic ulcer disease

PVC   premature ventricular contraction

PVR   pulmonary vascular resistance

PVR(I)   pulmonary vascular resistance index

PWP   pulmonary wedge pressure

PX   physical

q   every

Q   blood flow

qd   every day

qh   every hour

qhs   every bedtime

qid   four times a day

qns   quantity not sufficient

$\dot{Q}O_2$ oxygen transport

qod   every other day

QRS   part of electrocardiographic wave representing ventricular depolarization (stimulation)

qs   quantity sufficient

$\dot{Q}_s$ shunt blood flow

$\dot{Q}_s/\dot{Q}_T$ shunt fraction

r   right

R   respiratory rate (per min), respiratory quotient

RA   rheumatoid arthritis, right atrium

RAI   radioactive iodine

RAN   resident's admission note

RAP   right atrial pressure

Raw   airway resistance to air flow into the lung

RBBB   right bundle branch block

RBC   red blood cells

RDS   respiratory distress syndrome

RDW   red cell distribution width

R&E   round and equal

readm   readmission

REM   rapid eye movement

RF   rheumatoid factor

Rh   *Rhesus* blood factor

RIA   radioimmunoassay

RIND   reversible ischemic neurologic deficit

RL   Ringer's lactate

RLL   right lower lobe

RLQ   right lower quadrant

RML   right middle lobe

RN   registered nurse

RNA   ribonucleic acid

R/O   rule out

ROM   range of motion

ROS   review of systems

RPGN   rapidly progressive glomerulonephritis

RPI   reticulocyte production index

RPR   rapid plasma reagin

rpt   repeat

RQ   respiratory quotient

RR   recovery room

RSR   regular sinus rhythm

rt-PA   recombinant tissue plasminogen activator

R/T   related to

rT_3 reverse triiodothyronine

RTA   renal tubular acidosis

RTC   return to clinic

RUL   right upper lobe

RUQ   right upper quadrant

RV   right ventricle, residual volume

RVH   renovascular hypertension, right ventricular hypertrophy

Rx   therapy, treatment, prescription

S_1 first heart sound

S_2 second heart sound

S_3 third heart sound

S_4 fourth heart sound

$\bar{s}$ without

S/A   sugar and acetone

SA   sinoatrial

SAH   subarachnoid hemorrhage

Sao_2 percent saturation of hemoglobin with oxygen in arterial blood

sat   saturated

SB   stillbirth

SBE   subacute bacterial (infective) endocarditis

SBP   spontaneous bacterial peritonitis

SBT   serum bacterial titer

SC   subcutaneous

SCP   standard care plan

SDH   subdural hematoma

SGA   small for gestational age

SGOT   serum glutamic-oxaloacetic transaminase (aspartate aminotransferase, AST)

SGPT   serum glutamic pyruvate transaminase (alanine aminotransferase, ALT)

SI   Système Internationale

SIADH   syndrome of inappropriate secretion of antidiuretic hormone

SL   sublingual

SLE   systemic lupus erythematosus

SLR   straight leg raising

SMI   suggested minimum increment

SMS   somatostatin

SNF   skilled nursing facility

SO_2 oxygen saturation

SOB   short of breath

SOC   state of consciousness

sol   solution

S/P   status post

SQ   subcutaneous

SR   slow release

SRM   spontaneous rupture membranes

$\bar{ss}$ half

S/S   signs and symptoms

SS   Sjögren's syndrome

SSE   soap suds enema

SSKI   saturated solution potassium iodide

SSS   sick sinus syndrome

ST   segment part of electrocardiographic cycle representing the beginning of ventricular repolarization (recovery)

stat immediately
STD sexually transmitted disease
STS serologic test for syphilis
subcu, SC subcutaneous
supp suppository
Surg surgery
susp suspension
SV stroke volume
SVC superior vena cava
S̄v̄o₂ percent saturation of hemoglobin with oxygen in mixed venous blood
SVR systemic vascular resistance
SVT supraventricular tachycardia
Sx symptoms
syr syrup
T wave part of ECG cycle, representing a portion of ventricular repolarization (recovery)
T₃ triiodothyronine
T₄ thyroxine
T & A tonsillectomy and adenoidectomy
tab tablet
TAH total abdominal hysterectomy
TB tuberculosis
TBG thyroxine binding globulin, total blood gases
TBIL total bilirubin
TBNa total body sodium
Tbsp tablespoon
TBW total body water
T/C throat culture
temp temperature
TENS transcutaneous electrical nerve stimulation
Tg thyroglobulin
THBR thyroid hormone-binding ratio
TIA transient ischemic attack
TIBC total iron-binding capacity
tid three times daily
tinc tincture
TLC total lung capacity
TM tympanic membrane
TMP-SMX trimethoprim/sulfamethoxazole
TNM tumor-nodes-metastases
TO telephone order
top topical
TP total protein
tPA tissue plasminogen activator
TPI *Treponema pallidum* immobilization
TPN total parenteral nutrition
TPR temperature, pulse, and respiration

TR tricuspid regurgitation
TRAP tartrate-resistant acid phosphatase
TRF thyrotropin releasing factor
T₃RIA triiodothyronine level by radioimmunoassay
T₃RU T₃ resin uptake
TRH thyrotropin releasing hormone
TRIG triglycerides
TS tricuspid stenosis
TSAb thyroid stimulating antibodies
TSH thyroid stimulating hormone
tsp teaspoon
TT thrombin time
TTP thrombotic thrombocytopenic purpura, ribothymidine 5′triphosphate
TTS transdermal therapeutic system
TU tuberculin unit
TUR transurethral resection
TURP transurethral resection prostate
TV tidal volume
Tx therapy
U unit
UA umbilical artery
U/A urinalysis
UGI upper gastrointestinal
ung ointment
U/P urine/plasma ratio (concentration)
URAC uric acid
URI upper respiratory tract infection
USP United States Pharmacopeia
UTI urinary tract infection
UV ultraviolet
v̄ mixed venous
V volume
V_A alveolar gas volume
vag hyst vaginal hysterectomy
VAMP vincristine, doxorubicin (Adriamycin), methylprednisolone
VAT ventricular activation time
VC vital capacity
V̇_CO rate of carbon monoxide uptake per min
VD venereal disease
VDRL Venereal Disease Research Laboratories (test for syphilis)
V_D/V_T ratio of dead-space volume to tidal volume
VER visual evoked response
VF ventricular fibrillation
VIP vasoactive intestinal polypeptide
VLDL very low density lipoprotein
VMA vanillylmandelic acid
VPC ventricular premature contraction

V̇O   verbal order
V̇O₂   oxygen consumption
V̇O₂(I)   oxygen consumption index
V/Q scan   ventilation/perfusion scan
VR   venous return
vs   visit
VS   vital signs
VSD   ventricular septal defect
V$_T$ tidal volume
VT/VF   ventricular tachycardia/fibrillation
W   white
WBC   white blood (cell) count

w/c   wheel chair
WD   well developed
WF   white female
WHO   World Health Organization
WM   white male
WN   well nourished
WNL   within normal limits
WPW   Wolff Parkinson White
wt   weight
y/o   years old
X   times
ZDV   zidovudine
Z-E   Zollinger-Ellison (syndrome)

SYMBOLS

@   at
++   moderate amount
+++   large amount
0   zero, none
°   degree
♀   female
♂   male
number
↑   increased
↓   decreased

>   greater than
<   less than
μ or **μm**   micron (micrometer)
″   seconds
′   minute
∅   absence of
✔   check
−   negative, absence
△   changes

NOTICE: The science of medicine is constantly evolving. Every attempt has been made by the author and consultants to ensure that this manual includes the latest recommendations from the medical literature. Doses of drugs and treatment recommendations have been carefully reviewed. **However, it is strongly recommended that the reader become completely familiar with the manufacturer's product information when prescribing any of the drugs described in this manual.** This recommendation is especially important with new or infrequently used drugs. As new information becomes available, changes in treatment modalities invariably follow; therefore when choosing a particular treatment, the reader should consider not only the information provided in this manual but also any recently published medical literature on the subject.

Approach to the Intensive Care Unit

3

Joseph Varon

3.1 WELCOME TO THE ICU

What is an intensive care unit?

An intensive care unit (ICU) is an area of a hospital that provides aggressive therapy, state-of-the-art technology, and both invasive and noninvasive monitoring for critically ill and high-risk patients. In these units, the patient's physiologic variables serve as feedback to the practitioner on a continuous basis so that titrated care can be provided.

As a medical student, resident physician, and attending physician, one is likely to spend several hundred hours in these units caring for very sick patients. Knowing the function and organization of these specialized areas will help the practitioner in the understanding of critical care.

Historical development of the ICU

The origin of the ICU is controversial. In 1863, Florence Nightingale wrote: "In small country hospitals there are areas that have a recess or small room leading from the operating theater in which the patients remain until they have recovered, or at least recover from the immediate effects of the operation. . . ." This is probably the earliest example of what would become the ICU. Recovery rooms were developed at the Johns Hopkins Hospital in the 1920s. The first well-organized postoperative ICU was developed in Germany in the 1930s. In the United States more specialized postoperative recovery rooms were implemented in the 1940s at the Mayo Clinic. In the late 1950s, the first shock unit was established in Los Angeles. The initial surveillance unit for patients after acute myocardial infarction was started in Kansas City in 1962.

Economic impact of the ICU

Since the initial development of the ICU, there has been a rapid and remarkable growth of ICUs in the United States. There are presently an estimated 50,000 ICU beds in the United States and critical care consumes approximately 1.5% of the gross national product.

Organization of the ICU

ICUs in the United States may be *open* or *closed*. Open ICUs may be utilized by any attending physician with admitting privileges in that institution and many subspecialists may manage the patient at the same time. These physicians do not need to be trained in critical care medicine. In closed ICUs, management of the patient upon admission to the unit is provided by the ICU team and orchestrated by physicians with specialized training in critical care medicine. While there may be consultants on the case, all orders are written and all decisions are approved by the ICU team.

ICUs may be organized also by the types of patients the units are designed to treat. Examples include the neurosurgical ICU (NICU), the pediatric ICU (PICU), the cardiovascular surgery ICU (CVICU), the surgical intensive care unit (SICU), the medical intensive care unit (MICU), and the coronary care unit (CCU).

Most ICUs in the United States have a medical director who, with varying degrees of authority, is responsible for bed allocation, policy making, and quality assurance. The medical director may also be the primary attending physician for patients admitted to the ICU, particularly in closed ICUs.

3.2 TEAMWORK

Care of the critically ill patient has evolved into a discipline that requires specialized training and skills. When not at the patient's bedside, the physician in the ICU is dependent upon the nursing staff for accurate charting and assessment, as well as for the provision of the full spectrum of nursing care. This includes psychological and social support, and the administration of ordered therapies.

Complex mechanical ventilation devices need appropriate monitoring and adjustment. This expertise and other functions are provided by a professional team of respiratory therapy practitioners. The wide spectrum of the pharmacopeia used in the ICU is greatly enhanced by the assistance of pharmacy colleagues. Many institutions find it useful to have a pharmacist with advanced training help practitioners in determining the appropriate pharmacologic management of the critically ill patient. Additionally, experienced technicians may help in obtaining physiologic data and in maintenance of the monitoring equipment. Without these additional health care professionals, optimal ICU management would not be possible.

3.3 THE FLOWSHEET

By virtue of the critical illness, the ICU patient presents with complex pathophysiology and symptomatology. In many cases, these patients are endotracheally intubated and have mental status depression, and are therefore unable to provide historic information. In these cases, the physical examination, as well as the monitoring of physiologic and laboratory data, provides the information on which to base a diagnosis and initiate appropriate treatment.

The flowsheet is the repository of information necessary for the recognition and management of severe physiologic derangements in critically ill patients. A well-organized flowsheet not only provides around-the-clock information regarding the vital signs, but also about the different organ systems. In some institutions these flowsheets are computerized, theoretically to improve accessibility and allow real-time data. However, these devices are complex and expensive, and to date, no studies have proven that electronic flowsheets decrease charting time or improve care. Thus, caution in their adoption is warranted.

Major categories appropriate for an ICU flowsheet include the following:

- Vital signs
- Neurologic status
- Hemodynamic parameters
- Ventilator settings
- Respiratory parameters
- Inputs and output
- Laboratory data
- Medications

3.4   THE CRITICALLY ILL PATIENT

In general, ICU patients are not only very ill, but they may also have disease processes that involve a number of different organ systems. Therefore, the approach to the critically ill patient needs to be systematic and complete (see below).

Several issues need to be considered in the initial approach to the critically ill patient. The initial evaluation consists of assessment of airway, breathing, and circulation (ABC) with interventions performed as needed. An organized and efficient history and physical examination should then be obtained for all patients entering the ICU, and a series of priorities for therapeutic interventions established.

How to conduct rounds and how to write the ICU progress note

In the ICU accurate transmission of clinical information is required. It is important to compulsively follow every detail. The mode of presentation during ICU rounds may vary according to institutional tradition. Nevertheless, because of multiple medical problems, a systematic gathering and presentation of data are needed for proper management of patients. Some prefer presenting and writing notes in a "head-to-toe" format (see Box 3-1).

The ICU progress note is system-oriented. This differs from the problem-oriented approach commonly utilized on general medicine-surgery wards. The assessment and plan are formulated for each organ system as an aid to organization, and similar to the non-ICU chart, each progress note should contain a list of problems that is addressed daily. This problem list allows the health-care provider to keep track of multiple problems and enables the physician unfamiliar with a given case to understand its complexities should the need arise.

The art of presenting cases during rounds is perfected at the bedside over many years, but the following abbreviated guide may get the new member

Minimum Amount of Information Necessary for Presentation During Rounds

1. Identification/problem list
2. Major events during the last 24 hr
3. Neurologic
   Mental status, complaints, detailed neurologic exam (if pertinent)
4. Cardiovascular
   Symptoms and physical findings, record BP, pulse variability over the past 24 hr, ECG
   If CVP line and/or Swan-Ganz catheter in place, check CVP and hemodynamics personally
5. Respiratory
   Ventilator settings, latest ABGs, symptoms and physical findings, CXR daily if the patient is intubated. Other calculations (e.g., compliance, minute volume)
6. Renal/Metabolic
   Urine output (per hr and during the last 24 hr), inputs/outputs with balance (daily, weekly), weight, electrolytes, and if done, creatinine clearance. Acid-base balance interpretation
7. Gastrointestinal
   Abdominal examination, oral intake, coffee grounds, diarrhea. Abdominal X-rays, liver function tests, amylase, etc.
8. Infectious diseases
   Temperature curve, WBC, cultures, current antibiotics and number of days on each drug, and antibiotic levels
9. Hematology
   CBC, PT, PTT, TT, BT, DIC screen (if pertinent), peripheral smear. Medications altering bleeding
10. Nutrition
    TPN, enteral feedings, rate, caloric intake, and grams of protein.
11. Endocrine
    Do you need to check TFTs or cortisol? Give total insulin needs per hour and 24 hr
12. Psychosocial
    Is the patient depressed or suicidal? Is the family aware of his/her present condition?
13. Other
    Check the endotracheal tube position (from lips or nostrils in cm), and check CXR position. Check all lines, transducers. Note position of the catheter, skin insertion sites
    All medications and drips must be known. All drips must be renewed before or during rounds

of the ICU team off to a good start. Remember that for each system, there should be a full assessment of data, and a management plan should be provided.

Upon arrival in the morning:

1. Ask the previous night's residents and nurses about the patients.
2. Go to each patient's room. Review the flowsheet. Then proceed by reviewing each organ system as follows:

Identification

Provide name, age, and major diagnosis; day of entry to the hospital; day of admission to the ICU

Major events over the past 24 hours

Mention or list in the progress notes any significant medical event or diagnostic endeavor and treatment; e.g., major thoracic surgery, cardiopulmonary arrest, CT scan of the head, reintubation, or changes in mechanical ventilation

| 3.5 | SYSTEMS REVIEW |

Neurologic

- *Mental status:* Is the patient awake? If so, can a mental status examination be performed? If comatose, is the patient spontaneously breathing?
- *Glasgow Coma Scale score*
- Perform a detailed neurologic examination in patients with major neurologic abnormalities or where major disease process involves the central nervous system
- Consider the results of any neurologic evaluation in the past 24 hr; e.g., a lumbar puncture or CT scan

Cardiovascular

- *Symptoms and physical findings:* It is important to inquire specifically for symptoms of dyspnea and chest pain or discomfort. The physical examination should be focused on the cardiac rhythm, presence of congestive heart failure, pulmonary hypertension, pericardial effusion, and valvulopathies
- *ECG:* It is recommended that an ECG be considered in every ICU patient on a frequent basis. Since many ICU patients cannot communicate chest pain or other cardiac symptoms, an ECG may be the only piece of information that indicates cardiac pathology
- If the patient has a central venous line and/or a pulmonary artery (Swan-Ganz) catheter in place, check the central venous pressure (CVP) and hemodynamics *personally*. Hemodynamic calculations of oxygen consumption and delivery should be noted. (A detailed list of hemodynamic parameters useful in the management of critically ill patients can be found in the Appendix.)
- Note the blood pressure (BP) and pulse variability over the past 24 hr

Respiratory

- If the patient is on mechanical ventilation, the current ventilator settings need to be charted, including ventilatory mode; tidal volume; preset respiratory rate and the patient's own respiratory rate; amount of oxygen being provided (FIo_2); whether or not the patient is receiving positive end expiratory pressure (PEEP) and/or pressure support (PS); and when pertinent, peak flow settings and inspiration:expiration (I:E) ratio

Mechanically ventilated patients should have a daily measurement of the static and dynamic compliance, minute volume, and other parameters (see Appendix)

- Compare the most recent measurements of arterial blood gases (ABG) with previous measurements. Perform the calculation of the alveolar-arterial oxygen gradient (see Appendix)
- Note any symptoms or physical findings and, if pertinent, mention sputum characteristics
- Obtain a daily portable chest X-ray (CXR) in all intubated patients. Attention should be paid to CVP lines, endotracheal tubes, chest tubes, pericardiocentesis catheters, opacities in the lung fields (infiltrates), pneumothoraces, pneumomediastinum, and subcutaneous air

Renal/metabolic

- Urine output is quantified per hr during the past 24 hr. In patients requiring intensive care for more than 2 days, it is important to keep track of inputs, outputs, and overall daily and weekly fluid balance
- Daily weights
- Note electrolytes, including magnesium, phosphorus, calcium (ionized), and if performed, creatinine clearance, urine electrolytes, etc. Any changes in these values need special consideration
- The ABGs are used for acid-base balance interpretation. (The formulas most commonly used for these calculations are depicted in Chapter 16.)

Gastrointestinal

- *Abdominal examination:* A detailed abdominal examination may uncover new pathology or allow the assessment of changes in recognized problems
- If the patient is awake and alert, mention oral intake (e.g., clear liquids well tolerated)
- Mention the characteristics of the gastric contents or stool (e.g., coffee grounds, diarrhea)
- Review *abdominal x-rays,* if pertinent, paying special attention to the presence of feeding tubes, free air under the diaphragm, and bowel gas pattern.
- Note *liver function tests* (e.g., transaminases, albumin, coagulation measurements), pancreatic enzymes (e.g., amylase, lipase) when pertinent, as well as any changes since previous measurements

Infectious diseases

- *Temperature curve:* Note changes in temperature (e.g., "fever spike" or hypothermia), as well as the interventions performed to control the temperature. Note fever character, maximum temperature (T-max), and response to antipyretics
- The total white blood cell count (WBC) is mentioned, when pertinent, with special attention to changes in the differential
- *Cultures:* Culture (e.g., blood, sputum, urine) results should be checked daily with the microbiology laboratory and recorded. Those positive cultures should include the antibiotic sensitivity profile when available

- *Current antibiotics:* Mention current dosages and routes of administration as well as the number of days on each drug. Report any adverse reaction related to the administration of antibiotics
- For many antibiotics with known pharmacokinetics, antibiotic levels should be drawn to adjust their dosage (e.g., peak and trough levels for gentamicin)
- If the patient is receiving a new drug, either investigational or FDA-approved (e.g., antiendotoxin, newer antibiotics), side effects and/or benefits should be mentioned

Hematology

- *Complete blood cell count (CBC):* When presenting the results, it is important to be aware of the characteristics of the peripheral blood smear
- *Coagulation parameters:* The prothrombin time (PT), partial thromboplastin time (PTT), thrombin time (TT), bleeding time (BT), and disseminated intravascular coagulation screen (e.g., fibrinogen, fibrin split products, d-dimer, platelet count), should be addressed when pertinent
- Special attention should be paid to all medications that directly alter bleeding (e.g., heparin, desmopressin acetate), as well as those that indirectly alter it (e.g., ticarcillin-induced thrombocytopathy, ranitidine-induced thrombocytopenia)

Nutrition

- *Total parenteral nutrition (TPN):* State what kind of formula the patient is receiving, the total caloric intake provided by TPN with the percentage of fat and carbohydrates given. The total amount of protein should be mentioned with an assessment of the anabolic or catabolic state (see Appendix)
- *Enteral feedings:* These are similarly presented with mention of gastrointestinal intolerance (e.g., diarrhea)
- For both of the above, state the infusion rate, the nutritional needs of the patient, and what percentage of those needs is actually being provided

Endocrine

- Special attention should be paid to the pancreatic, adrenal, and thyroid functions. If needed, tests should be performed for the cortisol level or thyroid function. In most situations these determinations are not appropriate in the ICU, but under special circumstances they are necessary (e.g., hypotension refractory to volume resuscitation in a patient with disseminated tuberculosis should make you suspect Addisonian crisis). The results are not usually available immediately
- *Insulin:* Give the total insulin needs and blood sugar values (per hr and per 24 hr). Specify the type of insulin preparation being used
- For patients with hyperosmolal states and diabetic ketoacidosis it is necessary to determine calculated and measured serum osmolality, as well as ketones. The values for these should be charted and compared with those from previous days

Psychosocial

- Patients in the ICU tend to be confused and on occasion disoriented. Although these symptoms and signs are reviewed as part of the neurologic

examination, it is important to consider other diagnoses (e.g., depression or psychosis)
- In cases of drug overdose or depression, ask specific questions regarding the potential of new suicidal or homicidal ideations

Other

There are other parameters that must be checked daily prior to the morning or evening rounds:
- Check the endotracheal tube size and position (from the lips or nostrils in centimeters). Check its position on the CXR as mentioned earlier
- If the patient has a nasotracheal or orotracheal tube, perform a detailed ear, nose, and throat examination (e.g., patients with nasotracheal tubes may develop severe sinusitis)
- Check all lines with their corresponding equipment (e.g., transducers should be at an adequate level). Note the position of the catheter(s) both in the physical examination and on the X-ray. Also note the appearance of the skin insertion site(s) (e.g., in case of infection)
- Proper concentrations and infusion rates must be known for all medications and continuous infusions
- At the time of "pre-rounding" all infusions must be renewed. TPN orders need to be written early, with changes based on the most recent laboratory findings
- After rounds every morning it is important to prepare a list of the things that need to be done that day; e.g., changes in central venous lines or arterial lines or performing a lumbar puncture

3.6 DO NOT RESUSCITATE (DNR) AND ETHICAL ISSUES

Ethical issues arise every day in the ICU. For example, should a particular patient be kept on mechanical ventilation when there is an underlying malignancy? Should the patient with acquired immune deficiency syndrome (AIDS) receive CPR in the event of a cardiorespiratory arrest? Should the family be permitted to terminate mechanical ventilation or tube feedings?

These and similar questions are frequently asked and, in reality, may have no single correct answer. Although patients may express their wishes about resuscitation, ICU physicians need to discern the difference between the patient's wishes and futile attempts at care. Physicians are not obliged to provide life-support interventions that are useless.

DNR orders have become widely used in American hospitals in the past decade. A DNR order specifically instructs the patient's health-care provider to forego cardiopulmonary resuscitation should the patient undergo cardiac or respiratory arrest. Various levels of support may be agreed upon by patients, their physicians, and their families.

Different institutions have distinct categories of support. Examples include:
- *Code A:* full support, including CPR, vasopressors, mechanical ventilation, and surgery
- *Code B:* full support except CPR (no endotracheal intubation or chest compressions). However, vasopressor drugs are utilized in these cases
- *Code C:* comfort care only. Depending on the policies of the institution, intravenous fluids, antibiotics, and other medications may be withheld

A patient who has a DNR order may be in either of the last two groups. It is important that a full description of a particular triage status is provided, carefully explained to the patient and/or family, and discussed as needed.

As mentioned, the level of resuscitative efforts will depend on the patient's wishes. When the patient is unable to express those wishes, then the closest family member or another designated individual will make these decisions. For example, does the patient want full mechanical ventilatory support in the event of a cardiopulmonary arrest? Have provisions been made for a health-care surrogate should the patient become incompetent?

Ethical problems often can be resolved by seeking consultation with a group of individuals experienced in dealing with these issues. In many institutions an ethics committee is available to provide consultation to the practitioner regarding moral and ethical dilemmas.

Selected readings

Ayres SM, Combs AH: A tale of two intensive care units? All intensive care units are not the same! Crit Care Med 1992;20(6):727-8.

Bedell SE, Delbanco TL: Choices about cardiopulmonary resuscitation in the hospital. When do physicians talk with patients? N Engl J Med 1984;310(17):1089-93.

Engelhardt TH, Rie MA: Intensive care units, scarce resources and conflicting principles of justice. JAMA 1986;255(9):1159-64.

Piergeorge AR, Cesarano FL, Casanova DM: Designing the critical care unit: a multidisciplinary approach. Crit Care Med 1983;7(11):541-5.

Strauss MJ, LoGerfo JP, Yeltatzie JA, et al: Rationing of intensive care unit services: an everyday occurrence. JAMA 1986;255(9):1143-6.

Varon J, Sarinas P, Combs AH: Predictors of outcome in the intensive care unit. Hosp Physician 1991;27(5):19-22.

The Basics

4

Arthur H. Combs and Joseph Varon

Critical care medicine is an integrated discipline that requires the clinician to examine a number of important basic interactions. These include the interactions among organ systems, between the patient and the environment, and between the patient and life-support equipment. For example, gas exchange within the lung is dependent on matching ventilation and perfusion in quantity, space, and time. Thus, neither the lungs nor the heart is solely responsible; rather, the cardiopulmonary interaction determines the adequacy of gas exchange.

Many times critical care entails providing advanced life-support through the application of technology. Mechanical ventilation is a common example. Why is it that positive pressure ventilation and PEEP can result in oliguria or reduction of cardiac output? Many times clinical assessments and therapeutic plans will be directed at the interaction between the patient and technology; this represents a unique physiology in itself.

4.1 CARDIAC ARREST AND RESUSCITATION

Resuscitation from death is not an everyday event but is no longer a rarity. The goal of resuscitation is restoration of normal or near-normal cardiopulmonary function without deterioration of other organ systems.

1. Etiology
   The most common causes of sudden cardiac arrest are depicted in the Box on the facing page.
2. Pathogenesis
   a. Ventricular fibrillation (VF) or pulseless ventricular tachycardia (VT)
   b. Asystole
   c. Pulseless electrical activity (PEA) (electromechanical dissociation): Patients arresting with PEA can have a cardiac rhythm but no effective mechanical systole; thus, BP is unobtainable
   d. Cardiogenic shock: No effective cardiac output is generated
   e. The central nervous system (CNS) will not tolerate more than 6 min of ischemia at normothermia
3. Diagnosis
   a. Unexpected loss of consciousness in the unmonitored patient
   b. Loss of palpable central arterial pulse
   c. Respiratory arrest in a patient previously breathing spontaneously

---

Common Causes of Sudden Nontraumatic Cardiac Arrest

1. Primary cardiac event
   a. Coronary artery disease (CAD)
   b. Dysrhythmias due to
      (1) Hyperkalemia
      (2) Severe acidemia
      (3) Other electrolyte disturbances
   c. Myocarditis
   d. Tamponade
2. Secondary to a respiratory arrest (e.g., children)
3. Secondary to acute respiratory failure
   a. Hypoxemia
   b. Hypercapnia
4. Extreme alterations in body temperature
5. Drug effects
   a. Digitalis
   b. Quinidine
   c. Tricyclic antidepressants
   d. Cocaine

---

4. Differential diagnosis
   a. Syncope or vasovagal reactions
   b. Coma
   c. Collapse
   d. Seizures
5. Management
   a. Cardiopulmonary resuscitation
      (1) The main indications for CPR in the ICU include
         (a) Cardiovascular collapse
         (b) Respiratory arrest with or without cardiac arrest
      (2) Mechanisms of blood flow during CPR
         (a) Direct compression of the heart between the sternum and vertebral column "squeezes" blood from the ventricles into the great vessels
         (b) Changes in intrathoracic pressure generate gradients between the peripheral venous and arterial beds resulting in forward flow
         (c) During CPR, the dynamics of the chest compression process may play a major role in determining the outcome of the resuscitation effort
      (3) Technique
         (a) Establish an effective airway (see Chapter 15)
            (i) Assess airway and breathing first (open airway, look, listen, and feel)
            (ii) If respiratory arrest has occurred, the possibility of a

foreign body obstruction needs to be considered and
measures taken to relieve it
(iii) If endotracheal intubation is to be performed, the maximum interruption of ventilation should be 30 seconds
(iv) The respiratory rate during cardiac or respiratory arrest
should be 10 to 12 breaths/min. Once spontaneous circulation has been restored, 12 to 15 breaths/min

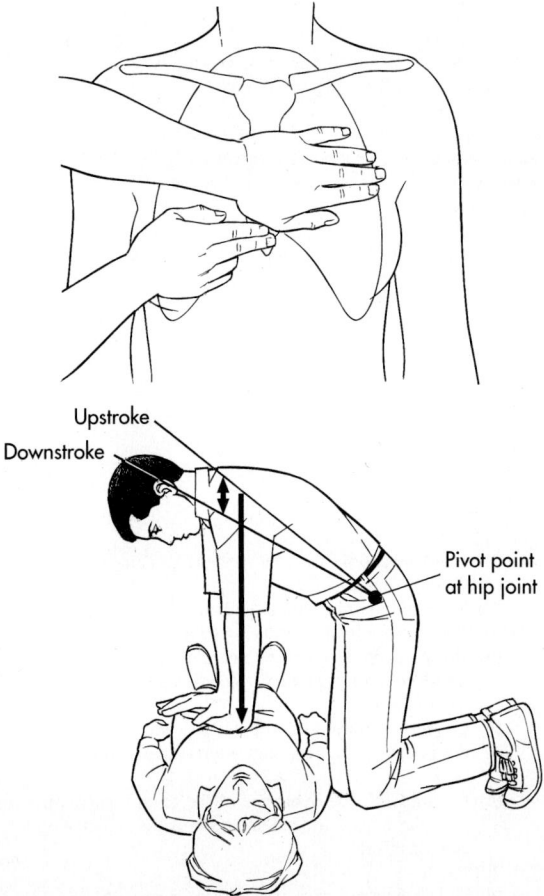

Figure 4-1
External chest compressions. *Top,* locating the correct hand position on the lower
half of the sternum. *Bottom,* correct position. (From American Red Cross: *First aid-
responding to emergencies.* ed 1, St. Louis, 1991, Mosby.)

(v) Ventilations should be performed with a tidal volume of 10-15 mL/kg of ideal body weight

(vi) The highest possible concentration of oxygen (100%) should be administered to all patients receiving CPR

(b) Determine pulse. If no pulse, start CPR immediately

(c) Chest compressions. Current basic and advanced cardiovascular life support (ACLS) recommendations:

  (i) Rescuer's hand located in the lower margin of sternum (see Fig. 4-1)

  (ii) Heel of one hand is placed on the lower half of the sternum; the other hand is placed on top of the hand on the sternum so that the hands are parallel

  (iii) Elbows are locked in position, the arms are straightened, and the rescuer's shoulders are positioned directly over the hands, providing a straight thrust (see Fig. 4-1)

  (iv) The sternum is depressed 1½ to 2 inches in normal-sized adults with each compression at a rate of 80 to 100/min

  (v) Current areas of investigation:
   • Mechanical versus manual CPR
   • High-impulse CPR
   • Interposed abdominal compressions
   • Active compression-decompression
   • Vest CPR

  (vi) Determinants of efficacy of CPR:
   • Systolic pressure of at least 60 mm Hg

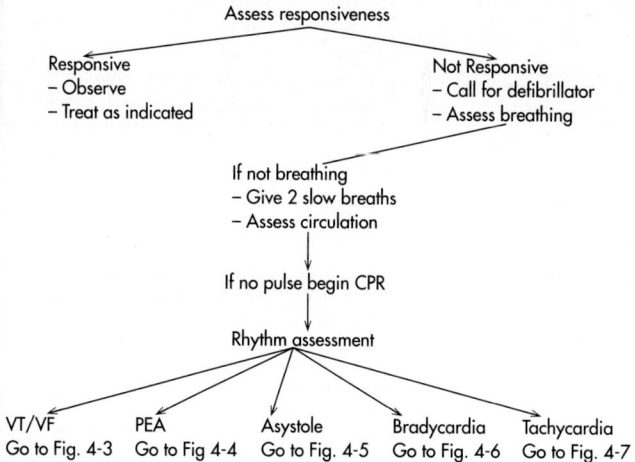

Figure 4-2

The algorithm approach. (Modified from *JAMA* Emergency Cardiac Care Committee and Subcommittees, American Heart Association. *Guidelines for cardiopulmonary resuscitation and emergency cardiac care, III: Adult advanced cardiac life support.* 1992; 268:2216.)

- End-tidal CO_2 ($ETCO_2$): Initial $ETCO_2$ values may predict whether or not the patient will regain a perfusing rhythm during resuscitation

(d) Cardiac monitoring and dysrhythmia recognition (see Chapter 5)
  (i) Distinguish between ventricular and supraventricular rhythms

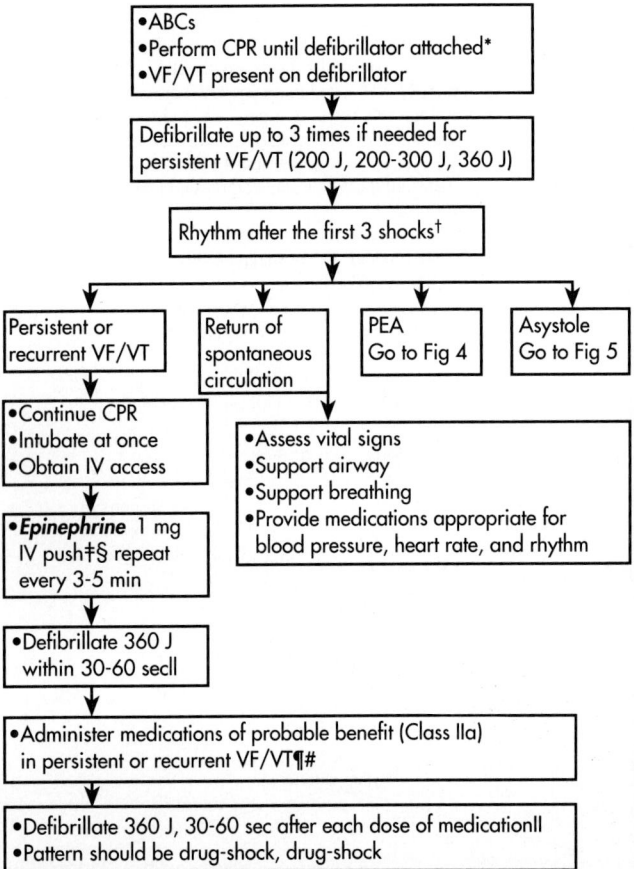

```
•ABCs
•Perform CPR until defibrillator attached*
•VF/VT present on defibrillator
        │
        ▼
Defibrillate up to 3 times if needed for
persistent VF/VT (200 J, 200-300 J, 360 J)
        │
        ▼
Rhythm after the first 3 shocks†
```

| Persistent or recurrent VF/VT | Return of spontaneous circulation | PEA Go to Fig 4 | Asystole Go to Fig 5 |

```
•Continue CPR
•Intubate at once
•Obtain IV access
        │
        ▼
•Epinephrine 1 mg
 IV push‡§ repeat
 every 3-5 min
        │
        ▼
•Defibrillate 360 J
 within 30-60 sec‖
        │
        ▼
•Administer medications of probable benefit (Class IIa)
 in persistent or recurrent VF/VT¶#
        │
        ▼
•Defibrillate 360 J, 30-60 sec after each dose of medication‖
•Pattern should be drug-shock, drug-shock
```

Return of spontaneous circulation:
- Assess vital signs
- Support airway
- Support breathing
- Provide medications appropriate for blood pressure, heart rate, and rhythm

Figure 4-3

Algorithm for ventricular fibrillation (VF) and pulseless ventricular tachycardia (VT). (From *JAMA* Emergency Cardiac Care Committee and Subcommittees, American Heart Association. *Guidelines for cardiopulmonary resuscitation and emergency cardiac care, III: Adult advanced cardiac life support.* 1992; 268:2217.)   *Continued.*

- Most rapid, wide QRS rhythms are VT
- Initiate therapy immediately (see below)

(e) Defibrillation is the major determinant of survival in cardiac arrest resulting from ventricular fibrillation

    (i) The energy requirements for different conditions vary (see below)

    (ii) Electrodes should be properly placed to maximize the current through the myocardium

(f) Drug therapy during CPR may given by the following routes

---

Class I: definitely helpful

Class IIa: acceptable, probably helpful

Class IIb: acceptable, possibly helpful

Class III: not indicated, may be harmful

*Precordial thump is a Class IIb action in witnessed arrest, no pulse, and no defibrillator immediately available.

†Hypothermic cardiac arrest is treated differently after this point. See section on hypothermia.

‡The recommended dose of **epinephrine** is 1 mg IV push every 3-5 min. If this approach fails, several Class IIb dosing regimens can be considered:
- Intermediate: **epinephrine** 2-5 mg IV push, every 3-5 min
- Escalating: **epinephrine** 1 mg-3 mg-5 mg IV push (3 min apart)
- High: **epinephrine** 0.1 mg/kg IV push, every 3-5 min

§**Sodium bicarbonate** (1 mEq/kg) is Class I if patient has known preexisting hyperkalemia

‖Multiple sequenced shocks (200J, 200-300J, 360J) are acceptable here (Class I), especially when medications are delayed.

¶•**Lidocaine** 1.5 mg/kg IV push. Repeat in 3-5 min to total loading dose of 3 mg/kg; then use
- **Bretylium** 5 mg/kg IV push. Repeat in 5 min at 10 mg/kg
- **Magnesium sulfate** 1-2 g IV in torsades de pointes or suspected hypomagnesemic state or severe refractory VF
- **Procainamide** 30 mg/min in refractory VF (maximum total 17 mg/kg)

#•**Sodium bicarbonate** (1 mEq/kg IV):

Class IIa
- if known preexisting bicarbonate-responsive acidosis
- if overdose with tricyclic antidepressants
- to alkalinize the urine in drug overdoses

Class IIb
- if intubated and continued long arrest interval
- upon return of spontaneous circulation after long arrest interval

Class III
- hypoxic lactic acidosis

Figure 4-3, cont'd

(i) Peripheral vein (antecubital or external jugular are preferred)
(ii) Central venous line (subclavian or internal jugular). On occasion a long line that extends above the diaphragm can be started in the femoral vein
(iii) Endotracheal: Medications should be administered at 2-2.5 times the recommended IV dose and should be diluted in 10 ml of normal saline or distilled water. A catheter should be passed beyond the tip of the endotracheal

PEA Includes
- Electromechanical dissociation (EMD)
- Pseudo-EMD
- Idioventricular rhythms
- Ventricular escape rhythms
- Bradyasystolic rhythms
- Postdefibrillation idioventricular rhythms

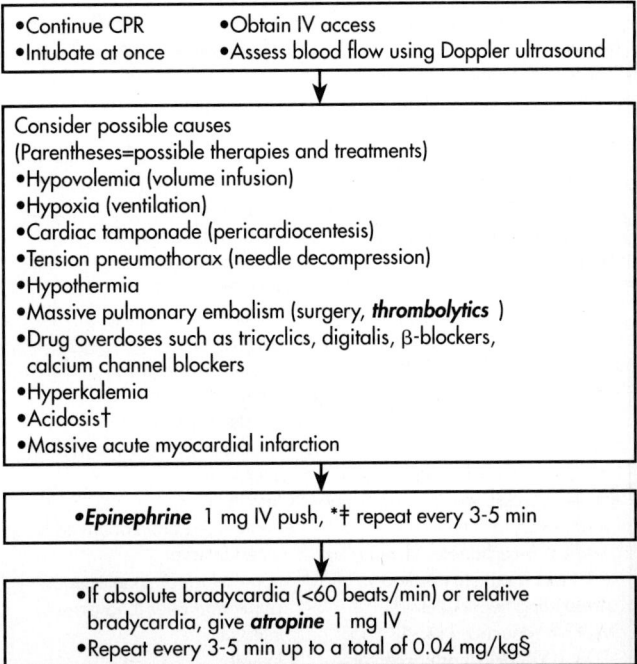

- Continue CPR
- Intubate at once
- Obtain IV access
- Assess blood flow using Doppler ultrasound

↓

Consider possible causes
(Parentheses=possible therapies and treatments)
- Hypovolemia (volume infusion)
- Hypoxia (ventilation)
- Cardiac tamponade (pericardiocentesis)
- Tension pneumothorax (needle decompression)
- Hypothermia
- Massive pulmonary embolism (surgery, *thrombolytics*)
- Drug overdoses such as tricyclics, digitalis, β-blockers, calcium channel blockers
- Hyperkalemia
- Acidosis†
- Massive acute myocardial infarction

↓

- *Epinephrine* 1 mg IV push, *‡ repeat every 3-5 min

↓

- If absolute bradycardia (<60 beats/min) or relative bradycardia, give *atropine* 1 mg IV
- Repeat every 3-5 min up to a total of 0.04 mg/kg§

Figure 4-4
Algorithm for pulseless electrical activity (PEA) Also known as electromechanical dissociation. (From *JAMA* Emergency Cardiac Care Committee and Subcommittees, American Heart Association. *Guidelines for cardiopulmonary resuscitation and emergency cardiac care, III: Adult advanced cardiac life support.* 1992; 268:2219.)

Continued.

tube and the medication sprayed quickly, followed by several quick insufflations

(iv) Intraosseous: particularly useful in pediatric patients

(v) The different drug dosages utilized during CPR and in the immediate post-resuscitation period are depicted in the Appendix

(g) The algorithm approach (see Fig. 4-2):

(i) ABCs

(ii) Call for defibrillator

(iii) If no circulation start CPR (as above)

(iv) Assess rhythm (see Appendix)

(v) If VT/VF are present, follow the algorithm presented in Fig. 4-3

(vi) If PEA is present, follow the algorithm in Fig. 4-4

(vii) If asystole is present, follow the algorithm in Fig. 4-5

(viii) For bradycardia follow the algorithm in Fig. 4-6

(ix) For tachycardia follow the algorithms presented in Figs. 4-7 and 4-8   *Text continued on p. 34.*

Class I: definitely helpful
Class IIa: acceptable, probably helpful
Class IIb: acceptable, possibly helpful
Class III: not indicated, may be harmful

*Sodium bicarbonate 1mEq/kg is Class I if patient has known preexisting hyperkalemia

†*Sodium bicarbonate* 1 mEq/kg:

Class IIa
- if known preexisting bicarbonate-responsive acidosis
- if overdose with tricyclic antidepressants
- to alkalinize the urine in drug overdoses

Class IIb
- if intubated and long arrest interval
- upon return of spontaneous circulation after long arrest interval

Class III
- hypoxic lactic acidosis

‡The recommended dose of *epinephrine* is 1mg IV push every 3-5 min.
If this approach fails, several Class IIb dosing regimens can be considered.
- Intermediate: *epinephrine* 2-5 mg IV push, every 3-5 min
- Escalating: *epinephrine* 1mg-3 mg-5 mg IV push (3 min apart)
- High: *epinephrine* 0.1mg/kg IV push, every 3-5 min

§Shorter *atropine* dosing intervals are possibly helpful in cardiac arrest (Class IIb).

Figure 4-4, cont'd

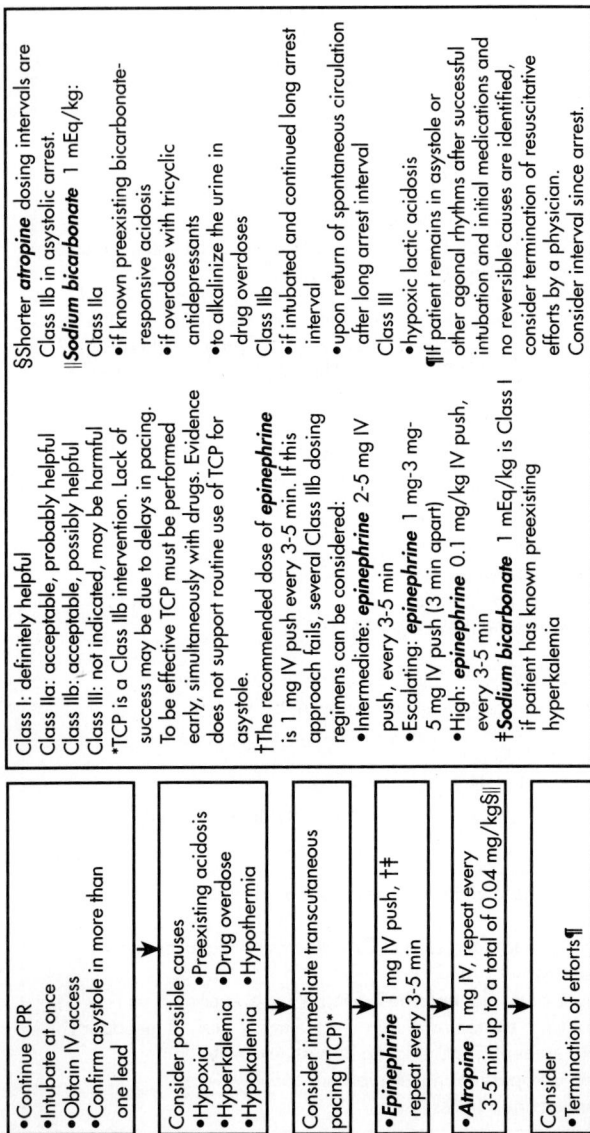

Figure 4-5

Asystole treatment algorithm. (From *JAMA* Emergency Cardiac Care Committee and Subcommittees, American Heart Association. *Guidelines for cardiopulmonary resuscitation and emergency cardiac care, III: Adult advanced cardiac life support. 1992; 268:2220.*)

- Assess ABCs
- Secure airway
- Administer oxygen
- Start IV
- Attach monitor, pulse oximeter, and automatic sphygomanometer

- Assess vital signs
- Review history
- Perform physical examination
- Order 12-lead ECG
- Order portable chest roentgenogram

Too slow (<60 beats/min)

Bradycardia
Either absolute (<60 beats/min) or relative

Serious signs or symptoms?*†

No

Yes

Type II second-degree AV heart block? or Third-degree AV heart block?‖

Intervention sequence
- *Atropine* 0.5-1.0 mg ‡§ (I & IIa)
- TCP, if available (I)
- *Dopamine* 5-20 μg/kg per min (IIb)
- *Epinephrine* 2-10 μg per min (IIb)
- *Isoproterenol*¶

No

Yes

- Observe

- Prepare for transvenous pacer
- Use TCP as a bridge device#

*Serious signs or symptoms must be related to the slow rate. Clinical manifestations include:
 symptoms (chest pain, shortness of breath, decreased level of conciousness) and
 signs (low BP, shock, pulmonary congestion, CHF, acute MI).
†Do not delay TCP while awaiting IV access or for *atropine* to take effect if patient is symptomatic.
‡Denervated transplanted hearts will not respond to *atropine*. Go at once to pacing, catecholamine infusion, or both.
§*Atropine* should be given in repeat doses in 3-5 min up to total of 0.04 mg/kg. Consider shorter dosing intervals in severe clinical conditions. It has been suggested that atropine should be used with caution in atrioventricular (AV) block at the His-Purkinje level (type II AV block and new third-degree block with wide QRS complexes) (Class IIb).
‖Never treat third-degree heart block plus ventricular escape beats with *lidocaine*.
¶*Isoproterenol* should be used, if at all, with extreme caution. At low doses it is Class IIb (possibly helpful); at higher doses it is Class III (harmful).
#Verify patient tolerance and mechanical capture. Use analgesia and sedation as needed.

Figure 4-6

Bradycardia treatment algorithm. (From *JAMA* Emergency Cardiac Care Committee and Subcommittees, American Heart Association. *Guidelines for cardiopulmonary resuscitation and emergency cardiac care, III: Adult advanced cardiac life support.* 1992; 268:2221.)

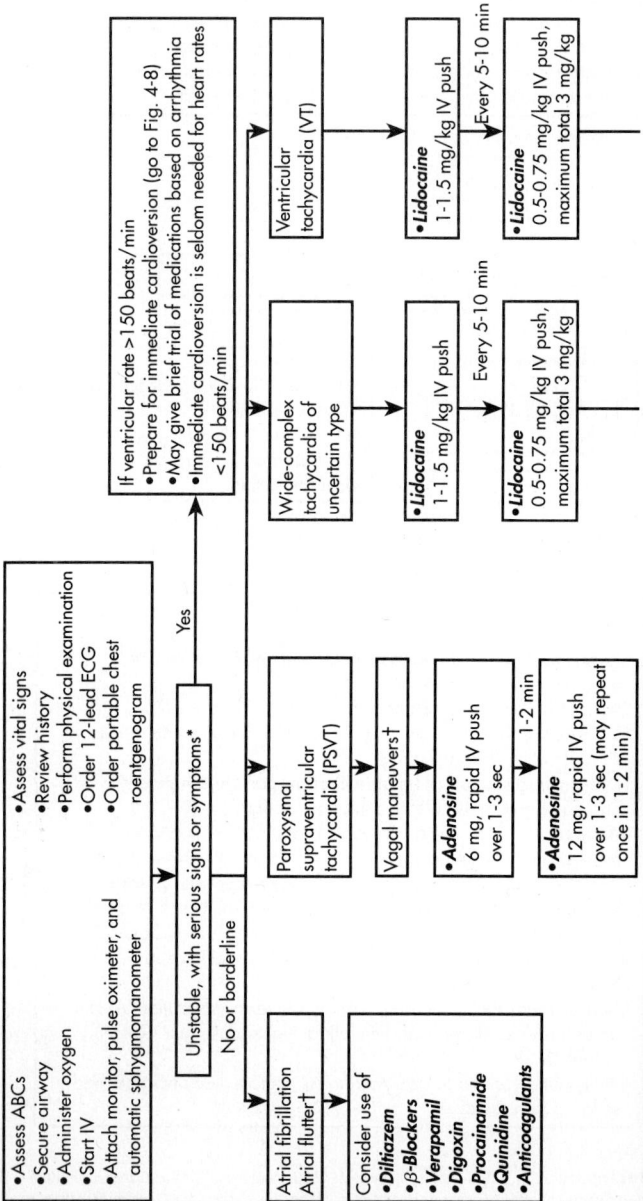

- Assess ABCs
- Secure airway
- Administer oxygen
- Start IV
- Attach monitor, pulse oximeter, and automatic sphygmomanometer

- Assess vital signs
- Review history
- Perform physical examination
- Order 12-lead ECG
- Order portable chest roentgenogram

↓

Unstable, with serious signs or symptoms*

No or borderline ↓   Yes →

No or borderline path:

Atrial fibrillation
Atrial flutter†

Consider use of
- *Diltiazem*
- *β-Blockers*
- *Verapamil*
- *Digoxin*
- *Procainamide*
- *Quinidine*
- *Anticoagulants*

Paroxysmal supraventricular tachycardia (PSVT)

→ Vagal maneuvers†

→ •*Adenosine* 6 mg, rapid IV push over 1-3 sec

1-2 min

→ •*Adenosine* 12 mg, rapid IV push over 1-3 sec (may repeat once in 1-2 min)

Yes path:

- Prepare for immediate cardioversion (go to Fig. 4-8)
- May give brief trial of medications based on arrhythmia
- Immediate cardioversion is seldom needed for heart rates <150 beats/min

If ventricular rate >150 beats/min

Wide-complex tachycardia of uncertain type

→ •*Lidocaine* 1-1.5 mg/kg IV push

Every 5-10 min

→ •*Lidocaine* 0.5-0.75 mg/kg IV push, maximum total 3 mg/kg

Ventricular tachycardia (VT)

→ •*Lidocaine* 1-1.5 mg/kg IV push

Every 5-10 min

→ •*Lidocaine* 0.5-0.75 mg/kg IV push, maximum total 3 mg/kg

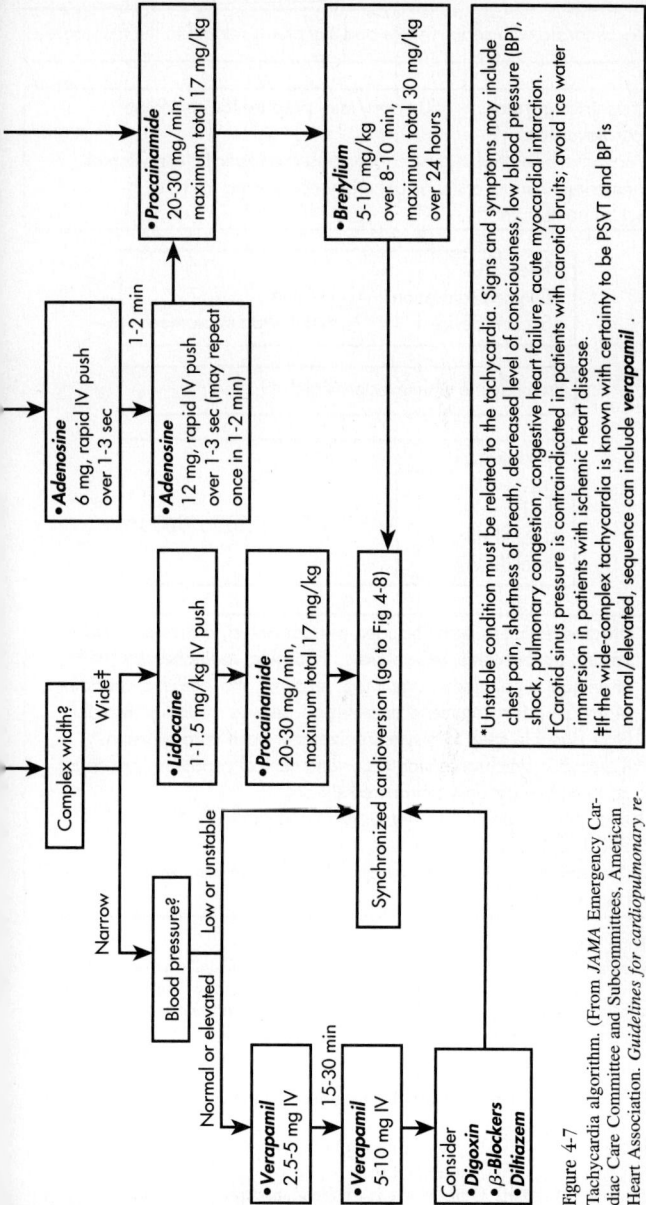

Figure 4-7
Tachycardia algorithm. (From *JAMA* Emergency Cardiac Care Committee and Subcommittees, American Heart Association. *Guidelines for cardiopulmonary resuscitation and emergency cardiac care, III: Adult advanced cardiac life support.* 1992; 268:2223.)

*Unstable condition must be related to the tachycardia. Signs and symptoms may include chest pain, shortness of breath, decreased level of consciousness, low blood pressure (BP), shock, pulmonary congestion, congestive heart failure, acute myocardial infarction.

†Carotid sinus pressure is contraindicated in patients with carotid bruits; avoid ice water immersion in patients with ischemic heart disease.

‡If the wide-complex tachycardia is known with certainty to be PSVT and BP is normal/elevated, sequence can include *verapamil* .

Complex width?

Wide‡

Narrow

Blood pressure?

Low or unstable

Normal or elevated

• *Lidocaine*
1-1.5 mg/kg IV push

• *Procainamide*
20-30 mg/min,
maximum total 17 mg/kg

Synchronized cardioversion (go to Fig 4-8)

• *Verapamil*
2.5-5 mg IV

15-30 min

• *Verapamil*
5-10 mg IV

Consider
• *Digoxin*
• *β-Blockers*
• *Diltiazem*

• *Adenosine*
6 mg, rapid IV push
over 1-3 sec

• *Adenosine*
12 mg, rapid IV push
over 1-3 sec (may repeat
once in 1-2 min)

1-2 min

• *Procainamide*
20-30 mg/min,
maximum total 17 mg/kg

• *Bretylium*
5-10 mg/kg
over 8-10 min,
maximum total 30 mg/kg
over 24 hours

Tachycardia with serious signs and symptoms related to the tachycardia

---

If ventricular rate is > 150 beats/min, prepare for immediate cardioversion.
May give brief trial of medications based on specific arrhythmias.
Immediate cardioversion is generally not needed for rates <150 beats/min.

Check
- Oxygen saturation
- Suction device
- IV line
- Intubation equipment

Premedicate whenever possible*

Synchronized cardioversion†‡
VT§
PSVT‖
Atrial fibrillation
Atrial flutter‖   ⎯ 100 J, 200 J, 300 J, 360 J‡

---

*Effective regimens have included a sedative (eg, *diazepam, midazolam, barbiturates, ethomiolate, ketamine, methohexital*) with or without an analgesic agent (eg, *fentanyl, morphine, meperidine*). Many experts recommend anesthesia if service is readily available.
†Note possible need to resynchronize after each cardioversion.
‡If delays in synchronization occur and clinical conditions are critical, go to immediate unsynchronized shocks.
§Treat polymorphic VT (irregular form and rate) like VF:
  200 J, 200-300 J, 360 J.
‖PSVT and atrial flutter often respond to lower energy levels (start with 50 J).

Figure 4-8
Electrical cardioversion algorithm (with the patient not in cardiac arrest). (From *JAMA* Emergency Cardiac Care Committee and Subcommittees, American Heart Association. *Guidelines for cardiopulmonary resuscitation and emergency cardiac care, III: Adult advanced cardiac life support.* 1992; 268:2224.)

(h) Selected areas of investigation in drug therapy in ACLS include
   (i) High-dose epinephrine
   (ii) Aminophylline
   (iii) Other alpha agents (e.g., norepinephrine, methoxamine)
   (iv) Amiodarone for patients with refractory VT/VF

(v) Magnesium sulfate
(vi) Buffer therapy
- Sodium bicarbonate
- Trisaminomethane (THAM)
- Carbicarb

(4) Cerebral resuscitation
  (a) The best way of preserving neurologic function is obviously the early and effective restoration of cardiopulmonary function
  (b) Using standard closed-chest compressions, cerebral survival is minimal if circulation is not restored promptly
  (c) Autoregulation of cerebral blood flow is lost after an extended period of hypoxemia or hypercarbia. Thus, prompt correction of these variables is of extreme importance
  (d) Optimize cerebral perfusion pressure by maintaining a normal or slightly elevated mean arterial pressure and by reducing intracranial pressure, if increased (see Chapter 11)
  (e) The use of selective calcium-channel blockers (e.g., nimodipine, lidoflazine) to preserve cerebral function following a cardiac arrest is currently under investigation

b. Predictors of poor outcome in resuscitation
  (1) Preterminal illness (e.g., sepsis, malignancies)
  (2) Catastrophic events (e.g., massive pulmonary embolism, ruptured aneurysms, cardiogenic shock)
  (3) Delayed performance of BLS(basic life support)/ACLS
  (4) Initial rhythm
    (a) Asystole or PEA: prognosis grim
    (b) VT: good prognosis, but rarely encountered
    (c) VF: ability to prevent deterioration to asystole is dependent on amount of time elapsed before defibrillation

4.2 THE ALVEOLAR AIR EQUATION

1. Dalton's law states that the partial pressure of a mixture of gases is equal to the sum of the partial pressures of the constituent gases. Thus, the total pressure of alveolar gases must equal the sum of its constituents and, in turn, equilibrate with atmospheric pressure. The most frequent concern is with the respiratory gases, O_2 and CO_2.

2. The *alveolar air equation* is based firmly on Dalton's law but is expressed in terms that emphasize alveolar O_2 and CO_2

$$P_AO_2 = (P_{ATM} - P_{H_2O})\, FiO_2 - PCO_2/RQ$$

P_AO_2 = partial pressure of O_2 in the alveolus under present conditions.
P_{ATM} = current, local atmospheric pressure.
P_{H_2O} = vapor pressure of water at body temperature and 100% relative humidity.
FiO_2 = fraction of inspired O_2. PCO_2 = partial pressure of CO_2 in arterial blood. RQ = respiratory quotient.

3. Many clinical and environmental influences are immediately obvious when considering the terms of the equation:
  a. P_{ATM}: Altitude per se can clearly result in hypoxemia. A patient's PO_2

must be considered in the context of location. A "normal" arterial Po_2 is not the same in Denver (average = 73 mm Hg) as it is at sea level (average = 95 mm Hg)

b. Fio_2: While atmospheric air is uniformly about 21% O_2, one must ask: 21% of what? The Fio_2 on a mountaintop at 11,000 feet is 21%, but there is not enough total O_2 in the rarefied air to sustain an arterial Po_2 above 60 mm Hg

c. Pco_2: although CO_2 coming into the alveolus does not displace O_2 (this would not obey Dalton's law), the blood Pco_2 does equilibrate with alveolar gases. Simultaneously, O_2 is taken up from the alveolus. When patients hypoventilate, not only does CO_2 accumulate, alveolar O_2 becomes depleted. Thus, elevated Pco_2 is associated with low $P_{A}o_2$ and sometimes hypoxemia. Similarly, hyperventilating patients (excess CO_2 elimination, low Pco_2, frequent replenishment of alveolar O_2) can have higher than normal $P_{A}o_2$ and arterial Po_2. (See example 3 below)

d. RQ is the ratio of CO_2 production to O_2 consumption. The ratio of alveolar gas exchange—CO_2 coming into the alveolus and O_2 leaving the alveolus—also reflects the RQ. Given a particular ratio of alveolar gas exchange, the ultimate value for $P_{A}o_2$ will also be affected by the rate of CO_2 elimination from the alveolus; i.e., alveolar ventilation

4. The A-a gradient

a. While the alveolar air equation predicts the partial pressure of O_2 in the alveolus ($P_{A}o_2$) under current conditions, it is not necessarily true that arterial blood will have an identical partial pressure of O_2 ($P_{a}o_2$). One can, however, measure the $P_{a}o_2$ directly and compare it with the calculated value for $P_{A}o_2$. When subtracting arterial from alveolar Po_2 it is possible to obtain the *A-a gradient*

Example 1: a healthy young adult breathing room air at sea level.

Arterial blood gases (ABGs): pH=7.40, $P_{a}co_2$=40, $P_{a}o_2$= 95 (assume RQ = 0.8)

$$P_{A}o_2 = (760 - 47).21 - 40/0.8$$
$$P_{A}o_2 = 150 - 50 = 100$$
A-a gradient = $P_{A}o_2 - P_{a}o_2$
A-a gradient = $100 - 95 = 5$ mm Hg

This person has an A-a gradient of 5 mm Hg, which is normal (0-10).

Example 2: an elderly patient in respiratory distress secondary to pulmonary edema breathing 40% O_2 ($Fio_2 = 0.4$).

ABGs: pH = 7.43 $P_{a}co_2 = 36$ $P_{a}o_2 = 70$

$$P_{A}o_2 = (760-47).40 - 36/0.8$$
$$P_{A}o_2 = 285 - 45 = 240$$
A-a gradient = $P_{A}o_2 - P_{a}o_2$
A-a gradient = $240 - 70 = 170$ mm Hg

This person has an A-a gradient of 170 mm Hg, which is markedly elevated.

b. *Significance:* The presence of an A-a gradient indicates that *something is wrong; gas exchange is impaired.* It does not tell what is wrong; nor does it tell the etiology of hypoxemia when present. A widened A-a gradient simply indicates that alveolar O_2 tension is not successfully reflected in arterial blood

(1) Note that at a given Fio_2, $P_{A}o_2$ varies inversely as the $P_{a}co_2$. Thus at any A-a gradient a high $P_{a}co_2$ is associated with a low $P_{A}o_2$ and vice versa. A patient who hyperventilates (low $P_{a}co_2$) may do so purposely to improve $P_{A}o_2$ and thus $P_{a}o_2$

Example 3: an emergency room patient breathing room air.

ABGs: pH = 7.50 Pco_2 = 30 Po_2 = 65

What would the patient's $P_{a}o_2$ be with the same A-a gradient and a $P_{a}co_2$ of 40?

Room air:

$$P_{A}o_2 = (760 - 47).21 - \mathbf{30}/0.8 = 150 - 35 = 115$$

A-a gradient = 115 − 65
A-a gradient = 50

Now, what if the Pco_2 were 40:

$$P_{A}o_2 = (760 - 47).21 - \mathbf{40}/0.8 = 150 - 50 = 100$$
$$P_{A}o_2 = 100$$
A-a gradient = **50**
Therefore $P_{a}o_2$ = **50**

$P_{a}o_2$ would be **50** if the patient were not hyperventilating. "Normal" ventilation ($P_{a}co_2$ = 40) would be associated with hypoxemia, but with *hyperventilation* the patient's Po_2 is above 60. Note that it is also possible for a patient to have hypoxemia *without* a widened A-a gradient. There are two important examples: *high altitude* and *alveolar hypoventilation*

Example 4: a normal adult breathing room air at an altitude of 11,000 feet

A-a gradient = 0
$$P_{a}o_2 = (\mathbf{510} - 47).21 - 40/0.8 = 47$$
A-a gradient = 0
$$P_{a}o_2 = 47$$

This patient has hypoxemia *without* an A-a gradient
Example 5: a patient with pure alveolar hypoventilation secondary to narcotic overdose breathing room air

$$Pco_2 = 80; \text{A-a gradient} = 0$$
$$P_{A}o_2 = (760 - 47).21 - \mathbf{80}/0.8$$
$$P_{A}o_2 = 50$$
A-a gradient = 0
$$P_{a}o_2 = 50$$

This patient has hypoxemia *without* an A-a gradient

c. Summary
   (1) The alveolar air equation shows the relationships among atmospheric pressure, Fio_2, P_aco_2, and alveolar O_2 tension (P_Ao_2)
   (2) When alveolar O_2 tension (P_Ao_2) is not reflected faithfully in arterial blood (P_ao_2) (i.e., a widened A-a gradient), the calculation indicates that gas exchange is impaired, but it does not tell how or why
   (3) Calculation of the A-a gradient is a useful bedside tool for evaluation of patients with respiratory distress or abnormal ABGs, and for following their progress
   (4) It is possible to have hypoxemia without a widened A-a gradient; for example, high altitude and hypoventilation (elevated P_aco_2)

4.3   OXYGEN TRANSPORT

1. Oxygen delivery: calculations
   a. Calculation of oxygen delivery (Do_2) and oxygen consumption (Vo_2) are useful bedside techniques in the ICU.
   b. $Do_2 = CO \times Cao_2$
      Oxygen delivery = cardiac output $\times$ arterial o_2 content
   c. $Cao_2 = Hb \times Sao_2 \times K$
      Arterial O_2 content = Hb $\times$ arterial O_2 saturation $\times$ a constant
      The following uses 1.34 ml O_2/g Hb:
   d. Resolving the units

      DO_2 [ml O_2/min] = CO [ml/min] $\times$ Hb [g/100 ml] $\times$
      $$1.34 \text{ [ml } O_2/\text{g] } \times Sao_2 \text{ [scalar]}$$

   e. Normal values (70 kg man at rest)

      DO_2 = 5000 ml/min [CO] $\times$ 15 g/100 ml [Hb] $\times$
      1.34 ml O_2/g [constant] $\times$ 1.00 [SaO_2] DO_2 [ml O_2/min] = CO [ml/min] $\times$ Hb [g/100 ml] $\times$ 1.34 [ml O_2/g] $\times$ SaO_2 [scalar]

      $$Do_2 = 1005 \text{ ml } O_2/\text{min}$$

   f. This value does not take into account dissolved O_2 in the plasma: 0.003 ml O_2/100 cc/mm Hg Pao_2 which adds another 15 ml O_2 of arterial O_2 content
   g. Values to remember:

      Normal Cao_2 (15 g Hb, 100% Sao_2) = 20.4 ml O_2/100 cc (20.4 vol %)

      Normal Do_2 (70 kg man, at rest, CO = 5000 ml/min) = 1020 ml O_2/min

2. Oxygen transport: *concepts*
   There are only three clinical variables that can affect Do_2: cardiac output, Hb, and oxygen saturation. Note that what looks very simple is *not:*
   a. Cardiac output entails all of the normal cardiodynamics (preload, afterload, contractility), hemodynamics, state of hydration, blood gas and electrolyte influences, the influence of mechanical ventilation and other technology, intrinsic cardiac disease, dysrhythmias, etc.
   b. Hemoglobin is largely a quantitative problem (i.e., oxygen-carrying

capacity), but also includes the effects of abnormal hemoglobins, massive transfusions, pH and temperature, other causes of shift in the oxyhemoglobin-dissociation curve, and hemoglobin substitutes

c. Arterial oxygen saturation embodies the pathophysiology of acute and chronic lung disease, management of mechanical ventilation, cardiopulmonary interaction, venous admixture, intrapulmonary or intracardiac shunting, etc.

d. If this is not complicated enough, remember that what is done to support the lungs may have a detrimental effect on cardiac output (see below). Similarly, failure to correct severe blood gas abnormalities may adversely affect cardiac function. This makes the bedside management of oxygen delivery in critically ill patients straightforward, although at times very difficult

   (1) Support oxygenation so that

   $Po_2 > 60$, $Sao_2 > 0.9$ on nontoxic Fio_2 (≤ 0.5)

   (2) Ensure Hb concentration of at least 10 g/100 cc

   (3) Optimize CO *under current conditions* (i.e., current ventilator settings)

3. Physiologic maintenance of oxygen delivery. Since Do_2 is dependent on only three variables, how does a normal person respond to abnormalities of one of the values?

a. Fall in Sao_2

   If Sao_2 falls to *0.5*, a person can achieve normal O_2 delivery by *doubling* CO:

   $Do_2 = CO \times Hb \times Sao_2$
   $Do_2 = 2CO \times Hb \times \frac{1}{2} Sao_2$

   (1) Therefore, in the short term, increased CO can compensate for even severe hypoxemia

   (2) Note that when $Sao_2 = 0.5$, $P_ao_2 = 27$! This is the definition of P_{50} for normal adult hemoglobin A, namely the P_ao_2 at which hemoglobin is 50% saturated (27 mm Hg). Thus even *severe* hypoxemia can be well tolerated as long as Hb is normal and CO can be enhanced

   (3) In patients with chronically low Sao_2 (e.g., high altitude, chronic lung disease, cyanotic heart disease) there also will be an increase in the Hb concentration

b. Fall in hemoglobin

   If Hb falls dramatically, Do_2 is again maintained by increasing CO

   (1) Note that Sao_2 can never increase beyond 100% and therefore *cannot compensate* for low hemoglobin. The ability to increase and maintain CO is an important mechanism by which anemia can be tolerated

   $Do_2 = CO \times Hb \times Sao_2$
   $Do_2 = 2CO \times \frac{1}{2} Hb \times Sao_2$

c. Fall in cardiac output

   If CO falls dramatically, how is Do_2 maintained? The answer is that Do_2, in totality, is *not* maintained, but tissue Do_2 is maintained by *enhanced extraction*

(1) If fewer liters of oxygenated blood are delivered, then the tissues must extract more from every liter that *is* delivered
(2) Normally, arterial blood is nearly 100% saturated with O_2. Venous blood returning to the heart is the same in terms of hemoglobin and quantitatively the same as CO. Thus, it is the *venous oxygen saturation* (S_vO_2) that reflects O_2 extraction. Normal $S_vO_2 = .75$. Therefore normal extraction is about 25%
(3) Under some circumstances, such as heart failure, looking at extraction (i.e., A-V O_2 difference) is therefore a good probe of the adequacy of CO. High extraction implies inadequate CO

d. Fall in oxygen delivery
Here is a general rule of thumb: A normal person can withstand a severe abnormality of any one of the O_2 delivery variables (CO, Hb, Sao_2) without developing lactic acidosis. Lactic acidosis would indicate cellular O_2 deprivation with resultant anaerobic metabolism
(1) During cardiac arrest lactate is generated not only because of hypoxemia, but also because the cardiac output is severely compromised and is unable to compensate for low P_aO_2 to maintain Do_2

4. Oxygen consumption ($\dot{V}o_2$)
a. Do_2 is what quantitatively and qualitatively leaves the heart. What returns to the heart should be quantitatively the same, with the same Hb concentration, different only in terms of oxygen saturation
b. If the $\dot{D}o_2$ (what left the heart) is known, and what has returned to the heart is calculated, then subtract to ascertain the amount consumed. Cvo_2 is the mixed venous O_2 content. ($Cao_2 - Cvo_2$) is the arteriovenous O_2 content difference.

$$\text{Oxygen consumption } (\dot{V}o_2) = CO \times (Cao_2) - CO \times (Cvo_2)$$
$$\text{what left} \qquad \text{what returned}$$
$$\text{the heart} \qquad \text{to the heart}$$

Thus, $\dot{V}o_2 = CO (Cao_2 - Cvo_2)$

This is the Fick equation
c. Cvo_2 is calculated in exactly the same way as the Cao_2. Svo_2 is the mixed venous O_2 saturation

$$Hb \times 1.34 \times Svo_2$$

d. If Vo_2 is known, the Fick equation can be used to calculate the cardiac output

$$CO = \frac{\dot{V}o_2}{(Cao_2 - Cvo_2)}$$

e. At the bedside, what is needed to calculate Vo_2?
(1) The patient needs a pulmonary artery (Swan-Ganz) catheter
(a) for CO determination
(b) to obtain a true mixed venous blood sample from the pulmonary artery (Svo_2)
(2) Arterial blood gas determination (or Sao_2 determination)
(3) Hemoglobin determination

f. Example of normal values (70 kg man at rest)

Cao_2 = 15 [Hb] × 1.34 [constant] × 1.00 [Sa_2] = 20.1
Cvo_2 = 15 [Hb] × 1.34 [constant] × 0.75 [Svo_2] = 15.1
CO = 5000 ml [5 liters/min]
Vo_2 = 5000 ml/min (20.1 ml O_2/100 ml − 15.1 ml O_2/100cc)
Vo_2 = 50 (20 − 15)

Vo_2 [normal, at rest] = 250 ml O_2/min

g. Bedside application in the ICU: Human life depends on oxygen. This is a good reason to assess the adequacy of Do_2 in critically ill patients. Where there is life, there is O_2 consumption
   (1) We are concerned about factors that increase resting O_2 consumption, e.g., fever. Febrile patients increase their resting O_2 consumption by 10-13%/°C, (approximately 7%/°F)
   (2) We are also concerned when calculated O_2 consumption is less than predicted for body surface area and temperature, as in sepsis. Many times, in spite of high Do_2, patients with sepsis have low calculated Vo_2, lactic acidosis, oliguria, and other signs of poor parenchymal organ function
   (3) It is better to look for physiologic end-points than for arbitrary end points. It is likely that DO_2 is adequate when measured O_2 consumption, the Svo_2, the (A-V) O_2 content difference, and the serum lactate are all normal. Satisfaction of the body's (tissues') needs is better evidence of the adequacy of Do_2 than any arbitrary number
   (4) Be sure to see Do_2 as an integrated variable. Changing ventilator settings (see below)—e.g., raising the PEEP to enhance Sao_2—in the process that causes a fall in CO may not achieve any overall benefit in terms of Do_2. CO, Hb, and Sao_2 require individual attention and management
   (5) Look for opportunities to get the best results for each intervention. For example, a transfusion of packed red blood cells may increase Hb *and* raise CO. This management may be substantially better than trying to raise CO with crystalloid IV fluids to compensate for a borderline Hb and/or Sao_2
   (6) Check CO and O_2 transport variables often, and measure the response to interventions. HR and BP are often recorded every hr, even though CO can vary widely irrespective of these more traditional signs. Cardiac output is a *vital sign*
   (7) The technology now exists to have continuous data for Sao_2, Svo_2, and even CO. This can obviate the necessity of repeated blood gas determinations and facilitate frequent assessment of O_2 transport variables

4.4   MECHANICAL VENTILATION

Humans breathe for two reasons: to take in oxygen (oxygenation) and to eliminate carbon dioxide (ventilation). A patient's inability to perform either or both of these functions defines respiratory failure.

1. Ventilation

   Normal people produce CO_2 continuously, thus there is a constant need for CO_2 elimination. CO_2 is eliminated by a process that entails breathing in fresh air (essentially devoid of CO_2), allowing it to equilibrate with the CO_2 dissolved in capillary blood, and then exhaling it laden with CO_2. People perform this process 10-14 times each minute with significant volumes of air so that, under normal conditions, arterial CO_2 ($P_a co_2$) is kept nearly constant at 40 mm Hg (torr).

   More precisely, people move a *tidal volume* (V_T) in and out at a certain *frequency* (f) or *respiratory rate* (RR). The product of rate and tidal volume is the *minute ventilation* (V_{min}). Thus it is the minute ventilation which is fundamentally responsible for CO_2 elimination.

   $$V_{min} = V_T \times RR$$

   a. The minute ventilation can be further divided into the gases that reach the alveoli and are therefore available for exchange (the alveolar ventilation, V_A), as well as those gases that fill the airways or that reach unperfused alveoli (see below) and therefore cannot exchange gases (the anatomical and physiological dead space, respectively, V_D)

   b. CO_2 elimination is therefore directly proportional to the minute alveolar ventilation at any level of CO_2 production or blood $P co_2$

   $$CO_2 \text{ elimination} = (V_A)_{min} \times P co_2$$

   c. Since any physiologic parameter (e.g., serum creatinine, platelet count, $P co_2$) is ultimately the result of the balance between production and elimination, it follows that $P co_2$ (under any condition affecting production) can be controlled by adjusting minute ventilation

2. Oxygenation

   The way people accomplish oxygenation is considerably different from the way they accomplish ventilation. Humans purposely inhale an oxygen-enriched atmosphere all the way down to their alveoli. This allows the oxygen to be taken up by the capillary blood, where it is dissolved in proportion to its partial pressure (obeying Henry's law) and in combination with hemoglobin. More precisely, the air inspired has a certain fraction that is oxygen; i.e., a certain fraction of inspired O_2 (Fio_2)

   Although people breathe only intermittently, they need to accomplish gas exchange continuously. If there were oxygen in the alveoli upon inhalation only, then blood would pass through the lungs unoxygenated between breaths. Thus, it is necessary to maintain volume in the lungs even at end-exhalation. This is accomplished by maintaining a pressure gradient across the lungs between breaths. The pressure in the pleural space (outside the lungs) is negative (approximately [$-$]5 cm H_2O) with respect to the atmospheric pressure present in the airways. With vectorial subtraction, there is a $0 - (-5) = +5$ cm H_2O pressure gradient across the lungs even at end-exhalation; in effect, a positive end-expiratory pressure (PEEP). Thus oxygenation is accomplished in normal people by purposely inspiring a certain Fio_2 and maintaining a certain PEEP.

3. PEEP and compliance
  a. Compliance: The volume in the lungs is related to the transpulmonary pressure. Indeed, volume and pressure are intimately related in many systems (e.g., ventilator tubing, cardiac filling, resting lung volume) through the variable of compliance (C):

$$C = \frac{V}{P}$$

Compliance is defined as the change in volume for a given change in pressure. Thus, in order to achieve a given volume change (e.g., a tidal volume) in the lungs, there must be a pressure change. The precise pressure necessary is determined by the lung (and chest wall) compliance

It is mathematically clear that as compliance falls (as may occur in pulmonary edema, ARDS, lung fibrosis, and many other conditions) it is necessary to achieve ever-increasing P just to achieve the same V. The ultimate cause of respiratory failure is often a patient's inability to do the work required to increase P to maintain an adequate tidal exchange (V).

There are many important clinical implications in the fundamental role lung compliance plays in determining the relationship between clinically significant lung volumes (e.g., tidal volume) and the pressures required to achieve them:
    (1) If there is no gradient of pressure (P = 0), there is no volume change. When a patient develops a pneumothorax, the pressure in the pleural space equals the pressure in the airways. As a result, there is no transpulmonary pressure (P) and thus no lung volume (i.e., the lung collapses) because of the lungs' intrinsic compliance and elastance (which is defined as 1/compliance). Pneumothorax results in no lung volume (zero V) because there is no transpulmonary pressure (zero P)
    (2) In order to create a volume change, it is necessary to effect a pressure change. Thus, tidal volume is determined by the P generated as the chest wall expands and the diaphragm contracts. Similarly, to increase tidal volume, it is necessary to generate a larger P, or if compliance falls, a larger P may be needed just to achieve the same tidal volume
    (3) In the case of low lung compliance (i.e., restrictive disease), normal resting negative intrapleural pressure (P) will result in lower resting lung volume (V)
    (4) In high lung compliance (i.e., emphysema with destruction of lung parenchyma), normal resting negative intrapleural pressure will result in high resting lung volume (e.g., "barrel chest" of emphysema)
    (5) Since the lungs are merely populations of alveoli, the relationships among pressure, volume, and compliance apply to individual alveoli and specific lung regions, as well as to whole lungs
    (6) Compliance contributes to the logical connection between the requirements of gas exchange and the respiratory work
        (a) CO_2 production demands minute ventilation

    (b) Minute ventilation requires a certain tidal volume

    (c) This change in volume requires a change in pressure

    (d) The amount of pressure for a given volume is determined by compliance

    (e) The amount of pressure that must be generated is a major determinant of the work of breathing

  b. PEEP: The description of oxygenation and ventilation should clarify the clinical concern with maintaining the adequacy of two important lung volumes: the tidal volume of each breath and the resting lung volume between breaths.

    During active inspiration, the pressure generated by the ventilator or the patient will determine the tidal volume (mediated, of course, through compliance). But what determines the resting lung volume?

    The answer is the *resting transpulmonary pressure*. In people with normal lung compliance the vectorial difference between airway and intrapleural pressures (P) determines the resting lung volume. This is known more precisely as the *functional residual capacity* (FRC)

$$P_{airway} - P_{pleural} = P_{transpulmonary}$$
$$0 - (-5) = +5$$
$$P = +5 \text{ cm H2O}$$

FRC is therefore determined by the P and compliance

$$C = \frac{V}{P}$$

$$C = \frac{FRC}{P_{transpulmonary}}$$

$$FRC = C\ (P_{transpulmonary})$$

Since P is positive and present at end-expiration, this refers to positive end-expiratory pressure (PEEP). It should be clear that PEEP directly determines FRC

    We have all had the experience of inflating a balloon. It is difficult at first, then suddenly gets easier once there is some volume inside. As the balloon reaches full inflation, it may again become difficult to inflate as we reach the limits of the balloon's compliance. If we let go, the balloon recoils (elastance) and collapses (see Fig. 4-9)

    The alveoli, in many ways, are similar to the balloon. If the alveoli start fully collapsed, they are at first difficult to inflate. Once there is some volume, it becomes easier. This point of change in compliance is referred to as *critical opening pressure* (COP).

    Unlike balloons, normal alveoli do not immediately lose all of their volume when pressure is released, but may maintain some volume (thanks in large measure to surfactant) and will not collapse until distending pressure is critically low. The point at which this occurs is *critical closing pressure* (CCP).

    If one could maintain PEEP above CCP, then alveoli would not collapse; their volume would be enhanced and in the aggregate, so would FRC. If low lung compliance results in high CCP, PEEP must be in-

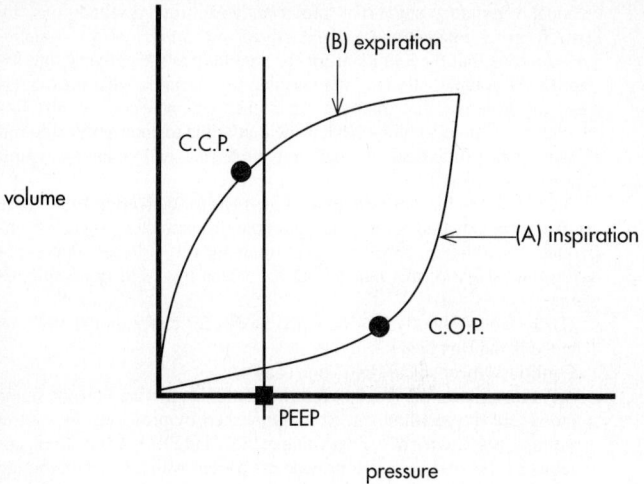

Figure 4-9
The rationale for PEEP. During inspiration, (A) as pressure increases, volume increases slowly until critical opening pressure (COP) is exceeded. During exhalation, (B) alveolar volume is well maintained as pressure dissipates until finally critical closing pressure (CCP) is reached and alveolar collapse ensues. If positive end-expiratory pressure (PEEP) is maintained above CCP, alveolar volume is also maintained, thus allowing gas exchange between breaths (shunt reduction) and a cumulative increase in resting lung volume (FRC).

creased above the CCP to prevent alveolar collapse. This is precisely the rationale for PEEP in the management of acute low compliance-lung diseases (e.g., ARDS)
   (1) Summary of the effects of PEEP:
      (a) PEEP increases FRC
      (b) PEEP increases compliance
      (c) PEEP reduces shunt fraction (see below) by maintaining volume for gas exchange in perfused lung units between breaths
      (d) PEEP increases dead space by overdistending normally compliant alveoli
      (e) PEEP increases intrathoracic pressure, which can impede venous return into the chest or specifically restrict cardiac filling; both may result in reduced cardiac output
      (f) PEEP may contribute to barotrauma because it represents the baseline (end-expiration) for all pressure changes, because it may cause overdistention of compliant lung regions, and because of the nature of the acute lung diseases in which PEEP is most frequently used
4. Modes of mechanical ventilation
   When a patient develops respiratory failure and is intubated, initial me-

chanical ventilatory support is provided, under routine conditions, by some form of conventional *volume-cycled ventilation* (VCV). *Volume-cycled* means that the end point for the ventilator is the delivery of a selected tidal volume, allowing the machine to determine what pressure is necessary to deliver that volume to a particular patient at a given time. Recent advances in technology have made it possible to control the required pressure while maintaining tidal volume as the end point (pressure-controlled ventilation).

In addition to the standard array of methods for delivering VCV, there are also modes that do not use quasiphysiologic parameters, such as high-frequency ventilation. These modes of mechanical ventilatory support are beyond the scope of this manual but have been reviewed in depth elsewhere.

There are essentially four common modes for conventional VCV, as depicted in the Box below.

a. Controlled mechanical ventilation (CMV)

From the discussion above, it follows that the basic functions of ventilation and oxygenation can be accomplished by providing four basic settings: respiratory rate, tidal volume, Fio_2, and PEEP. Given these parameters the ventilator will provide the patient with a constant minute ventilation and oxygen. These are the settings for CMV. The only gases the patient receives are from the machine breaths. The patient *cannot* initiate a breath, change the rate, or access any other source of fresh gases. Therefore CMV is useful in a limited number of settings. For example:

(1) When the patient is fully anesthetized in the operating room
(2) When the patient is apneic and likely to remain so
(3) When the patient is sedated/anesthetized and paralyzed in the ICU

It is important to remember that in CMV the patient absolutely cannot breathe without aid. A patient who awakens or attempts to breathe may become agitated and dyspneic. It is extremely frightening to be unable to breathe and essentially to experience a chronically occluded airway. It is worse yet if the patient becomes detached from the ventilator—an anesthetized and/or paralyzed patient will be functionally apneic and may soon experience full cardiopulmonary arrest

b. *Assisted/controlled mechanical ventilation (A/C)*

The four basic settings for A/C are the same ones used for CMV. There

---

Commonly Used Modes of Volume-Cycled Ventilation

1. Controlled mechanical ventilation (CMV)
2. Assisted/controlled mechanical ventilation (A/C)
3. Synchronized intermittent mandatory ventilation (SIMV)
4. Continuous positive airway pressure (CPAP)
5. Pressure support ventilation (PSV), which is not a separate mode, but rather an adjunct that can be used with other modes

is no difference between CMV and A/C in the anesthetized or apneic patient. For the patient who is not anesthetized or apneic, the singular difference is that in A/C mode the patient is able to initiate breaths. Unlike in healthy individuals, however, the amount of effort the patient makes does not determine the tidal volume. When the patient initiates a breath with sufficient force to trigger the ventilator, the tidal volume received is the one preset to be delivered as a *controlled* breath. Moreover, the machine will use whatever pressure is required to deliver the volume, and the patient's lungs and chest must then accommodate that tidal volume. The set rate in A/C is essentially a default control rate; i.e., the number of volume-cycled breaths the machine will deliver on its own, even if the patient is apneic. Thus the controlled aspect of A/C is the guaranteed minute volume delivered regardless of the patient's spontaneous efforts

While this mode has some value in its ability to relieve dyspnea in the immediate post-intubation period, it is not a good choice for prolonged mechanical support. There is now evidence that in accommodating assisted breaths, the respiratory muscles actually may be fatigued rather than rested, as was intended by the design. Better choices are available for routine use

c. Synchronized intermittent mandatory ventilation (SIMV)

SIMV is probably the most versatile of currently available modes, and therefore is the most widely used. What does the term mean?

(1) *Mandatory ventilation* represents the same guaranteed minute ventilation (respiratory rate × tidal volume) delivered by the machine as seen in CMV or A/C. Thus, should the patient become apneic while on SIMV, mandatory ventilation will be provided

(2) *Intermittent* is used to emphasize that the machine will deliver the desired number of breaths at intervals, leaving the patient free to breathe spontaneously in between. For example, if the set respiratory rate is 10 breaths/min, then the machine will deliver the selected tidal volume about every 6 seconds. The patient may need or desire to breathe more often than 10 times/min and is able to do so in the intervals between machine breaths

(3) *Synchronized* IMV is a relatively new refinement of the original IMV design. In the example above, the machine cycles every 6 seconds, but it is undesirable for the ventilator to attempt delivery of a new breath if the patient is in the process of exhaling a spontaneous breath. Without synchronization, this kind of collision could occur in the airways, causing very high airway pressure, a risk of barotrauma, ineffective ventilation, and enhanced (rather than relieved) dyspnea. The synchronizer looks at a "window" period when the next machine breath is due. If the patient is exhaling, the ventilator waits to begin inspiration. If the patient initiates a breath at the time the ventilator is due to cycle, the machine breath and the spontaneous breath will merge into one synchronized breath, similar to the triggered breaths in A/C mode. This represents a major improvement for IMV, especially in patients with prolonged expiratory times such as those with bronchial asthma

    (4) SIMV was introduced into wide usage as a weaning modality. Weaning from mechanical ventilation is discussed below, but in this context, the principle is simple. Initially the mandatory ventilation provides the entire minute ventilation necessary to maintain the patient's P_{CO_2} within normal limits. As the patient begins to breathe spontaneously, the mandatory ventilation is gradually reduced until the patient is essentially providing the entire minute ventilation (and therefore CO_2 elimination) through spontaneous efforts alone. At this point the patient no longer requires mechanical ventilatory support

    (5) It should be noted here that on SIMV, as in all of the modes thus far discussed, oxygenation is supported by the settings for PEEP and F_{IO_2}.

d. *Continuous positive airway pressure (CPAP)*

In the CPAP mode the machine provides only PEEP, F_{IO_2}, and humidification (maintained in all modes), but does not deliver any mechanical breaths. In this sense, it is the chosen mode if the patient is on either SIMV or A/C and the machine respiratory rate is set at zero. Its utility is limited to essentially two circumstances

    (1) Patients with no ventilatory difficulty who require PEEP to support oxygenation

    (2) Patients in the final stages of weaning who are being observed while breathing without ventilatory support

e. *Pressure support ventilation (PSV)*

Pressure support is not a mode of mechanical ventilation, but an adjunct to other modes. All people are able to inhale a certain tidal volume based on their ability to create a significant negative intrapleural pressure. As noted in the description of PEEP above, the vectorial result of the negative intrapleural pressure is a positive pressure gradient across the lungs. In the simplest terms, PSV is the delivery of gas flow (during a spontaneous breath) with a defined positive pressure that is selected on the ventilator. This positive pressure is vectorially summative with the negative pressure generated by the patient's effort. The net result is the enhancement of the positive pressure gradient across the lungs and, as a result, the spontaneous tidal volume is also enhanced

    No PSV:

    $0 - (-10) = +10$ H_2O transpulmonary pressure

    with PSV of +10

    $+10$ (PSV) $- (-10) = +20$ cm H_2O transpulmonary pressure

The above has many implications for the use of PSV

    (1) PSV has an effect only on spontaneous breaths

    (2) The effect of PSV can be measured as an enhancement of spontaneous tidal volume

    (3) In our basic description, then, PSV serves the function of ventilation

    (4) PSV can facilitate the reduction of mandatory machine breaths, since it increases the effectiveness of the patient's spontaneous efforts

(5) PSV can therefore be a very useful adjunct to ventilator weaning

(6) Patients may have significant relief of dyspnea with PSV because it enhances the efficacy of their own efforts, especially in low-compliance lung disease or when the respiratory muscles are fatigued

(7) PSV can help to overcome the additional work of breathing imposed by the endotracheal tube and the ventilator circuit

(8) Although the transpulmonary pressure is enhanced by PSV, the airway pressure is limited to the pressure support selected ($+10$ cm H_2O in the example above). This can have a significantly beneficial effect on hemodynamics

(9) Respiratory muscles do not benefit from rest (defined as *not contracting at all*). In fact, they may rapidly atrophy if not allowed to perform as they usually do. However, with acute lung disease, the work of breathing may result in fatigue. PSV should allow the respiratory muscles to perform a manageable amount of work without the risk of atrophy on the one hand or fatigue on the other

(10) If the PSV is set at more than 8-10 cm H_2O, it may have to be weaned gradually before mechanical ventilation is discontinued

(11) PSV can be used only in modes that allow the patient to breathe spontaneously; i.e., SIMV, CPAP

5. Initiation of mechanical ventilation
   a. Criteria for initiation of mechanical ventilation
      (1) *Physical assessment:* The patient is apneic, severely tachypneic, or in respiratory distress unresponsive to therapeutic interventions and supplemental oxygen
      (2) *Gas exchange:* hypoxemia (Po_2 <50) despite high-flow oxygen; hypercarbia (acute, Pco_2 >50 with acidic pH)
      (3) *Clinical judgement:* The constellation of laboratory and physical findings may be the most compelling—a Pco_2 of 60 and a respiratory rate of 35 may be the usual baseline for some patients but may represent a dire emergency in others
   b. Initial ventilator settings are depicted in the top Box on p.50

6. General principles of ventilator management (see the bottom Box on p.50)
   a. Therapeutic end points
      (1) *Pco_2:* Ventilatory parameters are adjusted to achieve a Pco_2 of 35-45 with the pH also in the normal physiologic range of 7.35-7.45
      (2) *Po_2:* a Po_2 >60 that corresponds to an Sao_2 >0.9 with the patient receiving nontoxic Fio_2 (≤0.5). If this is not achievable on physiologic PEEP, the PEEP can be raised in increments of $+2$ cm H_2O to achieve this end point.
         (a) This end point can be expressed as a Po_2/Fio_2 ratio 60/0.4 = 150 (Fio_2 = 0.4 is not associated with O_2 toxicity)
         (b) PEEP will be most beneficial in acute low-compliance lung disease. Patients with markedly asymmetrical lung disease, bullous emphysema, or asthma may actually have worsening gas exchange with significant PEEP

Initial Ventilator Settings

1. **Mode:** SIMV is the most versatile mode to use unless there is a compelling reason to do otherwise
2. **Respiratory rate:** generally between 8 and 12 breaths/min adjusted according to the P_{CO_2}
3. **Tidal volume:** in the ICU setting 12-15 ml/kg *lean* body weight. Do not count adipose tissue or edema
4. **Fio₂:** many people start with 1.00 (100% O_2), but often 0.8 (80% O_2) will suffice. There is a phenomenon called *absorption atelectasis* that increases proportionately with higher Fio_2. Regardless, the Fio_2 should be adjusted down as soon as possible
5. **PEEP:** normal people are able to create positive pressure in their airways with their lips, palate, and glottis. Since the endotracheal tube bypasses all of these structures, most initial setups include "physiologic" PEEP of +3 to +5 cm H_2O
6. **PSV:** 8-10 cm H_2O can usually overcome the additional work imposed by the endotracheal tube and ventilator circuit, but larger amounts may substantially reduce dyspnea. Remember PSV has relevance only for spontaneously breathing patients

---

Ventilator Principles

VENTILATOR PRINCIPLE 1: To reach a desirable clinical end point for the patient's P_{CO_2}, the ventilator settings to adjust are the respiratory rate (RR) and/or the tidal volume (V_T) delivered by the machine.

VENTILATOR PRINCIPLE 2: To reach a desirable clinical end point for a patient's P_{O_2}, the ventilator settings to adjust are the fraction of inspired O_2 (Fio_2) and/or the positive end-expiratory pressure (PEEP).

VENTILATOR PRINCIPLE 3: Patients do not buck or fight the ventilator; patients buck ill-conceived ventilator settings.

---

  b. When patients are in respiratory distress, it is acceptable to change any or all of the ventilator settings at one time. This does *not* apply to weaning
  c. Patient comfort
    (1) Having an endotracheal tube in place is not comfortable and is frustrating because the patient cannot speak
    (2) Patients who are going to be intubated for a short time should receive mild sedation with agents that do not have significant respiratory suppression

      (3) Patients requiring high ventilator settings and who are likely to be intubated for several days before weaning should receive more substantial sedation

      (4) It is the author's opinion that only a few selected patients require paralytic agents

  d. *Some simple rules of thumb*

      (1) Endotracheal tubes should be as large in diameter as possible, and cut as short as possible once the position is verified

      (2) Endotracheal tubes must be carefully secured and should not be between the patient's teeth

      (3) Suctioning is important but should be minimal or strictly as needed (prn) when the patient is on more than $+10$ cm H_2O PEEP. This minimizes the volume loss from within the lungs

      (4) When setting up the ventilator, the peak inspiratory flow rate is best kept relatively low (≤ 50 LPM), but must be at least *three times the minute ventilation* or the patient may become dyspneic

      (5) Generally, PSV of 8-10 cm H_2O overcomes the extra flow-resistive work of the endotracheal tube, but the optimal level usually results in a spontaneous respiratory rate <25 breaths/min and absence of accessory muscle use

      (6) Any intubated patient should have a nasogastric tube placed; this immediately empties the stomach of liquid contents and of the air that is often swallowed during respiratory distress. The tube can then be used for stress ulcer prophylaxis and enteral nutritional support

7. Weaning from mechanical ventilation

  The ultimate goal of placing the patient *on* mechanical ventilation is to take him or her *off* of mechanical ventilation.

  a. Reduction of the ventilator settings: It is acceptable to change two settings at once, but not two that serve the same function; e.g., reducing the Fio_2 and the respiratory rate at the same time is allowed because one serves oxygenation and the other serves ventilation; reducing the respiratory rate and the PSV at the same time is not allowed because both settings serve the minute ventilation

  b. Beginning to wean PEEP from its peak setting: It is prudent to reduce PEEP in 1 cm H_2O increments for the first few changes

  c. Weaning PEEP: Changes should not be made more than every 3-4 hr; some alveoli may destabilize and collapse rapidly, others may take time. It may not be clear for 3-4 hr if the patient will tolerate the change

  d. There are three sets of criteria a patient must meet to be successfully weaned from the ventilator and extubated (i.e., removed from the endotracheal tube): gas exchange, pulmonary mechanics, circumstantial

      (1) Gas exchange

         (a) The Fio_2 should be ≤ 0.5 and the PEEP physiologic before contemplating active weaning

         (b) The Pco_2 should be normal for the patient and the pH in the normal range (i.e., not acidic) before reducing parameters that serve ventilation

Table 4-1 Weaning parameters

Parameters	Desirable Values
Tidal volume	4-7 ml/kg
Respiratory rate	<30 breaths/min
Negative inspiratory force	more negative than (−)20 cm H_2O
Minute ventilation	<10 liters/min
Vital capacity	>10 ml/kg

      (c) The desirable therapeutic end points outlined above should, in general, be met before the settings are reduced

  (2) Pulmonary mechanics

      (a) Although often referred to as "weaning parameters," these are more correctly thought of as *extubation criteria*

      (b) The parameters to be measured and the desirable values are depicted in Table 4-1

  (3) Circumstantial criteria

      (a) If possible, the patient should be awake and alert for extubation

      (b) If the patient is neurologically impaired, careful testing of the gag and cough reflexes is necessary

      (c) Secretions should have been minimized or the patient should clearly demonstrate an ability to manage them

      (d) The airway should be patent and nonedematous. The patient should have control (voluntary or reflex) over the airway

      (e) Correct extraneous stresses placed on respiratory requirements (e.g., metabolic acidosis, anemia, fever, bronchospasm, and cardiac dysrhythmia)

      (f) Correct electrolyte abnormalities that compromise respiratory muscle function (e.g., low values for potassium, magnesium, phosphorus, and ionized calcium)

4.5 HEMODYNAMICS

The subject of hemodynamics has two major components: *cardiodynamics,* which is the physiology of heart function; and traditional *hemodynamics,* which is pertinent to the pulmonary circulation, the systemic circulation, and the right and left sides of the heart, respectively, as the functional pumps of these circuits.

    The most useful bedside tool is the pulmonary artery (Swan-Ganz) catheter, which provides continuous assessment of the cardiac pump function and management of the hemodynamic state of the circulation. Although much useful information can be derived from the measurements and calculations made possible through the use of this catheter, the most important reason to place one in a critically ill patient is to measure cardiac output. In the critical care unit, the principal rationale for placement of the catheter is the assurance of adequate cardiac output and its integral role in life-sustaining Do_2. Proper interpretation and manipulation of other values (e.g., the pulmonary capillary wedge pressure) depend on the cardiac output for context.

The PA catheter is not a therapy; it is a monitoring device. Like all interventions it carries an inherent risk: benefit ratio. Unless the catheter is used actively to assess the patient, to guide management, and to reassess the response to interventions, its placement is all risk and no benefit.

1. Physics and physiology

Conceptually, the flow of any fluid through a conduit is governed by the following general principle:

$$\text{Pressure} = \text{Flow} \times \text{Resistance}$$

This applies to airway pressure, inspiratory flow rate, and airway resistance. In the present discussion, it also applies to blood pressure, blood flow (cardiac output), and vascular resistance.

Specifically:

MAP mean arterial pressure	=	CO cardiac output	×	SVR systemic vascular resistance

or

PAP pulmonary artery pressure	=	CO cardiac output	×	PVR pulmonary vascular resistance

To solve these equations for the calculated resistances:

$$\text{SVR} = \frac{\text{MAP} \times 79.9^*}{\text{CO}}$$

$$\text{PVR} = \frac{\text{PAP} \times 79.9^*}{\text{CO}}$$

Vascular resistance: conceptually the resistance to flow of a fluid through a conduit is given by the equation of Poiseuille:

$$\text{Resistance} = \frac{8 \times \text{Length} \times \text{Velocity} \times \text{Viscosity}}{\pi \, (\text{Radius})^4}$$

2. Cardiodynamics

The pump function of the heart is the result of the interaction of three variables: preload, afterload, and contractility.

a. *Preload:* In simple terms, preload is the amount of cardiac filling during diastole. In this sense, think of it as the end-diastolic volume (EDV) that is either the cause or the result of end-diastolic pressure (EDP). In the purest terms, preload is the resting fiber length of the myofibrils and forms the fundamental basis for the Frank-Starling curve (see Fig. 4-10)

b. Afterload: Afterload is quite complicated, but can be thought of in simple terms as the impedance to cardiac ejection. For example, if the

*79.9 is a constant that converts the units according to Poiseuille's resistance equation.

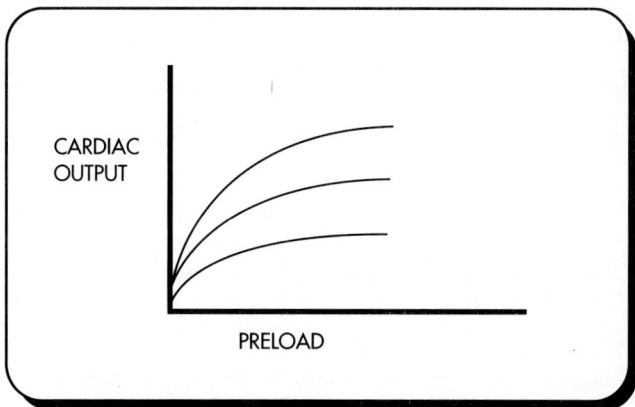

Figure 4-10

The Starling curve. The fundamental relationship between preload (end-diastolic volume) and cardiac putput. Volume (preload) enhancement can improve cardiac output on any function curve. There is no one Starling curve, but rather a family of curves which may represent different patients, or the same patient at different times or under different conditions.

diastolic blood pressure is high, the heart has to overcome that pressure just to open the aortic valve. In physiologic terms, afterload is the developed wall tension during systole and is affected by several factors. Generally speaking, anything that makes it easier for the heart to eject blood reduces afterload; anything that makes it more difficult increases afterload

c. Contractility: Contractility is literally the force with which the heart contracts. Given any amount of filling and a constant afterload, the amount of blood ejected by a given heartbeat will depend on the force of contraction

d. Cardiac output: The cardiac output is the product of the amount of blood pumped each time the heart contracts (stroke volume, SV) multiplied by the number of contractions/min (HR)

$$CO = HR \times SV$$

$$SV = \frac{CO}{HR}$$

A person can have a CO of 5 LPM (liters/min) with an HR of 70 or an HR of 140. Part of the clinical assessment of the CO includes looking at the efficiency of cardiac performance. In general, greater SV and lower HR represent greater efficiency

e. Indexing: Normal adults come in all shapes and sizes. The absolute CO for a healthy 45 kg woman may be the same as the value for an NFL football player in hemorrhagic shock. How can the values be compared? The answer is to *index* the values to body surface area (BSA). Thus, raw values for CO in adults may vary widely while indexed values are usually closely comparable

a. (45 kg female) CO = 4.0 LPM, BSA = $1.387 m^2$

$$CI = \frac{CO}{BSA} = \frac{4.0 \text{ LPM}}{1.387 \text{ m}^2} = 2.88 \text{ LPM/m}^2$$

b. 145 kg male: CO = 8.0 LPM, BSA = $2.77 m^2$

$$CI = \frac{CO}{BSA} = \frac{8.0 \text{ LPM}}{2.774 \text{ m}^2} = 2.88 \text{ LPM/m}^2$$

Notice that in the above example a 4 LPM CO yields an excellent index for the smaller patient but would result in a value (1.44) for the larger patient consistent with a diagnosis of shock

Any of the values calculated as part of a hemodynamic profile can be indexed; e.g., cardiac index (CI), stroke volume index (SVI), systemic vascular resistance index (SVRI). The normal values for these indices are useful since they are the standard for comparison of all patients, not just those of average size

3. Basic approach to hemodynamic management

Bedside pulmonary artery catheterization in the ICU is different from the procedure of diagnostic cardiac catheterization in the laboratory. The fundamental purpose in the ICU is to measure, monitor, and manage the CO as an integral part of oxygen delivery. Since many of the patients are intubated, on positive pressure ventilation (VCV), and may have multiple problems that affect cardiac performance (even if those problems are not of cardiac origin), the CO must be managed to meet O_2 transport end points, not to make the numbers look "textbook" normal.

a. Pulmonary artery catheter placement: The bedside methodology for catheter placement is reviewed elsewhere (see Chapter 17). The important principles to remember are as follows:

(1) The catheter is placed to measure CO; all other values and calculations are useful only for management within the context of a known CO

(2) Record and evaluate all values during placement of the catheter: right atrial pressure (RA); right ventricular pressure (RV); pulmonary artery pressure (PA systolic, diastolic, and mean); and the pulmonary capillary occlusion (wedge) pressure (PCWP). All of these can help in assessment, diagnosis, and most important, management

(3) Understand the clinical circumstances of the catheterization. Interpretation of the measured pressures in a patient on PEEP (see below) and positive pressure ventilation is markedly different from interpretation of the same values in a nonintubated, spontaneously breathing patient

b. If the CO is lower than desired for good O_2 transport, or is acceptable but achieved inefficiently (e.g., low SV and a significant tachycardia), then the following interventions are recommended (see Fig. 4-11)

(1) *Optimize the preload* (see *1.* in Fig. 4-11): In general, the higher

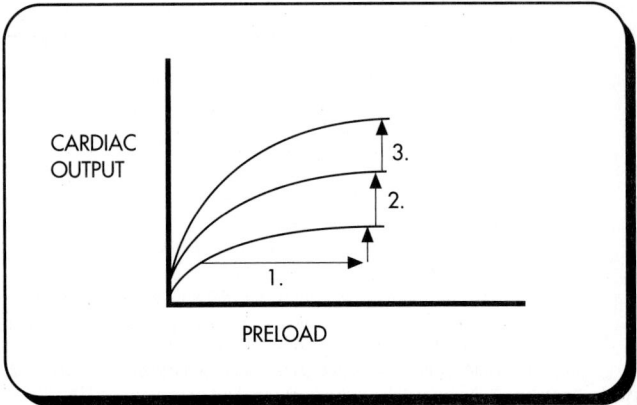

Figure 4-11

Optimization of cardiac output. *1,* Very low cardiac output is enhanced by volume loading to optimal preload. *2,* If cardiac output is still unacceptably low, addition of an inotrope can enhance cardiac out at the *same* preload (i.e., place the patient on a higher function curve). *3,* Further increase in cardiac output at the same preload may be achieved by afterload reduction.

the filling pressure (PCWP), the higher the end-diastolic volume (EDV), and thus, the higher the preload. Remember, the end point is optimized CO as part of optimized O_2 delivery. On any Starling curve, maximal CO (SV or stroke work index [SWI]) is achieved at an optimal filling pressure of about 18-22 mm Hg. This is true only as a general rule of thumb. It does not take into account other mitigating factors such as oncotic pressure, capillary permeability, or the transmural pressure, which may be markedly different in a patient on significant PEEP (see below)

(2) *Inotropic support* (see *2.* in Fig. 4-11): If CO is still inadequate or achieved inefficiently, the addition of an inotrope is justified. An inotrope enables the heart to achieve a higher function curve at the same filling pressure. A good choice for this intervention is dobutamine at 5-30 µg/kg/min

(3) Reduced afterload (see *3.* in Fig. 4-11): If CO is still less than desired, further enhancement may be achieved by afterload reduction. Dobutamine itself has some peripheral vasodilating properties. Amrinone is a phosphodiesterase-inhibitor with both inotropic and vasodilating properties, and may work well in tandem with dobutamine. If the patient's blood pressure is frankly elevated, afterload reduction can be achieved by adequate blood pressure control with a variety of agents

(4) Perform a 2-D echocardiogram: If available, a bedside 2-D echocardiogram can further enhance your assessment
   • Evaluate chamber size/ventricular volume

- Evaluate contractility/regional wall motion
- Evaluate valvular function, which may be hemodynamically important
- Estimate ejection fraction

(5) Re-evaluation: After each incremental intervention (volume loading, inotropic support, and afterload reduction) re-evaluate CO, oxygen transport, and the derived hemodynamic profile

c. Transmural pressures: The discussion of transpulmonary pressure addressed the gradient across the lungs from the airways to the pleural space. An exactly analogous gradient exists across the wall of the heart between intracavitary pressure (inside the atria or ventricles) and the intrathoracic (intrapleural) pressure (ITP). Again it is the vectorial difference across the wall of the heart that is the true transmural pressure and, therefore, the real determinant of ventricular volume. This concept has many important physiologic implications

(1) A normal filling pressure for the right ventricle of 5 cm H_2O (i.e., a normal CVP) is not really *5,* but rather *10;* i.e., 5 cm H_2O filling from *within* and $(-)5$ cm H_2O pulling from *without.*

$$CVP - ITP = P_{transmural}$$
$$5 - (-5) = +10 \text{ cm } H_2O$$

(2) This is a fundamental observation of the Starling relationship: When people inhale (more negative ITP), right ventricular filling is enhanced and, as a result, so is cardiac output

(3) Similarly, a normal PCWP, which serves as left ventricular filling pressure, is not the measured intracavitary pressure (normal $\approx$ 8-12 mm Hg), but rather the transmural pressure, which includes the effect of negative ITP

(4) The heart (or any of its chambers) has compliance. Just as transpulmonary pressure determines lung volume through compliance, so does transmural filling pressure determine ventricular volume (end-diastolic volume [EDV]; i.e., true preload)

(5) Since EDV is the preload and a major determinant of cardiac output, appreciation of transmural pressures may help in the management of CO and Do_2

d. Spontaneously breathing patients with negative ITP make it easy to use readily measured values for CVP or PCWP. When patients are on positive pressure ventilation (any conventional mode of VCV) and especially when they are on PEEP, ITP may no longer be negative and may be substantially positive. Thus, instead of *enhancing* transmural filling pressures, positive $(+)$ ITP may *reduce* transmural gradients, ventricular filling, and therefore, cardiac output

$$\text{No PEEP:}$$
$$CVP - ITP = P_{transmural}$$
$$+5 - (-5) = +10 \text{ cm } H_2O$$

$$PEEP = +10 \text{ cm } H_2O:$$
$$CVP - ITP = P_{transmural}$$
$$+12 - (+10) = +2 \text{ cm } H_2O$$

(1) Even though the measured CVP (inside the vena cava) is higher (+12) in the patient on PEEP, the transmural filling pressure is substantially lower and, as a result, so is the preload (and CO)

(2) If the CVP or PCWP rises, it is normally presumed that the RVEDV and the LVEDV also increase respectively. This is because the normally negative ITP vectorially enhances the transmural pressures and therefore the end-diastolic volumes

(3) If positive ITP actually squeezes the heart from without, the measured filling pressure within the chambers will go *up* as the volume (EDV) is going *down*

(4) A patient on high PEEP who has high measured values for CVP and PCWP may have any of the following

   (a) High end-diastolic volume, good preload, and therefore, good CO as normally would be predicted by elevated filling pressures

   (b) Less than the expected end-diastolic volumes and CO because of restricted cardiac filling secondary to increased ITP

   (c) Very small end-diastolic volumes because of squeezing from positive ITP with resultant poor CO

(5) No algorithm can tell to what degree PEEP is affecting the measured filling pressures or the degree to which positive airway pressure (PEEP) is transmitted to the pleural space and mediastinum. The best indicator of adequate filling pressures (CVP and/or PCWP) is a good CO achieved efficiently with a good SV

(6) A bedside echocardiogram may be of value to look at chamber size (EDV) and to correlate it with measured filling pressures from the PA catheter. This will help in the decision of whether or not a given PCWP yields a good preload (EDV) and whether or not the CO may benefit from further volume (preload) enhancement. The findings can also help to decide whether or not inotropic support should be added

4. *Summary*

   a. The PA catheter can tell a great deal about the patient's condition, but the most important information it gives pertains to the cardiac output

   b. The CO is one of only three parameters that can be manipulated to optimize life-sustaining oxygen delivery

   c. The derived hemodynamic calculations and profiles may help categorize shock states and suggest specific management (see Chapter 3)

   d. In the ICU setting, particularly with patients on positive pressure ventilation, *all* manipulations are likely to have hemodynamic effects; therefore, use the catheter as a monitoring device and frequently update data

   e. All of the following can and will affect cardiac performance, CO, and as a result, Do_2: ventilator setting changes, diuresis, IV fluids, fever, anemia, acidosis/alkalosis, electrolyte abnormalities, medications, and anesthetics/analgesics

4.6   THE CARDIOPULMONARY INTERACTION

1. Proper gas exchange within the lungs depends on the matching of ventilation (V) and perfusion (Q_t). It is immediately obvious that both the pulmonary and cardiac functions are intimately involved.

2. By far the most common cause of arterial hypoxemia is the mismatching of V and Q_t. If ventilation and perfusion are not matched in space, quantity, or time, then some mixed venous blood will pass from the right side of the heart to the left side of the heart without being oxygenated.

   a. Matching in space: If there is a region of lung that receives blood flow with little or no ventilation, the mixed venous blood flowing through that area will reach the left side of the heart without picking up oxygen. A good clinical example of this problem is acute atelectasis

   b. Matching in quantity: Suppose a region of lung receives normal capillary blood flow but a reduced amount of ventilation. When fresh gas is present in the alveoli, the capillary blood is initially well oxygenated, but because of reduced ventilation, the O_2 tension in the alveolus falls and subsequent blood flow is poorly oxygenated until alveolar gas is replenished. This kind of V/Q_t abnormality is very common in both acute and chronic lung disease. It follows that supplemental O_2, which allows capillary oxygen uptake to take place over a longer period of time, improves the hypoxemia resulting from this V/Q_t abnormality

   c. Matching in time: Imagine a region of lung that has ventilation during the inspiratory phase of respiration but no residual gas after exhalation (see discussion of PEEP above and Fig. 4-1). Gas exchange would take place only during inspiration. Ventilation and perfusion would not be present at the same time and mixed venous blood would be allowed to pass unoxygenated through the lungs between active inspirations. Such severe mismatch can occur in acute low-compliance lung disease such as hyaline membrane disease or adult respiratory distress syndrome (ARDS)

   d. Overall V/Q_t matching: Any of the above scenarios—V and Q_t in different places, unequal quantities, present at different times —could be represented mathematically as a low V/Q_t ratio. However, such a depiction would hide the individual pathogenesis and the accompanying rationale for therapy

   e. Venous admixture: In the above examples of mismatched V and Q_t, note that the low V/Q_t ratio means that some venous blood is not oxygenated and is returned as such to the left side of the heart. Thus, as the result of either disproportionately high perfusion for the ventilation (which exhausts available oxygen) or of blood that passes an alveolus that is only intermittently ventilated, *some* quantity of mixed venous blood is added to oxygenated blood. The result is a decrease in the final Po_2 or frank hypoxemia

   f. True shunt: This occurs when there is zero ventilation and some measurable perfusion. This shunted blood never comes in contact with air and thus, reaches the left side of the heart as unaltered mixed venous blood. No change in Fio_2 will improve the resultant hypoxemia, since oxygenated blood cannot saturate beyond 100% and a fixed quantity of unoxygenated blood (shunt) will be added to the final mix

3. General principles

   a. Venous admixture will show improvement in hypoxemia with enhanced Fio_2. The component of low V/Q will be corrected and the true shunt component will not

b. True shunt does not show any improvement of hypoxemia with enhanced Fio_2. If the Fio_2 is increased three times in 10% increments (.21 to .30 to .40 to .50) and the Po_2 increases <10 torr, there is a fixed shunt

c. Clinical end points: Po_2 >60 torr, Sao_2 >.90 achieved a nontoxic Fio_2 (≤0.5) are acceptable. If the patient either requires higher Fio_2 or fails to reach these end points regardless of Fio_2, then therapy directed at shunt reduction per se should be instituted

d. Shunt reduction may occasionally be achieved rapidly, as in relieving atelectasis or collapse, but often requires positive pressure ventilation and PEEP. The rationale for this approach is the recruitment and stabilization of alveoli so there is measurable ventilation in perfused lung regions where previously there was none

   (1) Normal people have <5% shunt resulting from some venous blood being returned directly to the left heart (most importantly, the bronchial circulation)

   (2) Patients with >15% usually require mechanical ventilation

   (3) It is interesting to note that the desirable clinical end points (Po_2 >60, Sao_2 >90 on Fio_2 ≤.5, and Po_2/Fio_2 ratio ≥150) are *all* achieved when Q_s/Q_t is reduced to <15%

   (4) Shunt reduction is often achieved by mechanical ventilation per se and sometimes by the application of PEEP (above physiologic), but ultimately depends on reversal of the pathologic condition (e.g., atelectasis, pulmonary edema, and ARDS)

e. Shunt equation can be used in a modified form at the bedside to calculate the shunt fraction and can be followed during the course of management

$$\frac{Q_s}{Q_t} = \frac{1 - Sao_2}{1 - Svo_2}$$

4. The cardiopulmonary interaction

   It is clear that management of V/Q_t means the management of V *and* the management of Q_t. It is of paramount importance to realize that the two are intimately and inextricably related.

a. Cardiac output and hypoxemia: As discussed previously, a typical response to low CO is enhanced peripheral extraction and low S_vo_2. If the patient has a significant *quantitative* shunt, it will be *qualitatively* enhanced by low S_vo_2. Improvement in CO can thus result in improvement in Po_2 without a single pulmonary intervention. There are also times when a fixed shunt flow (Q_s) represents a larger fraction of a low CO (Q_t), whereas the same Q_s may be a less significant fraction of an improved CO. The message is: Hypoxemia may improve significantly with enhancement of CO and, conversely, a low CO can have a serious adverse effect on oxygenation in the patient with respiratory failure and significant shunt

b. Ventilators and cardiac output: Patients who require shunt reduction to reach clinical end points are likely to be on positive pressure ventilation and PEEP. While positive airway pressure may help recruit and stabilize alveoli, it may also significantly impede venous return to the chest, restrict cardiac diastolic filling, and thus reduce CO (see discussion above). Note that raising the Sao_2 with a maneuver (e.g., raising PEEP), that results in loss of CO achieves *nothing* in terms of optimizing Do_2:

$$Do_2 = 10 \text{ (CO)} \times 12 \text{ (Hb)} \times 1.34 \times 0.80 \text{ } (Sao_2) = 1286$$
$$Do_2 = 8 \text{ (CO)} \times 12 \text{ (Hb)} \times 1.34 \times 0.99 \text{ } (Sao_2) = 1273$$

Do_2 is the same in both cases and what has been gained in Sao_2 has been lost in CO, perhaps secondary to the application of PEEP

4.7   INTEGRATED CARDIOPULMONARY MANAGEMENT PRINCIPLES

1. Below are some practical suggestions based on the acknowledged interdependence of ventilator management and hemodynamics.
   a. Adjust the ventilator settings to reach clinical end points as outlined previously
   b. If the patient requires PEEP >physiologic, and especially ≥10 cm H_2O, the patient should have a PA catheter placed to assist management
   c. CO (CI) should be optimized to at least within normal limits on the current ventilator settings
   d. Do not detach the patient from the ventilator to try to obtain "true readings." The relevant hemodynamics are those measured on the ventilator
   e. Optimize CO first by preload enhancement followed by the use of inotropes or afterload reducing agents as indicated in Fig. 4-3
   f. Reassess. ABGs may improve with good hemodynamic management and no further escalation of ventilator support will be needed
   g. If the filling pressures are elevated or suggest *high preload with poor cardiac output* in a patient on PEEP, an echocardiogram may help to define ventricular volume and ventricular function, and to interpret the measured filling pressures
   h. PEEP (like everything else) should be increased as much as necessary and as little as possible
   i. If the patient is breathing spontaneously, it is acceptable to reduce the number of IMV breaths as tolerated and maintain V_{min} with spontaneous (usually with appropriate PSV) breaths. The fewer positive pressure breaths, the less impedance to venous return, ventricular filling and, therefore, cardiac output
   j. There are 1440 min in a day. A reduction in IMV breaths from 10 to 8 spares the heart 2880 positive pressure breaths and translates into many liters of CO and Do_2
   k. Do not forget to make frequent measurements and calculations. Do_2, Vo_2, Q_s/Q_t, CO, PCWP, SV, SVR, and others can be assessed and reassessed anytime. These assessments give far more precise insights into the causes of hypoxemia or hypotension than the simple measure of Po_2 or blood pressure
   l. Patients on positive pressure ventilation and PEEP should receive dopamine at ≤3 mcg/kg/min to enhance renal blood flow

m. Patients with respiratory failure who are on mechanical ventilation should also receive
   (1) Stress ulcer prophylaxis
   (2) Nutritional support (preferably enteral)
   (3) DVT prophylaxis
   (4) Appropriate sedative/analgesic
n. Noninvasive and/or continuous monitors such as pulse oximetry, end-tidal Co_2 monitoring, and Svo_2 fiberoptic catheters all can help guide dynamic management, and reduce the need for arterial and mixed venous blood gas determinations
o. Invasive arterial and central venous lines are needed for monitoring, blood sampling, and administration of vasoactive substances, concentrated electrolytes, or emergency medications
p. Give such patients a daily chest X-ray (CXR) to verify positions of tubes and catheters, follow lung pathology, and monitor for complications such as barotrauma, atelectasis, or ICU-acquired disease

Selected readings

American Heart Association: Guidelines for cardiopulmonary resuscitation and emergency cardiac care. *JAMA* 1992; 268:2171-295.

Bone RC, Eubanks DH: The basis and basics of mechanical ventilation. *Dis Mon* 1991; 6:331-406.

Carlon GC, Combs AH, Groeger JS: Ventilation at supraphysiologic frequencies: theoretical, technical, experimental, and clinical basis. *Acute Care* 1983/84; 10:123-83.

Chandra NC: Mechanisms of blood flow during CPR. *Ann Emerg Med* 1993; 22:281-8.

Falk JL, Rackow EC, Weil MH: End-tidal carbon dioxide concentration during cardiopulmonary resuscitation. *Circulation* 1988; 77:234-9.

Hedges JR, Barsan WB, Doan LA, et al.: Central versus peripheral intravenous routes in cardiopulmonary resuscitation. *Am J Emerg Med* 1984; 2:385-90.

Kerber RE: Electrical treatment of cardiac arrhythmias: defibrillation and cardioversion. *Ann Emerg Med* 1993; 22:296-301.

Levine S, Levy S, Henson D: Negative-pressure ventilation. *Crit Care Clin* 1990; 6:505-31.

Luce JM: What to consider when choosing a positive-pressure ventilation mode. *J Crit Illness* 1991; 6:339-47.

Matthay MA: Invasive hemodynamic monitoring in critically ill patients. *Clin Chest Med* 1983; 4:233-49.

O'Quin R, Marini JJ: Pulmonary artery occlusion pressure: clinical physiology, measurement and interpretation. *Am Rev Respir Dis* 1983; 128:319-26

Ornato JP: Use of adrenergic agonists during CPR in adults. *Ann Emerg Med* 1993; 22:411-6.

Patel M, Singer M: The optimal time for measuring the cardiorespiratory effects of positive end-expiratory pressure. *Chest* 1993; 104:139-42.

Robin ED: The cult of the Swan-Ganz catheter. *Ann Intern Med* 1985; 103:445-446.

Robotham JL, Scharf SM: Effect of positive and negative pressure on cardiac performance. *Clin Chest Med* 1983; 4:161-87.

Safar P: Cerebral resuscitation after cardiac arrest: research initiatives and future directions. *Ann Emerg Med* 1993; 22:324-49.

Sanders AB, Kern KB, Otto CW, et al.: End-tidal carbon dioxide monitoring during cardiopulmonary resuscitation: a prognostic indicator for survival. *JAMA* 1989; 262:1347-51.

Sassoon CSH: Positive pressure ventilation: alternate modes. *Chest* 1991; 100:1421-9.

Schuster DP: A physiologic approach to initiating, maintaining, and withdrawing mechanical ventilatory support during acute respiratory failure. *Am J Med* 1990; 88:268-78.

Tuxen DV: Detrimental effects of positive end-expiratory pressure during controlled mechanical ventilation of patients with severe airflow obstruction. *Am Rev Respir Dis* 1989; 140:5-9.

Varon J, Fromm RE: Cardiopulmonary resuscitation: new and controversial techniques. *Postgrad Med* 1993; 93(8):235-42.

Varon J, Fromm RE: Aminophylline and cardiac arrest. *Ann Intern Med* 1993; 119(6):536.

Varon J, Sternbach GL: Cardiopulmonary resuscitation: lessons from the past. *J Emerg Med* 1991; 9:503-7.

Villar J, Slutsky AS, Hew E, et al: Oxygen transport and oxygen consumption in critically ill patients. *Chest* 1990; 98:687-92.

Vincent JL, Roman A, De Backer D, et al: Oxygen uptake/supply dependency. *Am Rev Respir Dis* 1990; 142:2-7.

Weisman IM, Rinaldo JE, Rogers RM: Positive end-expiratory pressure in adult respiratory failure. *N Engl J Med* 1982; 307:1381-4.

Yang KL, Tobin MJ: A prospective study of indexes predicting the outcome of trials of weaning from mechanical ventilation. *N Engl J Med* 1991; 324:1445-50.

Yu M, Levy MM, Smith P, et al.: Effect of maximizing oxygen delivery on morbidity and mortality rates in critically ill patients: a prospective, randomized, controlled study. *Crit Care Med* 1993; 21:830-8.

Cardiovascular Disorders

5

Robert E. Fromm, Jr. and Joseph Varon

Cardiovascular disease is the number one cause of death in the United States, killing more than 900,000 patients each year. Recent advances in the understanding of the pathogenesis of some of these disorders, as well as new therapeutic techniques, have greatly improved the ability to treat these patients.

5.1 ISCHEMIC HEART DISEASE

1. Unstable angina pectoris
   a. Definition
      Angina pectoris is chest discomfort that occurs when the demand for myocardial output exceeds supply. Unstable angina is the manifestation of coronary artery disease, falling somewhere between angina pectoris and myocardial infarction. It is characterized by one or more of the following:
      (1) Recent onset of ischemic chest pain
      (2) Increase of severity, duration, or frequency
      (3) Prolonged anginal pain
      (4) Anginal pain that occurs at rest
   b. Risk factors
      (1) Increasing age
      (2) Male sex
      (3) Family history
      (4) Smoking history
      (5) Hypertension
      (6) Diabetes mellitus
      (7) Hyperlipidemia
   c. Pathophysiology
      Coronary artery atherosclerosis most commonly underlies unstable angina. Some controversy exists as to what causes transformation of a stable angina picture into that of unstable angina. However, 7%-9% of hospitalized patients with unstable angina will develop myocardial infarction (MI). 12%-21% of these patients will suffer an acute myocardial infarction within 3 months. Coronary artery spasm, hemor-

rhage, atherosclerotic plaque, and increased platelet aggregation in coronary arteries have been argued to play a role in this syndrome.

d. Clinical presentation

Substernal pain—pressure, heaviness, tightness, and/or burning—that is new in onset, prolonged, or occurring at rest is common. Shortness of breath, diaphoresis, nausea, and pain in the left arm may be present. On occasion, back and jaw pain is the cardinal feature.

e. Differential diagnosis

(1) Acute MI

(2) Acute aortic dissection

(3) Pulmonary disorders, including pulmonary embolism, pleurisy, pneumothorax, and pneumonia

(4) Peptic ulcer disease, pancreatitis, esophageal reflux and spasm, cholecystitis, and biliary colic

(5) Musculoskeletal conditions, chest-wall pain, costochondritis

(6) Herpes zoster

f. Diagnostic studies

(1) Diagnosis is made primarily by history. Physical examination is usually unrevealing. However, look for evidence of hyperlipidemia, hypertension, congestive heart failure, and the presence of murmurs

(2) Electrocardiograms (ECG) during episodes of pain may show tangent repolarization abnormalities. Normal tracing may also be present. Obtain chest x-rays (CXR); these may show evidence of cardiomegaly and/or pulmonary edema

g. Treatment

A patient with unstable angina should be placed on bed rest in the ICU.

(1) Pharmacotherapy

(a) Nitrates

This class of agents causes relaxation of vascular muscle and venodilatation. Diastolic ventricular wall tension is reduced by decreased venous return following the administration of these agents, thus decreasing myocardial oxygen consumption. Therapy may be started with sublingual nitroglycerin, 0.4 mg (1/150) q5min × 3. Topical therapy with 2% nitroglycerin ointment (½-2 inches) q6hr may also be instituted. Recurrent bouts of pain should prompt institution of intravenous nitroglycerin beginning at 10 mcg/min and titrated upward to the desired effect (i.e., absence of pain, systolic blood pressure of 100-110 mm Hg)

(b) Beta-adrenergic blocking agents

These agents reduce myocardial oxygen demand by decreasing heart rate (HR), blood pressure (BP), and contractility. Patients with bradycardia of <50 bpm, systolic BP <100 mm Hg, CXR evidence of pulmonary edema, second- or third- degree atrioventricular (AV) block, or a PR interval ≥0.24 second, and those with bronchospastic lung disease should not receive these agents. Intravenous and oral beta-blocker dosage schedules are depicted in Table 5-1

Table 5-1   Commonly used beta-blockers in unstable angina

Drug	Acute Intravenous Dosage	Oral Dosage
Atenolol	5 mg over 5 min, repeat × 1 after 10 min	50 mg q12hr or 100 mg q24hr
Metoprolol	5 mg q5min × 3 doses	50 mg q6hr; after 48 hr 100 mg q12hr
Labetalol	20-80 mg bolus 2 mg/min infusion titrate to effect	100 mg bid
Nadolol		40-80 mg q day
Propranolol	0.5-3 mg slow IV bolus. Repeat as necessary	40-800 mg/day given bid to qid

Table 5-2   Oral calcium channel antagonists used in unstable angina

Agent	Oral Dosage
Nifedipine	10-120 mg/day
Verapamil	240-480 mg/day
Diltiazem	180-360 mg/day

(c) Calcium channel antagonists

These agents decrease myocardial ischemia by coronary and peripheral vasodilatation, negative effects on contractility, and HR

Oral dosages of representative calcium channel antagonists are noted in Table 5-2. Because of their negative inotropic effect, do not administer these agents in patients with congestive heart failure (CHF)

(d) Aspirin

Aspirin has been shown to decrease the rate of myocardial infarction and coronary death in patients with unstable angina. Various dosage regimens from 160-325 mg q day have been advocated. Some studies have demonstrated a 50% reduction in cardiovascular death or nonfatal MI with this regimen

(e) Anticoagulants

Intravenous heparin has been a useful adjunct in unstable angina, demonstrating reduced incidence of MI and refractory angina in some studies

(f) Thrombolytic therapy

Despite its benefits in treating acute MI, thrombolytic therapy has not been shown to improve outcome in patients with unstable angina. Its use at the current time cannot be advocated

(2) Nonpharmacologic therapy

Persistent chest pain despite maximal therapy with nitrates, beta-blockers, or aspirin may require early cardiac catheterization with the view toward potential mechanical intervention; (i.e., percutaneous transluminal coronary angioplasty [PTCA] or coronary bypass surgery). Perform intraaortic balloon pump (IABP) insertion with the goal of stabilizing the patient. The IABP relieves pain, and may provide relative stability for evaluation prior to intervention

5.2 MYOCARDIAL INFARCTION

1. Definition
   MI is necrosis of the cardiac muscle resulting from an insufficient supply of oxygenated blood.
   a. *Q-wave MI* presents with ST segment elevation and the subsequent development of pathologic Q waves in the ECG
   b. *Non–Q-wave MI:* More than 50% of acute MIs in the United States do not present with ST segment elevation but have nonspecific ECG changes or even normal ECGs
2. Risk factors
   Risk factors for coronary artery disease including MI are: 1. Age 2. Male sex 3. Family history 4. Smoking 5. Hypertension 6. Elevated cholesterol 7. Diabetes mellitus 8. Cocaine use
3. Pathophysiology
   a. MI is almost universally the result of coronary artery atherosclerosis
   b. Atherosclerotic lesions reduce and limit the flow through coronary arteries resulting in ischemic myocardial cells
   c. The formation of thrombi plays a significant role in acute MI and almost all ST segment elevation infarcts will have an occlusive thrombus in the infarct-related artery if examined early enough in the course of the MI
   d. Occlusion of the right coronary artery (RCA) generally results in inferior/posterior MI
   e. Occlusion of the left anterior descending artery (LAD) generally leads to anterior infarctions, while blockage of the left circumflex artery (LCA) results in lateral and/or inferior/posterior MI
   f. Spasm of the coronary arteries may also play a role in MI. As many as 2% of all MI patients, a significantly higher percentage of those patients less than 35 years of age, have angiograms that indicate normal coronary arteries and, presumably, spasm is a significant pathophysiologic event
4. Clinical presentation
   a. Chest pain, typically substernal, lasting 30 min or longer that is unrelieved by rest or nitroglycerin and pain that may radiate from the left or right arm into the jaw. The pain is typically nonpleuritic and may be associated with dyspnea, diaphoresis, nausea, or vomiting
   b. Approximately 20% of all MIs are painless
   c. Burning discomfort is as predictive of acute MI as pressure-type discomfort
5. Physical findings
   a. Skin may be cool. Diaphoresis may be evident
   b. Heart may demonstrate an apical systolic murmur, mitral regurgitation secondary to papillary muscle dysfunction. Third heart sound (S_3) or fourth heart sound (S_4) gallop sounds may be present

c. Advanced signs of congestive heart failure (CHF) with pulmonary edema may be present with rales auscultated in lung fields
d. In many instances the physical examination will not reveal specific abnormalities

6. Diagnostic studies
   a. The diagnosis of MI must be presumptive based on history, physical, and ECG
   b. ECG (see Table 5-3)
      (1) Q-wave MI: the classic description of the evolution of Q-wave MI includes
         (a) ST segment elevation: indicative of an area of injury (see Fig. 5-1).
         (b) T-wave inversion: a sign of ischemia
         (c) Q waves: indicative of areas of infarction. Development of Q waves may occur early or may not occur for several days during the evolution of an MI
      (2) Non–Q-wave MI: ST segment elevation/depression and T-wave inversion may be seen
   c. Enzyme studies
      Necrotic heart muscle cells release enzymes into the bloodstream. Classically, creatine kinase (CK), lactic dehydrogenase (LDH), and serum glutamic-oxaloacetic transaminase (SGOT or AST) have been used in laboratory diagnosis of MI
      (1) CK becomes elevated within 24 hr. This particular enzyme is the most sensitive enzyme for detection of myocardial damage. CK

Table 5-3 ECG localization of infarcts

Infarct Location	ECG Abnormality
Anterior	V_1-V_4
Anteroseptal	V_1-V_2
Anterolateral	I, aV_L, V_4, V_5, V_6
Lateral	I and aV_L
Inferior	II, III, aV_F
Posterior	$R > S$ in V_1

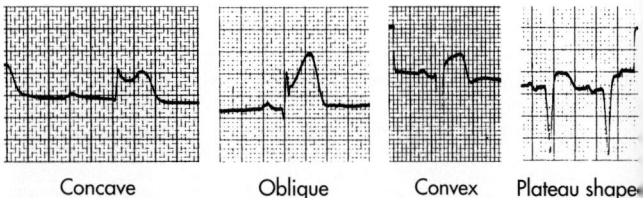

Concave   Oblique   Convex   Plateau shape

Figure 5-1
Different types of ST elevations in acute myocardial infarction. (From Conover MB: *Understanding electrocardiography,* ed 6, St. Louis, 1992, Mosby–Year Book.)

is also present in the skeletal muscle and brain; thus, it may be released in other clinical conditions. To increase specificity, the assay of the isoenzyme of cardiac origin (MB) of CK is used. This enzyme is found primarily in the myocardium

(2) LDH is elevated in the majority of patients with MI; however, it is less sensitive than CK and is elevated in many other clinical conditions. Isoenzyme determinations may show significant elevations of the LDH_1 isozyme that occurs primarily in myocardial cells

(3) SGOT (AST) levels become elevated in 8-12 hr, peaking in 24-36 hr, and, like LDH, are relatively nonspecific. The use of this test is declining

d. Nuclear medicine techniques

Thallium 201 is taken up by perfused viable cardiac myocytes and may indicate areas of infarction through the presence of "cold spots." Unfortunately this technique may not distinguish between acute MI and previous scar. ^{99m}Tc results in "hot spots" as the tracer accumulates in damaged myocardial cells

e. Other diagnostic studies that should be obtained in patients with suspected MI include blood counts, electrolytes, glucose, blood urea nitrogen (BUN), and creatinine

7. Treatment of acute MI

There are two goals in the management of acute MI: minimizing the amount of infarcted myocardium and controlling complications.

a. Give patients with suspected MI continuous ECG monitoring and establish an IV line. Such patients should also receive supplemental oxygen

b. If the patient's clinical condition permits, give sublingual nitroglycerin (0.4 mg SL q5min × 3) to help differentiate patients suffering from angina from patients with MI

c. Give aspirin (asa) to *all* patients without contraindications (160-325 mg PO)

d. Thrombolytic therapy

(1) Consider thrombolytic therapy, unless contraindicated, for patients with ST segment elevation who present within 6 hr of the onset of their symptoms

(2) Thrombolysis is indicated for patients presenting within 6-12 hr and perhaps up to 24 hr (ISIS II trial, LATE trial)

(3) Guidelines for thrombolytic agent administration

(a) Symptoms suggestive of acute MI that are unresolved with sublingual nitroglycerin and that last >20 min and <6 hr. Patients with symptoms lasting >6 hr may benefit as noted above

(b) ST segment elevation and 12-lead ECG consistent with acute MI

(c) Exclusion criteria

(i) Bleeding diathesis

(ii) Gastric or duodenal ulcers within the past 6 months

(iii) Significant surgery within 3 weeks

(iv) Severe trauma within 6 months

(v) History of cerebrovascular accident (CVA) or other central nervous sytem (CNS) processes with a potential for bleeding

(vi) Severe, poorly controlled hypertension is a commonly used exclusion criterion without great evidence

(vii) Poor underlying prognosis (i.e., malignancy) where risk/benefit assessment may not favor treatment

(4) Thrombolytic agents

(a) Tissue plasminogen activator (rt-PA) dosage: 100 mg (accelerated dosage appears to improve patency rates without increasing complications). Give 15 mg as an IV bolus followed by 50 mg infused over 30 min with the remaining 35 mg infused over 60 min. Heparin 5000 units intravenously and 1000 units/hr to be instituted to maintain the partial thromboplastin time (PTT) approximately 2 times control. HART trial evidence suggests unacceptable reocclusion rates if rt-PA is given without heparin. Give asa as well

(b) Streptokinase:
1.5 million units IV over 1 hr. Because of the systemic state induced by streptokinase and high levels of fibrin split products, the need for heparin therapy with streptokinase has been questioned

(c) Anistreptolase anisoylated (plasminogen/streptokinase activator complex): this drug is given as a bolus of 30 units over 5 min. Like streptokinase, heparin therapy is uncertain

e. PTCA
This should be considered in patients with contraindications to thrombolytic therapy. If facilities for rapid institution are available, the outcome of patients with primary PTCA appears to be equivalent to that obtained with thrombolytic therapy

f. Beta-blockers
Beta-blockers are useful in preventing tachydysrhythmias and reducing myocardial oxygen consumption. Early intravenous beta-blockade followed by oral maintenance therapy reduces recurrent ischemia and infarction, even in patients receiving thrombolytic therapy. Patients without contraindications should receive these agents (see Table 5-1)

g. The use of angiotensin converting enzyme (ACE) inhibitors and magnesium in the setting of acute MI is under clinical investigation at this time and is recommended by some authors. However, routine use of these agents cannot be advocated

h. Patients should be classified clinically for prognosis and to determine therapy (see Tables 5-4 and 5-5)

i. Additional management of patients may be based on hemodynamic subset

(1) Uncomplicated MI

(a) In addition to the therapeutic regimens mentioned above, use intravenous nitroglycerin in pain control. Clinical studies have suggested that mortality and infarct size may be reduced by the use of nitrates. Start therapy at 10 mcg/min and increase until the patient is free of pain, the systolic blood pressure

Table 5-4 Killip classification of acute MI

Class I	No heart failure: mortality <10%
Class II	Mild heart failure: mortality 10-20%
Class III	Severe heart failure: rales >50% of lung fields: Mortality 35-50%
Class IV	Cardiogenic shock: mortality 80%

Adapted from Killip T III, Kimball JT: Treatment of myocardial infarction in a coronary care unit: a two-year experience with 250 patients. *Am J Cardiol* 1967; 20:457-64.

Table 5-5 Hemodynamic subsets after acute MI

Subset	Cardiac Index (L/M^2)	Wedge Pressure (torr)
No pulmonary congestion or peripheral hypoperfusion	2.7 + 0.5	12 ± 7
Isolated pulmonary congestion	2.3 ± 0.4	23 ± 5
Isolated peripheral hypoperfusion	1.9 ± 0.4	12 ± 5
Pulmonary congestion and hypoperfusion	1.6 ± 0.6	27 ± 8

Adapted from Forrester JS, Diamond GA, Swan HJ: Correlative classification of clinical and hemodynamic function after acute myocardial infarction. *Am J Cardiol* 1977; 39(2):137-45.

        (BP) falls below 100 mm Hg, or a maximal dose of approximately 200 mcg/min has been achieved

(b) Morphine sulfate in 2 mg (IV) increments as needed for pain unrelieved by nitroglycerin.

(c) Heparin 5000 sq q8-12hr in patients without contraindications and who are not receiving the full dose of heparin. (Note: Patients with anterior wall MI have a lower incidence of left ventricular thrombosis if full heparinization is used)

(d) Strict bed rest for 24 hr followed by a gradual increase in activity

(e) Stool softener, commonly docusate sodium 100 mg PO q day

(f) A low-cholesterol, no-added-salt diet should be prescribed

(2) Complicated MI (see Table 5-5)

    (a) Left ventricular dysfunction manifested by pulmonary congestion

        (i) Decrease left ventricular end-diastolic pressure with intravenous nitroglycerin; consider dobutamine, diuretics, or other vasodilators (see dosages below)

    (b) Patients with hypoperfusion without pulmonary congestion

        (i) Careful intravenous hydration with normal saline. Pulmonary capillary wedge pressure is targeted at approximately 18 mm Hg

        (ii) Right ventricular MI accompanying inferior infarct may

present in this manner. Diagnosis may be made using right-sided precordial chest ECG leads. Significant volume administration may be required for adequate left ventricular (LV) preload

(c) Severe left ventricular dysfunction

Pulmonary artery cannulation should be performed

   (i) If the systolic BP is >100 mm Hg, start dobutamine up to 20 mcg/kg/min intravenously. If the patient demonstrates hypotension with systolic BP below 70-100 mm Hg, administer dopamine 2.5-20 mcg/kg/min IV. More profound hypotension may require norepinephrine 0.5-30 mcg/min intravenously

   (ii) Treat hypertensive patients with intravenous nitroglycerin beginning at 10 mcg/min and, if unsuccessful, sodium nitroprusside 0.5 mcg/kg/min titrated to effect. Thiocyanate accumulation is a potential problem with sodium nitroprusside. Exercise caution with prolonged administration and in patients with renal insufficiency

   (iii) Mechanical support with IABP may improve cardiac output and coronary perfusion while more definitive interventions are under consideration.

(3) Other complications following MI

(a) Mitral regurgitation

Characterized by the sudden appearance of a systolic murmur (radiating to the axilla) and worsening CHF.

   (i) Diagnostic studies: physical examination will demonstrate a systolic murmur and worsening pulmonary congestion. Cardiac catheterization will demonstrate giant V waves in the pulmonary wedge tracing. Echocardiography can be used as well.

   (ii) Therapy: afterload reduction (i.e., IV sodium nitroprusside) to decrease pulmonary capillary wedge pressure. Hypotensive patients may require catecholamines (i.e., dopamine and/or dobutamine)

   (iii) IABP may improve coronary perfusion and ventricular emptying

   (iv) Surgical repair

(b) Ventricular septal defect (VSD)

An event in <1% of Q-wave MIs that may occur at any point from several hours to several days after the onset of symptoms. VSD is most commonly seen during the first 7 days

   (i) Diagnosis: acute VSD results in a loud holosystolic murmur and sudden, severe CHF with cardiogenic shock. Right-heart catheterization with oxygen saturation measurements will exhibit an oxygen saturation step-up between the right atrium and the right ventricle. "Contrast" echocardiography will many times identify the defect

   (ii) Treatment: acute afterload reduction with IV sodium nitroprusside and IABP is required for acute VSD with subsequent surgical repair

(4) Dysrhythmias following MI

Dysrhythmias occur during the first 24 hr in 90% of patients suffering from acute MI

(a) Sinus bradycardia is the most commonly seen dysrhythmia in acute MI and should be treated only when signs of diminished cardiac output are present. Atropine 0.5-1 mg intravenously q3-5min until a total dose of 0.04 mg/kg. Should this prove ineffective, consider dopamine up to 20 mcg/kg/min or epinephrine 10 mcg/min

(b) Supraventricular dysrhythmias: address sinus tachycardia by treating the underlying cause. Pain relief and sedation are often all that is required. Patients with atrial fibrillation or flutter in emergent conditions may require acute cardioversion. Treat stable patients with calcium channel blockers, beta-blockers, etc

(c) Paroxysmal supraventricular tachycardia: approach initially with vagal maneuvers and, if this is unsuccessful, adenosine 6 mg, rapid IV push; if unsuccessful, adenosine 12 mg rapid IV push, followed by verapamil 2.5-5 mg IV push. (See also Chapter 4.)

(d) Ventricular dysrhythmias: prophylactic therapy with lidocaine does not result in improvement of overall survival and *is not indicated* in patients with acute MI. In the patient showing persistent ventricular activity (PVCs) or tachycardia, lidocaine at 1-1.5 mg/kg IV bolus up to a total loading dose of 3 mg/kg. A continuous intravenous drip of lidocaine at 2-4 mg/min may also be used. The second-line agent for ventricular dysrhythmias is procainamide administered at 20-30 mg/min to a maximum dose of 17 mg/kg. A continuous infusion of 1-4 mg/min should be started. End points for therapy include abolition of dysrhythmia, 50% widening of the QRS complex (part of electrocardiographic wave representing ventricular depolarization) and/or hypotension. Bretylium is a third-line pharmacologic agent for sustained ventricular tachycardia. Initial doses are 5-10 mg/kg over 10 min as an infusion, followed by a 1-2 mg/min drip. The most common side effect of bretylium is hypotension. Magnesium sulfate has been demonstrated to be useful also, particularly in polymorphic ventricular tachycardia; 1-2 g over 1-2 min, IV. (See also Chapter 4.)

(5) Conduction disturbances accompanying acute MI

(a) Atrioventricular conduction disturbances

(i) First-degree AV block occurs in 4%-14% of acute MIs

(ii) Second-degree AV block, Mobitz Type I: progressive prolongation of the PR interval with intermittent nonconduction of an atrial beat. Commonly seen in inferior infarction and rarely progresses to complete heart block

(iii) Second-degree AV block, Mobitz Type II: represents 10% of all second-degree blocks during acute MI. This is commonly seen in anterior infarction and infrequently progresses to complete heart block

(iv) Third-degree AV block occurs in 6% of patients. Mortality with inferior MI is 20%-25%, mortality with anterior MI is even greater

(v) Intraventricular block refers to abnormalities within the three divisions of the intraventricular conduction system. These blocks may progress to higher degrees of heart block. One in five patients with bundle-branch block in acute MI will develop second- or third-degree AV block. Mortality rates are double of those who do not

(vi) Complete heart block occurs frequently in MIs with right bundle-branch block plus block of the anterior fascicle or posterior fascicle and, less frequently, an isolated left or right bundle-branch. Similarly, instances of alternating the forms of bundle-branch block have a high incidence of complete heart block

(b) Therapy

(i) Atrioventricular block

(a) First-degree AV block: no specific therapy

(b) Mobitz Type I second-degree AV block: unless unusually slow ventricular rates occur, therapy is not needed. Give atropine (as for bradycardia) followed by temporary transvenous pacemaker insertion in symptomatic patients

(c) Mobitz Type II second-degree AV block should result in placement of transvenous pacemaker, particularly when associated with anterior MI

(d) Complete heart block: temporary transvenous pacemaker (some advocate pacemaker therapy in inferior MI for hemodynamic-compromised individuals only)

(e) Intraventricular conduction disturbances: Insert a transvenous pacemaker for right bundle-branch block and anterior fascicular, posterior fascicular, or alternating bundle-branch blocks. Also give transvenous pacing to patients with first-degree AV block and new onset right or left bundle-branch block

5.3   CARDIAC PACEMAKERS

1. Definition

Cardiac pacemakers are complicated devices that may be used to accelerate cardiac rate, bypass blocked conduction tissue, and/or disrupt dysrhythmias. Advancing technology has resulted in new modes of operation. A five-position code has been developed to describe clinical pacing mode (see Table 5-6).

2. Pacemaker evaluation

Rhythm strips and 12-lead ECGs can be useful in determining the mode of functioning of cardiac pacemakers placed in ICU patients. Examine patients for failure to sense (as indicated by inappropriate pacemaker spikes) and failure to capture (as indicated by pacemaker spikes without subsequent chamber depolarizations). More detailed information can be

Table 5-6 Pacemaker codes

Chamber Paced	Chamber Sensed	Response to Sensing	Programmability	Antitachycardic Functions
O=none	O=none	O=none	O=none	O=none
A=atrium	A=atrium	I=inhibited	S=simple programmable	P=antitachycardia
V=ventricle	V=ventricle	T=triggered	M=mutliprogrammable	S=shock
D=dual	D=dual	D=dual	C=communicating	D=dual
			R=rate modulation	

obtained by querying appropriately equipped pacemakers and examining pulse characteristics with appropriate devices.

3. Technique of pacemaker insertion: see Chapter 15

5.4   CONGESTIVE HEART FAILURE

1. Definition
   CHF is the clinical state that occurs when the heart is unable to pump sufficient oxygenated blood to meet the metabolic needs of the tissues.

2. Etiology
   CHF may result from the failure of either the left or right ventricle. In many instances both pumping chambers fail. Common causes of left ventricular failure include heart disease: aortic stenosis (AS), aortic regurgitation (AR), mitral regurgitation (MR), hypertension, ischemic heart disease, cardiomyopathy, and myocarditis. Common causes of right ventricular failure include pulmonary hypertension (primary and secondary), cardiomyopathy, and right ventricular infarction. Biventricular failure commonly results from left ventricular failure. Additional causes of CHF include dysrhythmias, anemia, thyrotoxicosis, medication-induced, and arteriovenous fistulas.

3. Clinical manifestations
   a. Shortness of breath
   b. Orthopnea: increased venous return associated with a recumbent position leads to worsening shortness of breath
   c. Paroxysmal nocturnal dyspnea: the result of a number of physiologic factors including the increased venous return in patients who are recumbent
   d. Fatigue and lethargy: due to low cardiac output

4. Physical examination
   Signs of left ventricular failure include tachycardia and tachypnea. Pulmonary venous congestion results in rales bilaterally. S_3 and S_4 gallop sounds may be heard. Patients with valvular heart disease may manifest cardiac murmurs. Signs of right heart failure include venous distinction in the jugular veins, peripheral edema, ascites, and congestive hepatomegaly with hepatojugular reflux.

5. Classification of CHF
   Functional classification is commonly reported *per* the New York Heart Association criteria (see Box below).

6. CXR: cardiomegaly with enlargement of involved heart chambers may be seen. Pulmonary vascular congestion progressing to alveolar edema.

New York Heart Association Classification of CHF

Class I: symptomatic with extraordinary activity
Class II: symptomatic with ordinary activity
Class III: symptomatic with minimum activity
Class IV: symptomatic at rest

7. Therapy
   a. Correct and identify the underlying cause (i.e., treat anemia, infections, hypertension)
   b. Decrease cardiac work load with bed rest
   c. Restrict sodium
   d. Reduce preload
      (1) Nitrates: venous dilatation associated with nitrates results in prompt improvement of symptoms in many patients with CHF. (See dosage recommendations)
      (2) Diuretic agents
         (a) Loop-acting agents
            (i) Furosemide: 10-240 mg IV, PO, or continuous IV infusion induces a prompt diuresis and results in venodilatation with rapid improvement in patient symptomatology
            (ii) Bumetanide: 0.5-1 mg IV or 4.5-2 mg PO
         (b) Non–loop acting agents
            (i) Thiazides: (i.e., hydrochlorothiazide 25-50 mg): less potent diuretics that may be of value in mild to moderate CHF
            (ii) Metolazone may potentiate the effect of loop-acting diuretics in doses of 2.5-10 mg
      (3) Morphine sulfate: traditionally used in the management of severe pulmonary edema because of its venodilatory properties and its anxiolytic effects. This agent may depress respirations; thus, other vasoactive substances may be preferable. If used, increments of 2 mg IV titrated to effect are recommended
   e. Arterial dilatation (afterload reduction)
      (1) ACE-inhibitors result in dilatation of the arteriolar-resistant vessels and increased venous capacity, affecting both preload and afterload. These agents decrease mortality in patients with CHF. Enalaprilat is available for intravenous administration (1.25 mg IV over several min). Oral enalapril and captopril are available
   f. Inotropic agents
      Intravenous infusions of dopamine and/or dobutamine have positive inotropic effects and may result in decreasing pulmonary capillary wedge pressures associated with an increase in cardiac output
   g. Digitalis glycosides
      These agents have limited value in the acute setting of pulmonary edema but may be useful in reducing heart rate (HR) of patients with atrial dysrhythmias and in the long-term management of patients with CHF
   h. Aminophylline
      This is used in patients with severe pulmonary edema. It is a weak diuretic and has a positive inotropic effect. Margin of safety with this agent is narrow and its routine use is discouraged
   i. Rotating tourniquets
      Recent clinical studies have questioned the utility of this intervention, though it was once advocated.
   j. Phlebotomy may be used in severe unresponsive cases or in cases where there is severe erythrocytosis

| 5.5 | CARDIOMYOPATHIES

1. Dilated congestive cardiomyopathy
   a. Etiologies: primary disorders of heart muscle in which dilatation of the ventricles and enlargement of the heart occurs (see Box below)
   b. Symptoms of CHF, dysrhythmias, pulmonary and systemic embolization
   c. Physical examination: signs of CHF are commonly seen. A laterally displaced point of maximum impulse (PMI) may be noted along with gallop sounds
   d. Diagnostic studies
      (1) CXR: cardiac enlargement may be seen, pulmonary congestion with interstitial edema, pleural effusion, etc
      (2) ECG: dysrhythmias may be seen as may conduction abnormalities, chamber enlargement/hypertrophy, and nonspecific repolarization abnormalities
      (3) Echocardiography: may demonstrate a low ejection fraction, global hypokinesis, and chamber enlargement
   e. Therapy
      (1) Treat underlying cause
      (2) Manage CHF as noted above
      (3) Prevent thromboembolism
      (4) Consider low-dose beta-blockade
      (5) Perform transplantation with potential mechanical support as bridging maneuver (i.e., left ventricular assist device)
2. Restrictive cardiomyopathy
   Myocardial disorder characterized by decreased ventricular compliance.
   a. Etiology: infiltrative disorders (e.g., sarcoidosis, hemochromatosis, amyloidosis), radiation, endocardial fibroelastosis, endomyocardial fibrosis, scleroderma
   b. Symptoms: right-sided CHF signs, fatigue, and weakness
   c. Specific diagnostic studies: echocardiogram or magnetic resonance imaging (MRI) may help distinguish restrictive cardiomyopathy from constrictive pericarditis (pericardial thickening). Cardiac catheterization and/or biopsy may be used
   d. Therapy

Etiologies of Dilated Cardiomyopathy

Idiopathic
Collagen vascular disease
Postmyocarditis
Peripartum
Familial
Toxins and nutritional deficiency
Radiation

Control of CHF as previously noted with special attention to volume status
3. Hypertrophic cardiomyopathy
Familial or sporadic disorder with marked hypertrophy of the myocardium. Focal or diffuse forms of hypertrophy may occur
   a. Symptoms: syncope, dyspnea, chest pain, palpitations, and sudden death
   b. Physical findings
      (1) Crescendo-decrescendo murmur at the left sternal border that increases with Valsalva's maneuver
      (2) S_4 gallop sound
   c. Diagnostic studies: CXR may be normal; ECG may show left ventricular hypertrophy, abnormal Q waves (anterior, lateral, and inferior leads); echocardiography demonstrates ventricular hypertrophy
   d. Treatment
      (1) Beta-blockers (e.g., propranolol 160-240 mg/day)
      (2) Verapamil
      (3) Surgical myectomy should be used only for failure of optimal medical therapy in appropriately selected patients
      (4) Digitalis, nitrates, diuretics, and vasodilators *may worsen the clinical condition* of this subset of patients

5.6   MYOCARDITIS

Definition
Inflammatory condition of the myocardium.
1. Etiology
   a. Infection
      (1) Viral (e.g., echovirus, adenovirus)
      (2) Bacterial
      (3) Mycoplasmal
      (4) Mycotic
      (5) Rickettsial
      (6) Spirochetal
      (7) Parasitic (*Trichinella*, *Trypanosoma cruzi*)
   b. Toxins
   c. Collagen vascular disease (scleroderma, systemic lupus erythematosus [SLE], rheumatic fever, sarcoidosis)
2. Symptoms
   a. Dyspnea
   b. Chest discomfort
3. Physical examination
   a. Tachycardia
   b. Pericardial friction rub (if coexistent pericarditis)
   c. Evidence of CHF
4. Therapy
   a. Supportive care
      (1) Treat CHF
      (2) Treat dysrhythmias as necessary
      (3) Treat with anticoagulant to prevent thromboembolism

b. Treat the underlying cause. The use of corticosteroids and immuno-suppressive therapy is not advocated, although some data support their use in selective populations with inflammatory infiltrates on endo-myocardial biopsy

5.7   PERICARDITIS

Definition
Inflammation of the pericardium is associated with many different etiologic factors.
1. Etiology (see Box below)
2. Symptoms
   a. Anterior chest pain commonly radiating to arms and back; classically increases with inspiration and is relieved by sitting up or leaning forward. Palpitations and tachycardia may also occur
3. Physical examination
   a. Pericardial friction rub best heard with the patient upright and leaning forward
   b. Tachycardia or other dysrhythmias may be auscultated
   c. If pericardial tamponade occurs, low BP, narrow pulse pressure, and accentuated *pulsus paradoxus* may be seen
4. Diagnostic studies
   a. ECG (see Fig. 5-2): an acute MI evolutionary pattern of ECG is seen with initial ST segment elevations with concavity upward; subsequent T-wave inversion and, finally, late resolution of the repolarization abnormalities. PR segment depression may also be seen
   b. Laboratory evaluation: MI should be ruled out as noted above. Other potential useful studies might include erythrocyte (ESR), antinuclear antibody (ANA), rheumatoid factor, viral titers, and purified protein derivative (PPD)
   c. Echocardiogram to document pericardial effusion, which may not be present

---

Etiologies of Pericarditis

1. Idiopathic
2. Infectious (e.g., tuberculosis, bacterial, viral, fungal, protozoal)
3. Collagen vascular disease
4. Drug-induced
5. Trauma
6. Acute MI and post-MI (Dressler's syndrome)
7. Uremic
8. Postradiation
9. Rheumatic fever
10. Neoplastic

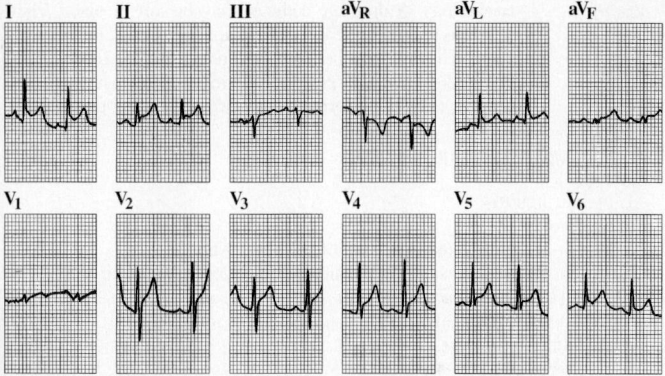

Figure 5-2
Acute pericarditis. (From Hurst JW: *Cardiovascular diagnosis: the initial examination,* St. Louis, 1993, Mosby-Year Book.)

5. Treatment
   a. Antiinflammatories; i.e., indomethacin 25-50 mg PO q8hr or salicylates 3-5 g/day. In severe cases, corticosteroids (i.e., prednisone 60 mg PO q day)
   b. Analgesic for pain unrelieved by antiinflammatories
   c. Observe for signs of cardiac tamponade
   d. Treat underlying causes
6. Complications
   a. Cardiac tamponade: accumulation of pericardial fluid may impair cardiac function mainly through inhibiting of diastolic filling
      (1) Symptoms: dyspnea, orthopnea, and fatigue
      (2) Physical findings
         (a) Neck pain
         (b) Distant heart sounds
         (c) Tachycardia
         (d) Pulsus paradoxus
         (e) Hypotension and a narrow pulse pressure
      (3) Diagnostic studies
         (a) ECG: decreased QRS amplitude and beat-to-beat changes in the R wave
         (b) Echocardiography demonstrates effusions and early right-ventricle diastolic collapse
         (c) Cardiac catheterization: right-heart catheterization reveals equalization of diastolic pressures that includes pericardial pressure if measured
      (4) Therapy
         (a) Pericardiocentesis (see Chapter 17): removal of a relatively small amount of pericardial fluid will improve diastolic filling in the ventricle and greatly improve the patient's symp-

tomatology. A drainage catheter may be left in place. Fluid obtained should be sent for protein, LDH, cell count, Gram's stain, acid-fast bacilli (AFB), culture/sensitivity, and cytology
(b) Pericardiectomy and pericardial window: these surgical procedures may be performed to relieve pericardial tamponade

5.8 VALVULAR HEART DISEASE

1. Aortic stenosis
   a. Etiology
      (1) Rheumatic inflammation of the aortic valve
      (2) Progressive stenosis secondary to congenital bicuspid valve
      (3) Congenital aortic stenosis
      (4) Idiopathic calcification stenosis of the aortic valve
   b. Pathophysiology
      Stenosis of the aortic valve results in increased resistance to ventricular ejection and increased left ventricular pressure. Hypertrophy of the ventricle occurs. Normal aortic valve area is approximately 3 cm^2. Aortic valves of <1 cm^2 generally produce symptoms and those with <0.5 cm^2 with pressure gradients of 50 mm Hg or higher are considered severe
   c. Symptoms
      (1) Syncope commonly occurs with exertion and is frequently associated with vasodilatation in muscle beds leading to cerebral ischemia
      (2) Transient dysrhythmias
      (3) Angina
      (4) CHF
   d. Physical findings
      (1) Slow-rising delayed carotid upstroke with decreased amplitude
      (2) Narrowing of pulse pressure
      (3) Loud systolic ejection murmur heard at the base of the heart and radiating to the neck often with a palpable thrill
   e. Diagnostic studies
      (1) ECG
         (a) Left-ventricular hypertrophy
         (b) Nonspecific repolarization abnormalities
      (2) CXR
         (a) Pulmonary congestion in patients with CHF
         (b) Aortic dilatation
         (c) Calcification of the aortic valve
      (3) Echocardiography
         (a) Hypertrophy of the left ventricular wall
         (b) Visualization of the abnormal aortic valve
      (4) Cardiac catheterization documents severity of disease and calculation of valve area
   f. Therapy
      (1) Judicious management for CHF and angina as they occur (see appropriate sections above). These patients may be very "preload sensitive"

        (2) Valve replacement (reserved as palliative therapy for poor surgical risks)

2. Aortic insufficiency
   a. Etiology
      (1) Infective endocarditis
      (2) Trauma with valvular rupture
      (3) Congenital bicuspid aortic valve
      (4) Rheumatic fibrosis
      (5) Myxomatous degeneration
      (6) Accompanying aortic dissection
   b. Pathophysiology
      Left ventricular pressure increases secondary to regurgitation of blood from aorta resulting in diastolic volume overload and subsequent decompensation
   c. Symptoms
      (1) Many patients remain asymptomatic for many years
      (2) During decompensation: dyspnea on exertion, syncope, chest pain, and CHF
   d. Physical findings
      (1) Widening pulse pressure with bounding pulses. Rapid rise and sudden fall in arterial pressure may result in head-bobbing, capillary pulsations in the nail beds (Quincke's pulse), and water-hammer pulse. In addition, a murmur can be heard over the femoral arteries
      (2) PMI may be displaced laterally and S_3 gallop may be heard. A diastolic blowing decrescendo murmur occurs along the left sternal border
      (3) Austin-Flint murmur: apical diastolic rumble of low pitch secondary to aortic regurgitation, affecting the anterior mitral leaflet
      (4) Systolic apical ejection murmur may also be heard
   e. Diagnostic studies
      (1) CXR may show LV and or aortic dilation
      (2) ECG: left ventricle hypertrophy is usually present
      (3) Echocardiogram: increased left ventricular dimensions and Doppler documentation of regurgitant aortic flow. Fluttering of the anterior mitral leaflet may also be seen
      (4) Cardiac catheterization: contrast study of the aortic root will demonstrate aortic regurgitation
   f. Therapy
      (1) Medical management of CHF as noted above
      (2) Surgical therapy for patients unresponsive to medical management or with acute aortic regurgitation, and for patients with left ventricular failure or a declining ejection fraction

3. Mitral stenosis
   a. Etiology
      (1) Rheumatic fever
      (2) Congenital defects
   b. Pathophysiology: the normal mitral orifice is 4-6 cm^2 in area. An obstruction of the orifice results in impedance of flow into the left ventricle. Symptoms appear when the orifice area approaches 1 cm^2

c. Symptoms
   (1) Dyspnea, orthopnea, and paroxysmal nocturnal dyspnea; pulmonary edema may develop following exertion
   (2) Systemic embolization secondary to thrombi forming in dilated left atrium
   (3) Dysrhythmias, particularly atrial fibrillation
   (4) Hemoptysis secondary to persistent pulmonary hypertension
d. Physical findings
   (1) Auscultation reveals an opening snap in early diastole
   (2) Apical presystolic or mid-diastolic rumble
   (3) Accentuated S_1, Graham-Steel murmur
   (4) Pulmonary regurgitation
e. Diagnostic studies
   (1) ECG: right ventricle hypertrophy, right axis deviation, left atrial enlargement, atrial fibrillation
   (2) CXR
      (a) Left atrial enlargement seen on the lateral chest and a double density on the PA CXR
      (b) Elevation of the left main stem bronchus and widening of the angle between the right and left main stem bronchi
      (c) Pulmonary arterial prominence
   (3) Echocardiography: abnormalities of the valve itself may be seen with calcification and reduction of the E-F slope of the anterior mitral leaflet during diastole
f. Treatment
   (1) Control ventricular rate in patients with atrial fibrillation and anticoagulation to prevent thromboembolism
   (2) Manage CHF as noted above
   (3) Surgical therapy if the valve orifice is less than approximately 0.8 cm^2 or if symptoms persist despite optimal therapy
   (4) Balloon valvuloplasty may be of value in poor surgical candidates
4. Mitral regurgitation
   a. Etiology
      (1) Papillary muscle dysfunction or rupture of the chordae tendineae; i.e., MI
      (2) Infective endocarditis
      (3) Left ventricle dilatation of any cause
      (4) Mitral valvular calcification
      (5) Rheumatic heart disease
      (6) Mitral valve prolapse
      (7) Idiopathic myxomatous degeneration of the mitral valve
      (8) Atrial myxoma
   b. Symptoms
      (1) Dyspnea, orthopnea, and CHF of varying severity
      (2) Hemoptysis
      (3) Atrial fibrillation
      (4) Systemic embolization
   c. Physical findings
      (1) Holosystolic murmur at the apex with radiation to the base or to the left axilla

    (2) Rarely, early to mid-diastolic rumble secondary to increased mitral blood flow
    (3) Signs of CHF
    (4) Left ventricular lift and apical thrill
  d. Diagnostic studies
    (1) ECG: left atrial enlargement, left ventricular hypertrophy, atrial fibrillation
    (2) CXR: left atrial enlargement, left ventricular enlargement, pulmonary congestion
    (3) Echocardiography
      (a) Hyperdynamic left ventricle with enlarged left atrium
      (b) Doppler studies demonstrating regurgitant flow
      (c) Flail leaflet in patients with ruptured chordae
  e. Therapy
    (1) Medical management of CHF as noted above with particular attention to afterload reduction and control of ventricular rate
    (2) Severity of acute disease may be temporized with IABP or surgical intervention

5.9 AORTIC DISSECTION

1. Definition
   Although commonly called *aneurysms,* this disorder is more appropriately termed *aortic dissection.* This condition is the result of a tear of the aortic intima, dissection of blood into the media, and stripping away of the vessel wall from the adventitia.
2. Etiology
   a. Hypertension is present in 90% of patients
   b. Connective tissue disorders; e.g., Marfan syndrome, Ehlers-Danlos syndrome
   c. Bicuspid aortic valve
   d. Granulomatous arteritis and syphilitic aortitis
   e. Pregnancy
   f. Aortic injury
3. Classification
   These lesions are commonly classified by their location: Type A dissections involve the proximal aorta from the aortic valve to the aortic arch and Type B dissections arise beyond the takeoff of the left subclavian artery.
4. Symptoms
   a. Chest pain is almost always present and usually abrupt, severe, and tearing or burning
   b. Syncope
   c. CHF
   d. Cerebrovascular accidents
5. Physical findings
   a. Hypotension or hypertension
   b. Pulse deficits
   c. Aortic regurgitation murmur
   d. Pericardial friction rub

    e. Neurologic signs
    f. Horner's syndrome and/or hoarseness
  6. Diagnostic studies
    a. CXR
      (1) Abnormal in 90% of aortic dissections
      (2) Widened aortic shadow
      (3) Pleural effusions
      (4) Aortic calcification
    b. ECG: usually abnormal (90%); however, nondiagnostic
    c. Computed tomography of the chest with or without contrast will reveal the lesion
    d. Echocardiogram: transthoracic and transesophageal studies may reveal the dissection
    e. Aortogram: the "gold standard" for diagnosis
  7. Therapy
    a. Surgical
      (1) Proximal dissections (Type A)
      (2) Distal dissection, particularly if vital organs are compromised or pain persists despite medical management
    b. Medical
      (1) Aggressive control of BP: typical regimen is administration of intravenous beta-blocker; traditionally, propranolol 1 mg IV q5min until beta-blockade is evident. This is followed by sodium nitroprusside to maintain systolic BP of approximately 100-120 mm Hg. The pharmacologic effects of labetalol infusion have not been well studied, but seem to make this agent ideal for aortic dissection

| 5.10 | SHOCK STATES

Definition
Shock can be defined as a state of inadequate tissue perfusion that, unless reversed, results in progressive organ dysfunction, damage, and death. Mortality rates for shock may exceed 50%. In early stages of shock the patient may be relatively asymptomatic. Sympathetic discharge and other compensatory mechanisms may cause tachycardia and mild peripheral vasoconstriction in attempts to maintain BP. If the state of shock worsens, organ hypoperfusion continues, and BP declines, then the following may be evident: signs of organ dysfunction, including restlessness and agitation; decreased urine output; and clammy skin.
  1. Classification and etiology
    A number of classification schemes for shock states have been devised.
        1. Cardiogenic
        2. Myopathic: reduced systolic function; i.e., acute MI
        3. Mechanical (mitral regurgitation, ventricular septal defect) extracardiac obstructive; i.e., pericardial tamponade, massive pulmonary embolus, or severe pulmonary hypertension
        4. Oligemic; i.e., hemorrhage or fluid depletion
        5. Distributive; e.g., septic shock, anaphylaxis, and neurogenic shock
  2. Diagnostic evaluation
    a. Physical examination: tachycardia, hypotension, and evidence of hypoperfusion (i.e., altered mental status, decreased urine output,

clammy skin) are generally present. Other manifestations may be seen depending on the etiology

  b. Laboratory evaluation
    (1) ECG: useful for identifying dysrhythmias and acute MI
    (2) CXR: pneumothorax, abnormal cardiac silhouette, and pulmonary edema
    (3) Hematology and chemistry: obtain complete blood cell count (CBC), BUN, creatinine, electrolytes, glucose, liver function tests (LFT), and arterial blood gases in the evaluation of any patient with shock
  c. Monitoring
    (1) Foley catheter: patients in shock without contraindication should receive catheter insertion to monitor urine output
    (2) Arterial line: to determine direct intraarterial pressure, to allow easy vascular access for laboratory, and to monitor arterial blood gases
    (3) Central venous pressure monitoring catheter or pulmonary artery catheter

3. Therapy
  Primary treatment goals: restore oxygen transport to normal (or supernormal levels in the cases of sepsis) and demonstrate adequate organ perfusion (i.e., urine output 0.5-1 ml/kg/hr and the absence of lactic acidosis)
  a. Airway, breathing, circulation (ABCs), as in all critically ill patients
  b. Supportive measures
    (1) Two large-bore intravenous catheters for those patients requiring volume resuscitation. Patients in whom fluid status is normal or elevated may require a central intravenous line for administration of medication. For patients not volume overloaded, volume administration is the initial management of hypotension and shock. Volume challenges of 250 cc to 1 L at a time should be rapidly administered with reassessment of the clinical condition
    (2) Supplemental oxygen appropriate for the patient's clinical status
    (3) Patients who are unresponsive to volume administration should receive beta-receptor stimulants. Dopamine is used commonly in hypotensive patients because of its positive inotropic effects at lower doses and its vasoconstrictor effect at higher doses. Initial doses are usually 5 mcg/kg/min
    (4) Mechanical support of the circulation may be necessary in patients with refractory cardiogenic shock and amenable lesions
    (5) Additional interventions and therapeutic goals for management of shock must be based on specific etiologies

5.11   INFECTIVE ENDOCARDITIS

1. Definition
  Infection of the endocardial structures of the heart.
2. Etiology
  a. *Streptococcus viridans:* streptococcus is the most common organism isolated, excluding prosthetic valve or right-side endocarditis
  b. *Staphylococcus aureus:* the most frequent organism isolated in right-side endocarditis

   c. *Staphylococcus epidermiditis*
   d. Others
     (1) Gonococci
     (2) Other bacteria
     (3) Fungi
3. Risk factors
  A number of disorders and behaviors are risk factors for the development of endocarditis.
   a. Valvular abnormalities
     (1) Rheumatic valvulitis
     (2) Bicuspid aortic valve
     (3) Aortic stenosis or insufficiency
     (4) Mitral stenosis, prolapse, or insufficiency
     (5) Mechanical heart valves
     (6) Previous endocarditis
   b. Intravenous drug abuse
   c. Marfan syndrome
   d. Instrumentation
4. Diagnosis
   a. History: elicit careful history for underlying risk factors
   b. Physical examination
     (1) Fever: generally present but may not be noted in elderly or immunocompromised patients
     (2) Cardiac murmurs: usually present but may not be detected, particularly in right-side endocarditis
     (3) Peripheral manifestations: these include painless erythematous papules and macules of the soles and palms (Janeway lesions); painful erythematous subcutaneous papules (Osler's nodes); and petechia and splinter hemorrhages of the nail beds
   c. Laboratory evaluation
     (1) Blood cultures: positive cultures are quite common (85%-95%) prior to antibiotic therapy. Reasons for negative cultures include prior antibiotic therapy, slow-growing or very fastidious organisms, or improper collection
     (2) Nonspecific laboratory findings
       (a) Decreased hemoglobin/hematocrit
       (b) Elevated, decreased, or normal white blood cell count with a left shift, hematuria on urinalysis, and an elevated sedimentation rate. Rheumatoid factor may be positive in half of the cases by 6 weeks. Assays of teichoic acid antibodies have been advocated for *Staphylococcus aureus* endocarditis
     (3) Echocardiography: transthoracic and transesophageal echocardiography may reveal valvular damage, impairments of left ventricular function, and valvular vegetations. Transesophageal echocardiography enhances sensitivity. Some patients will not demonstrate abnormal echocardiographic studies
5. Major complications
   a. CHF secondary to valvular destruction, dysrhythmias, or myocarditis
   b. Embolization
   c. Cardiac dysrhythmias

  d. Myocarditis and pericarditis
6. Therapy
  a. Antibiotics appropriate for the clinical setting: for a native valve en-
     docarditis, penicillin G IV (12-24 million U/day) and gentamicin (dos-
     age by body weight and renal function) are commonly advocated. For
     intravenous drug addicts, penicillinase resistant-penicillin, or vanco-
     mycin plus gentamicin is advocated
  b. Surgical therapy for endocarditis should occur if severe heart failure
     or valvular obstruction is present, or if uncontrolled infection exists.
     Relative indications for cardiac surgery include two or more embolic
     events, unusually large vegetations, extension of the infection to other
     intracardiac structures, or, in the case of prosthetic valve endocarditis,
     periprosthetic leak

| 5.12 | DYSRHYTHMIAS (also see chapter 4)

1. Supraventricular dysrhythmias
   A group of dysrhythmias in which the site of origin and pathway is not
   confined to the ventricles.
   a. Paroxysmal supraventricular tachycardia (PSVT) commonly origi-
      nates through a re-entrant mechanism in the AV node and is charac-
      terized by abrupt onset and termination. PSVT may occur in young
      patients without other evidence of cardiac disease, as well as in pa-
      tients with acute MI, Wolff-Parkinson-White syndrome, or other struc-
      tural heart diseases
      (1) ECG characteristics: regular tachycardia of 150-220 beats/min.
          Atrial activity (P waves) may be seen, depending on the rate and
          relationship between atrial and ventricular depolarization. QRS
          complex is frequently narrow; however, a wide QRS complex may
          be seen
          (a) Symptoms
              (i) Palpitations
              (ii) Possibly hypotension may precipitate CHF
          (b) Therapy
              (i) ABCs
              (ii) Synchronized DC countershock for patients demonstrat-
                   ing clinical instability; i.e., cardiogenic shock, ischemic
                   chest pain, or CHF
              (iii) Begin treatment of the stable patient with a vagal ma-
                    neuver. Valsalva or carotid sinus massage, following ex-
                    clusion of carotid disease, may abort the dysrhythmia
              (iv) Administer adenosine to patients who do not respond to
                   vagal maneuvers (6 mg rapid IV bolus). A second bolus
                   of 12 mg rapid IV may be given. Methylxanthines (e.g.,
                   theophylline, aminophylline, caffeine) are competitive
                   antagonists, and dipyridamole enhances the pharmaco-
                   logic effect of adenosine
              (v) Verapamil: 5-10 mg over 5 min (repeat if needed in 20-30
                  min) may be used if adenosine is ineffective. Pretreat-

ment with a slow injection of 10 ml of 10% calcium chloride may decrease the common hypotensive effects of this drug. Patients with wide complex tachycardia that cannot be confidently diagnosed as supraventricular should not receive verapamil

   (vi) Additional considerations include digoxin, beta-blockers, pace termination, and synchronized cardioversion

2. Atrial fibrillation is chaotic atrial activity without an organized atrial rhythm. This dysrhythmia may accompany coronary artery disease, mitral and aortic valvular disease, thyrotoxicosis, pericarditis, myocarditis, alcoholic heart disease, and MI without evidence of other organic cardiac disease.

   a. ECG: irregular, chaotic atrial activity without an organized rhythmic pattern. Conducted QRS complexes will have an irregular pattern; however, atrial ventricular block with emergence of a lower pacemaker site may result in a regular ventricular response

   b. Other diagnostic studies
      (1) Thyroid function tests
      (2) Echocardiography

   c. Therapy
      (1) DC cardioversion is indicated in unstable patients, as in PSVT
      (2) Digoxin loading: digoxin is the traditional therapy for new onset atrial fibrillation. 0.5 mg IV loading dose followed by 0.25 mg q 3-4 hr until the ventricular rate is controlled
      (3) Alternatives for rapid rate control
         (a) Verapamil 5 mg IV
         (b) Diltiazem 20-25 mg IV
         (c) Beta-blockers: propranolol 0.5 mg IV slowly followed by boluses of 1 mg q5min to a total of 5 mg
      (4) Only 15%-20% of patients treated with digitalization alone will convert to normal sinus rhythm. In the remainder of patients quinidine sulfate 300 mg q6hr is commonly employed, followed by elective cardioversion if normal sinus rhythm is not obtained
      (5) Anticoagulation is advisable pre- and postcardioversion, particularly in patients with mitral valve disease or a history of embolic phenomena

3. Atrial flutter: rapid regular atrial rate of 280-340 bpm, generally associated with varying degrees of atrioventricular block. This dysrhythmia may occur with coronary artery disease including MI, thyrotoxicosis, pulmonary embolism, and mitral valve disease.

   a. ECG: atrial depolarization classically has a sawtooth pattern with varying AV conduction block. Vagal maneuvers may slow the ventricular response rate and make atrial flutter waves more apparent

   b. Therapy
      (1) Atrial fibrillation: cardioversion with DC countershock is indicated in patient who are compromised
      (2) Commonly effective with the pharmacologic interventions previously denoted for atrial fibrillation. In addition, atrial pacing may terminate atrial flutter

4. Multifocal atrial tachycardia: a chaotic irregular atrial activity with rates

from 100-180 and varying P-wave morphology (three consecutive different P-wave morphologies). This disorder commonly accompanies chronic obstructive pulmonary disease, theophylline toxicity, hypoxemia, and/or other metabolic disturbances.

   a. ECG (see Fig. 5-3): varying P-to-P intervals and beat-to-beat variability in P-wave morphology

   b. Therapy: treat the underlying cause. Rate may be controlled, if necessary, with verapamil. In the absence of CHF, beta-blockers may be used. In addition, some authorities advocate intravenous magnesium

5. Bradycardias and AV-conduction blocks: low intrinsic rate from the sinus node or blockade of sinus impulses between the AV node results in slow ventricular rates.

   a. Etiology

      (1) Vagotonia

      (2) Ischemic heart disease

      (3) Cardiomyopathies

      (4) Drugs

      (5) Degenerative diseases of the AV-conduction system

   b. Treatment

     Patients who are symptomatic due to low ventricular response rate may be treated with the following:

      (1) Initially with atropine 0.5-1.0 mg intravenously, repeated every 3-5 min with a total dose of 0.04 mg/kg

      (2) Transcutaneous pacing, when available, may be employed

      (3) Pharmacologic therapy may include dopamine 5-20 mcg/kg/min IV infusion or epinephrine 2-10 mcg/min IV infusion titrated to heart rate. Consider urgent transvenous pacemaker placement in patients requiring transcutaneous pacers for high degrees of AV block

6. Ventricular tachycardia: three or more consecutive beats of ventricular origin. Common rates are 100-200 bpm. It may be difficult to differentiate ventricular and supraventricular dysrhythmias. A good rule of thumb is that wide-complex QRS tachycardia should be considered ventricular tachycardia until proven otherwise.

   a. Monomorphic ventricular tachycardia (a single QRS morphology) should be treated as noted in Chapter 4

   b. Polymorphic ventricular tachycardia or torsades de pointes may be caused by agents frequently used in the treatment of monomorphic

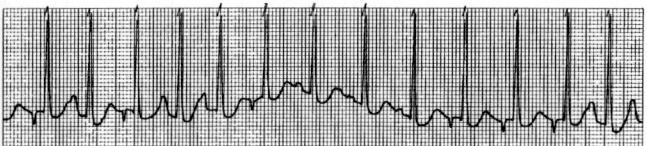

Figure 5-3
Multifocal atrial tachycardia (lead II). (From Conover MB: *Understanding electrocardiography,* ed. 6, St. Louis, 1992, Mosby–Year Book.)

ventricular tachycardia. Electrolyte disturbances including hypokalemia, hypomagnesemia, and the presence of cardiac and psychotropic
medications should be sought. Unstable patients should receive electrical therapy as previously outlined. Stable patients may respond to
overdrive pacing, intravenous magnesium, and correction of underlying causes

5-13   HYPERTENSIVE CRISIS

Definition
Potentially life-threatening situations that are the result of elevated blood
pressure. Manifestations include hypertension with end-organ dysfunction
(see Box below). Uncommonly occurs with BPs <130 mm Hg diastolic.
1. Treatment
   a. Promptly reduce BP. Many authorities recommend reductions of ap-
      proximately 15% in the first hr with gradual reduction to diastolic BPs
      of 100-110 mm Hg or a reduction of 25% of initial reading
   b. Reductions in BP may result in ischemia, thus, follow these patients
      carefully. Parenteral therapy with short-acting agents are initially rec-
      ommended (see Table 5-7)
   c. Patients receiving parenteral therapy should have continuous arterial
      pressure monitoring
      (1) Cyanide poisoning may occur with prolonged IV administration
          of sodium nitroprusside. Consider this if such patients develop

---

End-Organ Dysfunction in Hypertensive Emergencies

Hypertensive encephalopathy
Acute aortic dissection
Acute myocardial infarction
Acute cerebral vascular accident
Acute hypertensive renal injury
Acute congestive heart failure

Table 5-7   Intravenous antihypertensive medications

Medication	Dosage
Nitroprusside	0.5-10 mcg/kg/min
Labetalol	20 mg bolus, 2 mg/min (max 300 mg/day)
Trimethaphan	1-15 mg/min
Nitroglycerin	5 mcg/min (increase by 5-10 mcg every 3-5 min prn)
Diazoxide	25-150 mg IV over 5 min or infusion of 30 mg/min to effect
Nicardipine	5 mg/hr and increase by 2.5 mg/hr to effect (max 15 mg/hr)

CNS depression, seizures, lactic acidosis, or cardiovascular instability
    (a) May occur with infusion rate >2 mcg/kg/min
    (b) Infusion rates >10 mcg/kg/min should not be continued for
        prolonged periods of time because of this hazard
    (c) If cyanide intoxication is suspected, discontinue infusion and
        treat as described in Chapter 16
  d. Oral therapy with nifedipine (10 mg SL q5min × 2), clonidine (0.1
     mg PO q20min), or a host of other agents (e.g., nitroglycerin and cap-
     topril) may be used in ICU patients with less severe cases of hyper-
     tension

Selected readings

ACC/AHA Task Force: Guidelines for early management of patients with acute myocardial infarction. *J Am Coll Cardiol* 1990; 16:249-91.

American Heart Association: Guidelines for cardiopulmonary resuscitation and emergency cardiac care: chain of survival. *JAMA* 1992; 268:2171-302.

Angeli P, Chiesa M, Caregaro L et al.: Comparison of sublingual captopril and nife-
dipines in immediate treatment of hypertensive emergencies: a randomized, single-
blind clinical trial. *Arch Intern Med* 1991; 151:678-82.

Bregman D, Kaskel P: Advances in percutaneous intra-aortic balloon pumping. *Crit
Care Clin* 1986; 2:221-36.

Brown RW, Hunt D, Sloman JG, et al: The natural history of atrioventricular conduction defects in acute myocardial infarction. *Am Heart J* 1969; 78:460-66.

Cairns CB, Niemann JT: Intravenous adenosine in the emergency department
management of paroxysmal supraventricular tachycardia. *Ann Emerg Med* 1991;
20:717-21.

Calhoun DA, Oparil S: Treatment of hypertensive crisis. *N Engl J Med* 1990; 323:1177-
83.

Corrigall D, Bolen J, Hancock EW, et al: Mitral valve prolapse and infective endocarditis. *Am J Med* 1977; 63:215-22.

Crawford SE: The diagnosis and management of aortic dissection. *JAMA* 1990;
264:2537-41.

Forrester JS, Diamond G, Chatterjee MB et al: Medical therapy of acute myocardial
infarction by application of hemodynamic subsets. *N Engl J Med* 1976; 12:1356-
1412.

Gifford RW: Management of hypertensive crises. *JAMA* 1991; 266:829-35.

The GISSI Study Group: Long-term effects of intravenous thrombolysis in acute myocardial infarction: final report of the GISSI study. *Lancet* 1987; 10:871-4.

Hinton RC, Kistler JP, Fallon, JT et al: Influence of etiology of atrial fibrillation incidence of systemic embolism. *Am J Cardiol* 1977; 40:509-12.

Kastor JA: Multifocal atrial tachycardia. *N Engl J Med* 1990; 322:1713-17.

Levine HJ: Overview of results of randomized clinical trials in heart disease: treatments following myocardial infarction. *JAMA* 1988; 260:2088-93.

Nolan CM, Kane JJ, Grunow WA: Infective endocarditis and mitral prolapse: a comparison with other types of endocarditis. *Arch Intern Med* 1981; 141:447-50.

Smith MD, Kwan OL, DeMaria AN: Value and limitations of continuous-wave Doppler echocardiography in estimating severity of valvular stenosis. *JAMA* 1986;
255:3145-51.

Steinbeck G, Andresen D, Bach P, et al: A comparison of electrophysiologically guided
antiarrhythmic drug therapy with beta-blocker therapy in patients with symptomatic,
sustained ventricular tachyarrhythmias. *N Engl J Med* 1992; 327:987-92.

Tcheng JE, Jackman JD, Nelson CL, et al: Outcome of patients sustaining acute ischemic mitral regurgitation during myocardial infarction. *Ann Intern Med* 1992; 117:18-
24.

Théroux P, Ouimet H, McCans J, et al: Aspirin, heparin, or both to treat acute unstable angina. *N Engl J Med* 1988; 319:1105-11.

The TIMI Study Group: Comparison of invasive and conservative strategies after treatment with intravenous tissue plasminogen activator in acute myocardial infarction: results of the thrombolysis in myocardial infarction (TIMI) phase II trial. *N Engl J Med* 1989; 320:618-27.

Topol EJ: Coronary angioplasty for acute myocardial infarction. *Ann Intern Med* 1988; 109:970-80.

Varon J, Fromm RE: Cardiomyopathies in the ICU. *Hosp Physician* 1992; 28:23-9.

Zehender M, Kasper W, Kauder E, et al: Right ventricular infarction as an independent predictor of prognosis after acute inferior myocardial infarction. *N Engl J Med* 1993; 328:981-8.

Endocrinologic Disorders

Pamela R. Roberts

| 6.1 | **ADRENAL INSUFFICIENCY** |

1. Definition

   A deficiency of glucocorticoid production that can result from failure of the adrenal gland (primary adrenal insufficiency), or failure of hypothalamic-pituitary secretion of corticotropin releasing hormone (CRH) or adrenocortical trophic hormone (ACTH) (secondary adrenal insufficiency).

2. Pathophysiology

   a. Glucocorticoid synthesis is regulated by the hypothalamic-pituitary-adrenal (HPA) axis. Hypothalamus secretes CRH, stimulating the pituitary to release ACTH and increasing the release of cortisol by the adrenal cortex

   b. Cortisol is a negative feedback on further CRH and ACTH production

   c. Mineralocorticoid production is regulated primarily by the renin-angiotensin system, blood pressure (BP), and extracellular potassium level

   d. Catecholamines are synthesized by the adrenal cortex and medulla

   e. The adrenal cortex is composed of the *zona glomerulosa* (aldosterone synthesis), *zona fasciculata* (glucocorticoid synthesis), and *zona reticularis* (androgen and glucocorticoid synthesis)

   f. Primary adrenal insufficiency usually results in loss of both glucocorticoid and mineralocorticoid secretion

   g. Patients with secondary adrenal insufficiency maintain normal secretion of the mineralocorticoids

3. Etiology

   a. Infection (AIDS, TB, CMV, meningococcemia, fungus, *Pseudomonas* septicemia)

   b. Adrenal hemorrhage (coagulopathies, anticoagulant therapy, sepsis, trauma, pregnancy)

   c. Withdrawal of exogenous steroids or HPA axis suppression from recent (up to 1 year before) treatment with exogenous corticosteroids

   d. Drugs that interfere with adrenal steroid synthesis (ketoconazole, etomidate, aminoglutethimide)

      e. Tumor destruction

      f. Adrenal infarction (arteritis, thrombosis)

      g. Autoimmune disorders (sarcoidosis, amyloidosis)

4. Clinical manifestations

      a. Weakness

      b. Weight loss

      c. Anorexia

      d. Hyperpigmentation (only in primary adrenal insufficiency)

      e. Circulatory collapse

      f. GI disturbances (nausea/vomiting, abdominal pain, diarrhea, constipation)

      g. Dehydration

      h. Fever

      i. May have only vague symptoms (malaise, arthralgias)

5. Associated laboratory abnormalities

      a. Increased potassium and calcium

      b. Decreased sodium and chloride

      c. Decreased glucose

      d. Metabolic acidosis

      e. Increased blood urea nitrogen (BUN:Cr) ratio

      f. Normocytic, normochromic anemia, neutropenia, lymphocytosis, eosinophilia

6. Diagnostic evaluation

      a. Physical examination

         (1) Hypotension

         (2) Hyperpigmentation, except in acute or secondary adrenal insufficiency

         (3) Possible loss of axillary hair in females

      b. Laboratory evaluation

         (1) Measurement of a single plasma cortisol level usually does not allow reliable appraisal of pituitary and adrenal function; however, in stressed, critically ill patients it is sufficient to rule out or to suggest the diagnosis of adrenal insufficiency. A serum cortisol level ≥20 mcg/dL indicates adequate adrenal glucocorticoid secretion following stress, ACTH, or CRH

         (2) If the patient is hemodynamically unstable and adrenal insufficiency is suspected, draw a random cortisol level and initiate immediate treatment with hydrocortisone (see below).

         (3) If the patient is hemodynamically stable and adrenal insufficiency is suspected, a random cortisol level may be measured and the patient treated with dexamethasone (stress dose of 10 mg IV q6hr) until the result is available; then, if the cortisol level is <20 mcg/dL, a screening synthetic ACTH stimulation test may be performed

            (a) Measure baseline cortisol level

            (b) Give cosyntropin (synthetic ACTH) 0.25 mg IV

            (c) Measure cortisol level again after 60 min

            (d) An increase of <7 mcg/dL is suggestive of primary adrenal insufficiency if the basal cortisol level is <20 mcg/dL

            (e) If diagnosis of adrenal insufficiency is confirmed by plasma cortisol <20 mcg/dl, further testing (3-day ACTH infusion test) may be required to establish the exact etiology, but this should be done *only* when the patient is out of the ICU

(4) Diagnostic imaging may help determine the etiology. Bilaterally enlarged adrenal glands by CT scan suggest adrenal hemorrhage, neoplastic disease, TB, or fungal infection; small adrenal glands suggest autoimmune disease or lack of ACTH

(5) High ACTH levels associated with low cortisol levels or failure of the adrenal glands to respond to prolonged ACTH stimulation are consistent with primary adrenal insufficiency

(6) Measurement of the levels of plasma renin (PRA) and aldosterone (ALDO) may help distinguish primary from secondary adrenal insufficiency. (PRA : ALDO ratios are high in primary adrenal insufficiency and low in secondary adrenal insufficiency.)

(7) Patients with primary adrenal insufficiency have decreased 24-hr urinary cortisol, 17-hydrocorticosteroid (17-OHCS), and 17-ketosteroid (17-KS) and increased ACTH. Assessment of these substances is impractical in most ICU situations and should not be undertaken prior to or in lieu of treatment

7. Therapy

a. Treat immediately patients with circulatory collapse and suspected adrenal insufficiency. If possible, draw random cortisol level first, but do not wait to treat

b. Administer hydrocortisone 100 mg IV q6hr for 24 hr; if the patient shows a good clinical response or cortisol level confirms diagnosis, the dosage may be tapered gradually and changed eventually to oral

c. Provide adequate volume replacement with dextrose 5 normal saline (D5NS) until hypotension, dehydration, and hypoglycemia are corrected

d. Identify and treat any precipitating factors (infections, hemorrhage)

8. Complications

a. Short-term corticosteroid therapy is safe

b. When there is a question of adrenal insufficiency during an emergency, give short-term supplemental corticosteroids until adrenal integrity can be assessed

c. It is of the utmost importance to treat patients in these situations because adrenal crises will progress to death if untreated

| 6.2 | DIABETES INSIPIDUS |

1. Definitions

a. A disorder of fluid homeostasis resulting from inadequate vasopressin or antidiuretic hormone (ADH) secretion or action

b. Neurogenic diabetes insipidus may be caused by a lack of production of ADH precursor molecule by the hypothalamus or inadequate secretion of ADH by the posterior pituitary

c. Nephrogenic diabetes insipidus is caused by unresponsiveness of renal tubules to ADH

d. Both types of diabetes insipidus result in excretion of large volumes of hypotonic fluid

2. Etiology
   See Box below
3. Clinical manifestations
   a. Polyuria: urine volume usually >30 ml/kg/day
   b. Neurologic manifestations: seizures, profound central nervous system (CNS) dysfunction
   c. Dehydration
   d. Polydipsia: not likely to occur in the critically ill patient with limited access to water
4. Evaluation of polyuria
   a. History
      (1) Review clinical history for evidence of recent trauma, neurosurgical procedures, and pharmacologic causes
      (2) Rule out excess water administration
      (3) Rule out solute load
   b. Laboratory evaluation
      (1) Decreased urine specific gravity (≤1.010)
      (2) Inappropriately dilute urine (≤300 mOsm/kg H_2O)
      (3) Electrolytes: hypernatremia, hypercalcemia, hypokalemia
      (4) Increased plasma osmolality(>300 mOsm/kg H_2O)

Causes of Diabetes Insipidus

Neurogenic diabetes insipidus (ADH deficiency)
- Head trauma*
- Postoperative (e.g. secondary to neurosurgical procedures)*
- Neoplasms of the brain or pituitary fossa*
- Postanoxic/ischemic injury*
- Vascular injury (e.g. subarachnoid hemorrhage)*
- Meningoencephalitis*
- Infiltrative hypothalamic disorders (e.g. sarcoidosis, histiocytosis)
- Familial (autosomal dominant)
- Idiopathic

Nephrogenic diabetes insipidus (ADH resistance)
- Pharmacologic causes (e.g., lithium, amphotericin B)*
- Postobstructive*
- Metabolic disturbances (e.g., hypercalcemia, hypokalemia)*
- Pyelonephritis
- Polycystic kidney disease
- Sickle cell disease and trait
- Infiltrative diseases (e.g., sarcoidosis, amyloidosis)
- Familial (X-linked recessive)

Diabetes insipidus of pregnancy (secondary to ADH degradation by vasopressinase produced by the placenta): a rare form of diabetes insipidus and seen even less commonly in the ICU

---

*Designates causes likely to be seen in the critically ill.

c. Differential diagnosis
  (1) Diabetes insipidus
  (2) Solute diuresis (glucose, mannitol, urea, IV contrast media, sodium diuresis secondary to diuretic or dopamine administration)
  (3) Primary polydipsia
5. Diagnostic approach
  a. First exclude solute diuresis as etiology; check urine glucose, osmolality, and specific gravity
  b. The diagnosis of diabetes insipidus is made if the patient has hypernatremia and either an inappropriately low plasma ADH level or an inappropriately low urine osmolality. Further testing is needed only to distinguish the type of diabetes insipidus
    (1) Administer a therapeutic trial of 1 mcg desmopressin (DDAVP) subcutaneously
    (2) The diagnosis of neurogenic diabetes insipidus is confirmed and therapy can be instituted if urine osmolality increases ≥50%
    (3) Renal resistance to ADH is suggested and nephrogenic causes of diabetes insipidus should be addressed if urine osmolality does not increase in response to DDAVP
  c. A water deprivation test may be initiated if the plasma sodium is <145 mEq/L and the patient is hemodynamically stable. This stimulates secretion of ADH and determines if the patient will respond appropriately to ADH
    (1) Continue fluid restriction until plasma osmolality is ≥295 mOsm/kg or sodium level is ≥145 mEq/L. Attempt to decrease fluid intake to ≤1-2 L/day and follow serial urine output, osmolality, and plasma sodium
    (2) DDAVP may be given (as above) to distinguish between neurogenic and nephrogenic diabetes insipidus if plasma sodium ≥145 mEq/L while urine osmolality remains ≤300 mOsm/kg
    (3) Secondary diabetes insipidus is suggested (nondiagnostic) if plasma sodium ≥145 mEq/L and urine osmolality ≥300 mOsm/kg
    (4) Fluid restriction may be continued if the patient tolerated it well based on the suspicion that the cause is excessive water administration
    (5) DDAVP therapy may be started with close monitoring of water balance until further testing can be performed safely if the patient develops thirst or evidence of hypovolemia before polyuria resolves. This will distinguish between partial neurogenic diabetes insipidus and nephrogenic diabetes insipidus. Testing of plasma ADH levels may be needed when the patient is out of the critical care setting
6. Therapy
  a. Neurogenic diabetes insipidus
    (1) DDAVP (vasopressin analog desamino-D-arginine-8-vasopressin) is preferred because it can be administered easily (parenterally, intranasally, or directly onto the buccal mucosa). It has a relatively long duration of action and does not have vasoconstrictive or intes-

tinal motility effects. Others have advocated use of aqueous vasopressin in critically ill patients because of the shorter duration of
action allowing for flexibility as the patient's status changes. See
Table 6-1

(2) Regardless of initial sodium levels, avoid excess water administration and development of iatrogenic syndrome of inappropriate antidiuretic hormone (SIADH), especially after neurosurgical procedures that may have short duration of diabetes insipidus

(3) Withhold therapy every 3-5 days for assessment of potential
resolution of diabetes insipidus in patients with trauma- or
postoperative-related diabetes insipidus

(4) Many patients with neurogenic diabetes insipidus require long-
term hormone replacement

b. Incomplete neurogenic diabetes insipidus
   (1) DDAVP is the preferred agent in critically ill patients
   (2) Other options include medications that augment ADH action in the
       kidney or increase ADH release
       (a) Chlorpropamide 100-500 mg qd; concern is hypoglycemia
       (b) Clofibrate 500 mg q6hr; associated with increased risk of gall-
           stones
       (c) Carbamazepine 200-600 mg qd

c. Nephrogenic diabetes insipidus
   (1) Discontinue, if possible, all medications that could be causative
   (2) During critical illness, patients require fluid administration titrated
       against urine outputs and plasma sodium levels
   (3) These patients frequently respond well to chronic therapy with
       thiazide diuretics, which cause volume contraction, subsequent in-
       creased proximal tubule water and sodium reabsorption, decreased
       water delivery to the distal nephron, and ultimately decreased
       urine output

d. Diabetes insipidus of pregnancy
   (1) Due to its unique pathophysiology, this form of diabetes insipidus
       does not respond well to treatment with vasopressin (aqueous or in
       oil), but does respond well to DDAVP, which is resistant to vaso-
       pressinase action

Table 6-1 Replacement therapy for diabetes insipidus

Agent	Doseage	Route	Duration
Desmopressin (DDAVP)	1-4 mcg	Subcutaneous,	12-24 hr
	1-4 mcg	intravenous,	12-24 hr
	5-40 mcg	intranasal	8-20 hr
Aqueous vaso-pressin	5-10 U	Subcutaneous, intramuscular	2-8 hr
Vasopressin tan-nate in oil	2.5-5.0 U	Intramuscular	24-72 hr

| 6.3 | SIADH

1. Definition
   The syndrome of inappropriate antidiuretic hormone secretion is a state of euvolemic hyponatremia caused by excessive excretion of ADH.
2. Pathophysiology
   a. ADH secretion is independent of normal osmotic or hemodynamic stimuli
   b. Secretion of excess ADH may be ectopic or by the posterior pituitary
   c. Normal controls of sodium balance are maintained. High sodium intake increases urinary sodium excretion; low sodium intake reduces urinary sodium excretion, resulting in maintenance of extracellular volume within normal limits
   d. Free water cannot be excreted normally; persistent ADH secretion causes water retention, hyponatremia, and progressive expansion of intracellular fluid (ICF) and extracellular fluid (ECF)
   e. Expanded ECF stimulates natriuresis with an isotonic loss of ECF, bringing the extracellular compartment back to its baseline volume
   f. The intracellular compartment remains expanded
3. Etiology
   a. Postoperative (surgical stress, anesthetic agents, positive pressure ventilation)
   b. CNS disorders (head trauma, neoplasm, meningitis, encephalitis, brain abscess, hydrocephalus, intracranial hemorrhage)
   c. Pulmonary diseases (pneumonia, TB, bronchiectasis, chronic obstructive pulmonary disease [COPD], status asthmaticus)
   d. Drug-induced (vasopressin, DDAVP, chlorpropamide, carbamazepine, clofibrate, oxytocin, thiazide diuretics, vincristine, vinblastine, cyclophosphamide, phenothiazines, tricyclic antidepressants, narcotics, nicotine, monoamine oxidase inhibitors)
   e. Ectopic ADH production by tumors (carcinoma of lung, duodenum, pancreas, thymoma, lymphoma, hepatoma, carcinoid tumors, Ewing's sarcoma)
   f. Stress or pain
   g. Nausea
   h. Acute psychosis
   i. Endocrinologic disorders (myxedema, ACTH deficiency, panhypopituitarism)
4. Clinical manifestations
   a. Mental status changes may be present (confusion or lethargy)
   b. Seizures or coma may occur, especially if the hyponatremia is severe or of rapid onset
5. Diagnostic evaluation
   a. Physical examination
      (1) Evaluate for evidence of euvolemia
      (2) Note that edema may be absent
   b. Laboratory evaluation
      (1) Serum sodium ≤130 mEq/L
      (2) Urine osmolality >200 mOsm/kg (most reliable diagnostic test)

      (3) Urinary sodium usually >30 mEq/L due to increased atrial natri-
uretic hormone or suppressed ALDO

      (4) Plasma osmolality <280 mOsm/kg

      (5) Normal or decreased BUN, normal creatinine

      (6) Decreased uric acid

      (7) Normal thyroid, adrenal, and cardiac function

6. Differential diagnosis

   a. Factitious hyponatremia (substantial elevations of serum proteins or lipids, osmotically induced shifts of water into the intravascular space)

   b. Hypovolemic hyponatremia (gastrointestinal losses, renal dysfunction, diuretics, aldosterone deficiency)

   c. Hypervolemic hyponatremia (congestive heart failure [CHF], nephrotic syndrome, cirrhosis)

   d. Hypothyroidism

   e. Adrenal insufficiency

7. Therapy

   a. Therapy must be individualized

   b. Treat the underlying disease (antituberculous drugs for TB, evacuate subdural hematoma, etc.)

   c. Restrict fluids to 500-800 ml/day (difficult in the ICU; at least attempt to decrease free water intake)

   d. It is important to distinguish acute onset (<2-3 days) from chronic hyponatremia and to determine the presence or absence of neurologic symptoms

   e. Acute hyponatremia with symptoms may be treated with isotonic or hypertonic (3%) saline combined with a loop diuretic. Furosemide is usually added to diminish the ability of the renal tubules to concentrate urine and therefore increase free water excretion. This treatment is aimed at increasing the serum sodium by ≤1 mEq/L/hr; maximum safe increase of 10-12 mEq/L/day

   f. Infusion of isotonic saline alone seems to be reasonable, but since isotonic saline is hypertonic relative to the patient's plasma, the patient with SIADH can excrete the infused sodium in a more concentrated form than it was given. The net effect can be further retention of free water and exacerbation of hyponatremia

   g. Give hypertonic saline (3%) slowly (1-2 ml/kg/hr) until the sodium is at a "safe" asymptomatic level (usually 120-125 mEq/L); monitor serum sodium levels every 1-2 hr when using hypertonic saline to avoid dangerously rapid correction that can result in neurologic sequelae or death

   h. In chronic hyponatremia with minimal symptomatology, correct the sodium more slowly at approximately 0.5 mEq/L/hr to avoid central pontine myelinolysis that can result from aggressive sodium replacement and result in permanent neurologic impairment or death (see Chapter 16)

   i. Fluid balances should be measured every 4-8 hr until the serum sodium level is >125 mEq/L or is corrected halfway to normal

   j. Demeclocycline 300-600 mg PO bid may be useful in patients with chronic SIADH; it causes nephrogenic diabetes insipidus and counteracts the effects of the high ADH levels

8. Therapeutic precautions
   a. It is never necessary to raise rapidly the serum sodium to normal or even to a preconceived "safe" level if it requires an increase of >10-12 mEq/L/day
   b. Water moves freely across the blood-brain barrier in response to osmotic gradients; thus, even small increases in plasma osmolality will to some extent reduce brain edema
   c. Brain water can never increase by more than 10% due to constraints imposed by the skull; a 5%-10% increase in sodium concentration (6-12 mEq/L) can be expected virtually to eliminate cerebral edema. Clinical experience has shown this to be effective in symptomatic patients

---

| 6.4 | DIABETIC KETOACIDOSIS AND HYPEROSMOLAR NONKETOTIC COMA |

1. Definitions
   a. Diabetic ketoacidosis (DKA) and hyperosmolar nonketotic coma (HNKC) are hyperglycemic states in patients with diabetes mellitus and both are characterized by insulin deficiency and relative excess of glucagon and other counter-regulatory hormones
   b. DKA is also characterized by ketosis
2. Pathophysiology
   a. Insulin deficiency leads to
      (1) Increased glucagon, causing excessive hepatic glucose production (gluconeogenesis/glycogenolysis)
      (2) Decreased glucose clearance from peripheral tissues
      (3) Development of hyperglycemia causing an osmotic diuresis (loss of sodium [Na^+]/H_2O), hypovolemia, and decreased glomerular filtration rate (GFR)
      (4) Increased muscle proteolysis and decreased protein synthesis leading to loss of nitrogen and electrolytes from ICF to ECF to urine
   b. In DKA, insulin deficiency also leads to
      (1) Increased cortisol, epinephrine, and growth hormone that stimulate excessive adipose tissue lipolysis and free fatty acid delivery to liver, and subsequent ketogenesis and hyperketonemia (beta-hydroxybutyrate and acetoacetate) in DKA
      (2) Development of an anion gap metabolic acidosis (secondary to ketoacids that neutralize the bicarbonate buffering system) and loss of potassium (K^+) and Na^+ that buffer urinary excretion of keto-acids
   c. In HNKC, insulin levels may be sufficient to prevent lipolysis and ketogenesis
3. Etiology
   a. Common precipitating events include
      (1) Infection
      (2) Acute stress (myocardial infarction, stroke, trauma)
      (3) Discontinuation of insulin
      (4) Discontinuation of parenteral nutrition
      (5) Use of some medications (glucocorticoids, diphenylhydantoin, propranolol)

  b. In rare cases, nondiabetics develop HNKC
    (1) Iatrogenic (hypertonic intravenous hyperalimentation, hyperosmolar peritoneal dialysis)
    (2) Severe fluid losses in burned patients
    (3) Feeding infants hypertonic oral formulas
4. Diagnostic evaluation
  a. History
    (1) DKA develops in patients of all ages (75% adults) with insulin-dependent diabetes mellitus (IDDM) and infrequently with non–insulin dependent diabetes mellitus (NIDDM) in the setting of coexisting severe medical problems
    (2) HNKC patients are typically elderly with a history of NIDDM
    (3) Duration of symptoms averages 12 days in HNKC and 3 days in DKA
    (4) GI symptoms are common (abdominal pain occurs in 50% of patients, nausea or vomiting occurs in 75%)
    (5) Seizures are common in HNKC
  b. Physical examination
    (1) Altered mental status (severely depressed sensorium in HNKC associated with osmolalities of 340-350 mOsm/kg)
    (2) Dehydration (dry mucous membranes, orthostatic hypotension, tachycardia)
    (3) Patients with DKA may also have
      (a) Fruity breath
      (b) Hyperventilation (Kussmaul's respirations)
      (c) Abdominal tenderness
  c. Laboratory evaluation
    (1) Table 6-2 lists the common diagnostic laboratory findings in DKA and HNKC
    (2) DKA may also be associated with
      (a) Low serum Na^+ (if corrected for hyperglycemia may be normal or slightly elevated)
      (b) Normal to slightly elevated serum K^+ (note total body K^+ depleted)
      (c) Leukocytosis (with neutrophilia) may occur, secondary to stress or dehydration, instead of infection

Table 6-2 Laboratory values in DKA and HNKC

Lab Test	DKA	HNKC
Blood glucose (mg/dL)	200-2000	Usually >600
Blood ketones*	Present	Absent
Arterial pH	<7.4	Normal†
Anion gap	Elevated (usually >18)	Normal or elevated
Osmolality	Slightly elevated	Elevated
Urine dipstick	Glucose and ketones	Glucose

*Beta-hydroxybutyrate/acetoacetate.
†May be low if hypovolemia causes poor tissue perfusion.

    (d) Serum amylase often elevated even without pancreatitis
5. Management
  a. Initial evaluation
    (1) Rule out infection as precipitant
      (a) Complete blood cell count (CBC), urinalysis (U/A), chest x-ray (CXR), and appropriate cultures
      (b) Altered mental status: consider lumbar puncture (LP) to rule out meningitis
      (c) Abdominal pain: consider appendicitis, diverticulitis, pelvic inflammatory disease
    (2) Rule out myocardial infarction (ECG) in older patients or those with longstanding DM even without the complaint of chest pain
  b. Institute insulin therapy: 0.1 U/kg regular insulin IV bolus and begin infusion of regular insulin at rate of 0.1 U/kg/hr. If IV access unobtainable may use 0.1 U/kg IM q1hr
    (1) Expect blood glucose to decrease by approximately 75mg/dL/hr on this regimen
    (2) Follow blood glucose q1hr
    (3) If blood glucose levels do not begin to decrease after 4 hr of insulin therapy, increase insulin dosage every hr until blood glucose begins to decrease. Doses of >100 U/hr have occasionally been required in rare, extraordinarily insulin-resistant patients
    (4) Continue infusion until blood glucose level is approximately 250 mg/dL and serum ketones are negative (or positive only in undiluted serum), or until urine ketones are small or moderate; anion gap should be decreasing to near normal range unless there is an additional cause of persistent metabolic acidosis
    (5) Lower insulin infusion to 2 U/hr and change intravenous fluid (IVF) to D_5 0.45% normal saline (NS) or D_5NS (add K^+ if appropriate). Aim for blood glucose levels 150-200 mg/dL until patient can eat and drink
    (6) Give regular insulin dose to avoid recurrence of hyperglycemia and ketosis (5-10 U subcutaneous [SQ]) *before* stopping continuous infusion, (because half-life of insulin via infusion is only 6-8 min)
  c. Immediately begin volume repletion
    (1) Restore circulating volume (isotonic fluid: NS or lactated Ringer's [LR])
      (a) First L IV over first 30 min
      (b) Second L IV over next hr
      (c) Reassess volume status and continue as clinical situation warrants
      (d) If patient presents in shock:
        (i) May use colloid for volume expansion
        (ii) May require 2-3 L over first 1-2 hrs
    (2) Replace intracellular and total body fluid losses
      (a) Patients typically lose water and sodium at around 100 mL H_2O/kg and 7 mEq Na^+/kg so 0.45% NS is a good choice at this stage

(b) Gradual replacement is appropriate (150-300 mL/hr × 12-24 hr)

(c) Patients continue to have excessive urinary losses via osmotic diuresis while hyperglycemia persists

(d) Follow fluid balance every 1-2 hr and maintain positive fluid balance; adjust rate of IV replacement as needed

(e) Average patient in DKA requires 5-7 L positive balance during treatment

(f) When blood glucose level is ≤250 mg/dL IVF should contain 5% dextrose

d. Monitor patient

(1) CBC, Na^+/K^+/chloride (Cl^-)/bicarbonate (HCO_3^-)/creatinine (Cr), U/A, CXR, ECG, and appropriate cultures on admission

(2) Follow vital signs

(3) Record cumulative patient intake and output q1hr

(4) Check blood glucose q1hr while on continuous insulin infusion and q4hr after changed to SQ insulin

(5) Check serum potassium 2 hr after insulin treatment started and q2-4hr thereafter

(6) Check serum electrolytes (Na^+/HCO_3^-/Cl^-) and determine anion gap q4-6hr

(7) Check serum ketone level q4hr

(8) Check arterial blood gas (ABG) on admission and repeat q1-2hr until pH > 7.2 or as clinical situation warrants

(9) Check serum phosphate, magnesium, and ionized calcium level on admission. If low, repeat in 4 hr, otherwise repeat in 8-12 hr

(10) Check urine dipstick q1hr for presence of glucose/ketones until negative/small

e. K^+ supplementation

(1) Serum K^+ level decreases as soon as insulin action begins

(2) K^+ administration should begin when serum K^+ ≤5.0 mEq/L and urine output is documented

(3) Goal of K^+ supplementation at this point is to keep serum K^+ ≥3.5 mEq/L to prevent cardiac arrhythmias

(4) Patients typically have average total K^+ deficit of approximately (~) 5 mEq/kg (but it can be much greater)

(5) Total K^+ repletion can be completed gradually after DKA is resolved

(6) If admission K^+ is <3.5, immediately add 40 mEq potassium chloride (KCl) to each L IVF. KCl is usually used initially; if phosphate is low, monobasic potassium phosphate may be used

(7) Use IV K^+ until DKA is reversed and the patient can take potassium orally

f. Metabolic acidosis

(1) Insulin inhibits lipolysis and ketogenesis

(2) Fluid replacement restores perfusion

(3) Bicarbonate administration has not been shown to accelerate resolution of acidosis and is not generally advisable. Exception:

severe hyperkalemia with characteristic ECG changes; i.e., widened QRS or peaked T waves

    (a) If needed, use 50-100 mEq sodium bicarbonate ($NaHCO_3$) in 500-1000 mL 0.45% saline over 1-2 hr

    (b) The main risk of bicarbonate therapy is the induction of severe hypokalemia as potassium enters cell in exchange for hydrogen ions

g. Phosphate supplementation

    (1) Phosphate depletion in DKA averages $\sim$ 1.0 mmol/kg

    (2) Prospective randomized studies showed no beneficial effect of phosphate treatment on recovery from DKA

    (3) Phosphate levels frequently plummet to $\sim$ 1.5 mg/dL with insulin treatment

    (4) IV replacement is usually not essential

    (5) However, replacement is warranted if phosphorus $\leq$1.0 mg/dL, since severe hypophosphatemia may cause respiratory failure. Potassium phosphate IV is usually the best choice with concomitant hypokalemia

h. Magnesium supplementation

    (1) Mild magnesium depletion occurs in DKA and with insulin treatment

    (2) Typically does not need supplementation

    (3) If patient develops ventricular irritability with hypomagnesemia, magnesium sulfate 1-2 g IV may be given

6. Complications

Cerebral edema may develop; its therapy is not clear, but mannitol may be helpful

---

6.5   **MYXEDEMA**

1. Definition and epidemiology

  a. Severe thyroid hormone deficiency that can lead to a decreased level of consciousness and even coma

  b. Reported fatality rate as high as 80%

  c. Actual coma associated with severe hypothyroidism is rare; there are only about 200 cases reported in the literature

  d. Incidence is three times higher in females than in males; elderly females seem most susceptible to myxedema coma

2. Pathophysiology

  a. Thyroid hormone is essential for normal metabolism of all cells

  b. Thyroid-stimulating hormone (TSH) secreted by the pituitary is under regulation of the hypothalamus and stimulates the thyroid to secrete thyroxine (T_4) as well as smaller amounts of triiodothyronine (T_3), the active form of thyroid hormone

  c. Most T_3 is produced in the peripheral tissues by monodeiodination of circulating T_4

  d. T_3 and T_4 circulate bound to serum proteins; the free T_3 and T_4 are metabolically active

  e. T_3 feeds back on the pituitary gland to inhibit production of TSH

f. In myxedema coma the cause of coma is multifactorial (i.e., decreased cerebral perfusion associated with low cardiac output from bradycardia and reduced stroke volume, decreased circulating levels of thyroid hormones resulting in decreased mental responsiveness)

g. Hypothermia may result from decreased T_3 or T_4 leading to reduced metabolic rate in addition to an inability to shiver

h. Hypoventilation (alveolar) is secondary to respiratory center depression (exacerbated by use of analgesics, sedatives, and anesthesics), defective respiratory muscle function, and occasionally airway obstruction (enlarged tongue)

i. Hyponatremia often accompanies myxedema and may have associated hypochloremia (which may contribute to altered mental status)

j. Decreased plasma volume and intense peripheral vasoconstriction are typical

3. Etiology

a. Myxedema occasionally may be the result of chronic, severe, primary thyroid failure; patients with classic signs and symptoms lapse into stupor, coma, and death

b. May be precipitated in patients with moderate or unrecognized hypothyroidism by a superimposed acute illness (e.g., infection) or following administration of narcotics or sedatives

c. See Box below

4. Risk factors

a. Infection

b. Surgery

c. Anesthesia

d. Myocardial infarction

e. Sedating drugs

f. Cerebrovascular accidents

g. Bleeding

h. Cold exposure

i. Trauma

j. Hyponatremia

Causes of Hypothyroidism

1. Autoimmune thyroid disease (i.e., Hashimoto's thyroiditis)
2. Thyroid ablation (radioactive iodine or surgical)
3. Surgical thyroid resection
4. Pituitary disease (secondary hypothyroidism)
5. Hypothalamic disease (tertiary hypothyroidism)
6. Chemical agents: antithyroid drugs (e.g., lithium, organic goitrogens); iodine-containing drugs (e.g., amiodarone)
7. Congenital thyroid agenesis
8. Iodine deficiency or excess
9. Thyroid hormone resistance

5. Symptoms
   a. Decreased mental acuity
   b. Hoarseness
   c. Increased somnolence
   d. Cold intolerance
   e. Dry skin
   f. Brittle hair
6. Diagnostic evaluation
   a. History
      (1) Usually a long history of gradual deterioration
      (2) Gradual weight gain or inability to lose weight
      (3) May have been noncompliant with thyroid replacement therapy
      (4) May have history of Graves' disease or other thyroid dysfunction
   b. Physical examination
      (1) Hypothermia (core or rectal temperature <35° C)
      (2) Bradycardia
      (3) Hypoventilation (slow respiratory rate, shallow breaths)
      (4) Hypotension
      (5) Physical features consistent with long-standing hypothyroidism
         (a) Skin appears thick and doughy; may have an orange or yellow tint
         (b) Facial and general puffiness, periorbital edema
         (c) Large tongue
         (d) Alopecia, loss of lateral aspects of eyebrows
      (6) Palpable thyroid (present in <50%) or thyroidectomy scar
      (7) Cardiac examination may be consistent with pericardial effusion (e.g., muffled heart tones, cardiomegaly)
      (8) Neurologic exam rarely reveals focal findings
         (a) Altered level of consciousness
         (b) Delayed relaxation phase of deep tendon reflexes may be present but difficult to detect
         (c) Disorders of muscular function (paralytic ileus, urinary retention, atonic bowel with fecal impaction)
   c. Laboratory evaluation
      (1) Confirmation of diagnosis relies on thyroid function tests to document hypothyroidism. Measure TSH, T_4, free T_4, reverse T_3, T_3 resin uptake (RU). (See Table 6-3)
         (a) TSH level is elevated in primary hypothyroidism
         (b) TSH is not elevated in secondary and tertiary hypothyroidism and diagnosis will rely on other laboratory parameters and clinical judgement
      (2) Serum cortisol level should be drawn initially to evaluate for concomitant adrenal insufficiency
      (3) CBC, U/A, blood and urine cultures should be sent
      (4) Serum cholesterol is usually elevated
      (5) CXR may reveal signs of pleural or pericardial effusion, or infection
      (6) ECG is often abnormal (sinus bradycardia, small-voltage QRS complexes, prolonged Q-T intervals, isoelectric T-wave changes, supraventricular tachycardia)

Table 6-3 Thyroid function tests in thyroid disorders

Test	Hypothyroid	High T_4 Syndrome	Hyperthyroid	Low T_3 Syndrome	Low T_3/T_4 Syndrome
TSH	High*	Nl/low	Low	Low to sl ↑	Low to sl ↑
Total T_4	Low	High	High	Nl	Low
Total T_3	Low to low Nl	Low/Nl/high	High	Low	Low
Reverse T_3	Nl/low	Nl/high	High	High	High
Free T_4	Low	Nl/high	High	Nl	Nl
T_3RU	Low	Nl/low	High	Nl/high	High

Nl = normal; sl = slight.

* = except TSH is low in hypothyroidism of secondary and tertiary causes.

   (7) ABG may reveal hypoxemia, hypercapnia, and respiratory acidosis
   (8) Serum glucose or sodium may be low
   (9) Normochromic, normocytic anemia is typical
7. Differential diagnosis
   a. Other causes of altered mental status (e.g., stroke, electrolyte disturbances such as hyponatremia)
   b. Sepsis
   c. Hypothermia, especially with associated anemia
   d. Hypopituitarism
   e. Hypoglycemia
   f. Renal failure
8. Therapy
   a. Initiate thyroid hormone replacement upon suspicion, as awaiting confirmation of the diagnosis may be too late
      (1) Intravenous administration of replacement hormone is necessary due to unreliable gastrointestinal absorption in the myxedematous state
      (2) The authors prefer T_3 and T_4 combination therapy: T_3 20 mcg IV bolus, followed by 10 mcg q8hr with T_4 200 mcg IV, followed by 100 mcg IV q24hr for 1-2 days, followed by T_4 alone
      (3) T_3 for intravenous administration recently became available in the United States, so many references recommend treatment with IV T_4 alone or with oral T_3 plus IV T_4
      (4) Peripheral conversion of T_4 to T_3 requires the presence of some T_3 for enzyme activity
      (5) Advantages of IV T_3 include a more rapid onset of action than T_4 and that peripheral conversion of T_4 is not required for activity
      (6) T_3 is more arrhythmogenic than T_4 and careful cardiac monitoring is essential, especially since the risk of coronary artery disease is high in these patients
      (7) If IV T_3 is not immediately available, IV T_4 (as noted above) may be given with oral T_3 (25 mcg q12hr) until the patient can be treated with oral T_4 alone
      (8) Previously, T_4 was frequently used alone (200-500 mcg IV bolus followed by 50-100 mcg IV q24hr)
      (9) Controversy exists regarding the best therapeutic regimen and controlled trials will probably never be performed because the disease is so rare
      (10) Monitor T_3 and T_4 levels after 5 days and adjust the dosage accordingly if the patient remains unconscious
   b. Metabolic support
      (1) Hypothermia is best treated with passive rewarming, as active rewarming can cause peripheral vasodilatation and worsening of shock. See Chapter 7
      (2) Hyponatremia generally responds well to free water restriction
      (3) Treat hypoglycemia with IV dextrose
      (4) Seizures may be treated with standard anticonvulsant drugs
      (5) Identify and treat precipitating causes (e.g., infection, stroke, myocardial infarction, narcotics, gastrointestinal bleeding)

c. Supportive care
   (1) Respiratory support with mechanical ventilation may be required
   (2) Treat hypotension aggressively with IV fluids (avoid free water) and vasopressor therapy. Dopamine is preferable to norepinephrine as it may better maintain coronary blood flow and renal/mesenteric blood flow
   (3) Hypotension responds poorly to vasopressors until thyroid hormone replacement is initiated
   (4) Give hydrocortisone (100 mg IV q8hr) until initial cortisol level is available. Therapy may be stopped if this indicates a normal stress response to the acute medical illness. Otherwise, continue therapy for 3-7 days followed by a rapid taper in the absence of hypothalamic-pituitary-adrenal disease. This therapy may be life-saving in patients with secondary/tertiary hypothyroidism
   (5) Monitor for the presence of arrhythmias; if they occur, decrease the dosage of thyroid hormone replacement. Hypothyroidism is associated with a high incidence of coronary artery disease and these patients should be monitored for evidence of myocardial ischemia exacerbated by increased myocardial oxygen consumption with T_3/T_4 treatment
   (6) Avoid sedatives
9. Complications
   a. Euthyroid patients tolerate well the short-term administration of thyroid hormone
   b. Delay of treatment in a myxedematous patient can make the difference between survival and death
   c. This treatment regimen should *not* be routinely instituted in hypothyroid patients without clinical evidence of myxedema coma because of potential cardiac complications (myocardial infarction, arrhythmias)
   d. Severe hypothermia ($<32°$ C) is thought to have prognostic significance

6.6 THYROTOXIC CRISIS

1. Definitions
   a. *Thyrotoxic crisis,* or *thyroid storm,* is a life-threatening complication of hyperthyroidism characterized by a severe, sudden exacerbation of thyrotoxicosis
   b. The term *thyrotoxicosis* generally refers to the clinical and biochemical manifestations of excess thyroid hormone at the tissue level
   c. *True hyperthyroidism* refers to disorders of thyroid glandular hyperfunction with increased synthesis and secretion of thyroid hormone
   d. There are states of thyrotoxicosis without true hyperthyroidism (e.g., factitious ingestion of thyroid hormone, chronic thyroiditis with transient thyrotoxicosis, ectopic thyroid hormone production, and subacute thyroiditis). These states are associated with decreased thyroidal synthesis of new hormone; and are rare in the critically ill patient with the possible exception of T_4 or T_3 overdose (see Table 6-4)
2. Pathophysiology
   a. Actual mechanisms by which a patient with thyrotoxicosis decompensates into thyroid crisis are poorly understood

b. A crisis develops most often after a stressful precipitating event (e.g., trauma, infection, DKA, surgical emergency, parturition, or myocardial infarction)

c. Whatever the cause, the resulting syndrome resembles that of prolonged, severe beta-adrenergic agonist overload

d. Catecholamine levels appear to be normal despite the hypermetabolic state

3. Etiology
   a. Undiagnosed hyperthyroidism (most commonly Graves' disease or toxic multinodular goiter) in a patient with major stress
   b. Other etiologies of thyrotoxicosis may be distinguished by a 24-hr radioactive iodine uptake study (RAIU) when the patient is stable (see Table 6-4)
   c. Hyperthyroid patient on inadequate therapy

4. Symptoms
   a. Abnormal mental states (agitation, confusion, psychosis)
   b. Fever (T > 38.3° C) almost always present
   c. Heat intolerance and diaphoresis
   d. Palpitations (sinus tachycardia and atrial fibrillation are the most common dysrhythmias)
   e. Gastrointestinal disturbances (diarrhea, nausea, vomiting, abdominal pain)
   f. Muscle wasting and weakness
   g. Dyspnea

5. Diagnostic evaluation
   a. History
      (1) Marked, rapid recent weight loss may warn of impending storm
      (2) Unexplained fever in a thyrotoxic patient may precede storm
      (3) Precipitating event may be evident

Table 6-4 Thyrotoxicosis: etiologies and differentiation by RAIU

RAIU: High	RAIU: Low	RAIU: Low or High
TSH excess (e.g., pituitary tumors)	Destructive thyroid disease (e.g., subacute thyroiditis, postpartum thyroiditis)	Iodine-induced thyrotoxicosis (e.g., food or medication such as radiocontrast dye or amiodarone)
Abnormal thyroid stimulators (e.g., thyroid stimulating antibodies Graves' disease)	Ectopic thyroid tissue (e.g., metastatic follicular carcinoma)	
Thyroid autonomy (e.g., toxic multinodular goiter or toxic adenoma)	Exogenous sources (e.g., medication or food)	

   b. Physical examination
      (1) Goiter: palpate cautiously since vigorous massage may cause release of more hormone into the circulation
      (2) Tachycardia: may have tachydysrhythmias
      (3) Hyperthermia
      (4) Mental status changes
      (5) Tremor
      (6) Warm, moist skin
      (7) Ophthalmic signs of hyperthyroidism (proptosis, lid lag, lid retraction)
      (8) Signs of congestive heart failure (high output failure or cardiomyopathy)
   c. Laboratory evaluation
      (1) Confirmation of the diagnosis relies on thyroid studies (see Tables 6-3 and 6-4)
         (a) Elevated T_4
         (b) Elevated T_3
         (c) Decreased TSH
      (2) Routine studies include CBC, electrolytes, U/A, CXR, and ECG
      (3) Evaluate for infection as indicated by history and physical examination
      (4) Associated laboratory abnormalities
         (a) Hypercalcemia
         (b) Hypokalemia
         (c) Hyperglycemia
         (d) Hypocholesterolemia
         (e) Mild microcytic anemia
         (f) Lymphocytosis
         (g) Granulocytopenia
         (h) Hyperbilirubinemia
         (i) Elevated alkaline phosphatase
6. Differential diagnosis
   a. Hypermetabolic states (sepsis, pheochromocytoma, Cushing's syndrome)
   b. Thyrotoxicosis without crisis/storm
7. Therapy
   Do *not* wait for lab values to begin treatment; diagnosis is made on clinical suspicion and treatment should be initiated immediately
   a. Supportive measures
      (1) IV fluids for volume replacement
      (2) Acetaminophen for hyperthermia; avoid aspirin since it displaces T_4 from thyroid-binding globulin, thereby increasing the level of free T_4
      (3) Cooling blankets
   b. Inhibition of thyroid hormone synthesis
      (1) Propylthiouracil (PTU): 200-300 mg PO or via NG tube q6hr
      (2) Methimazole: 20-25 mg PO or via NG tube q4hr
   c. Inhibition of thyroid hormone release with iodide therapy beginning 1 hr after PTU therapy
      (1) Sodium iodide: 1 g IV q8hr

    (2) Potassium iodide and iodine (i.e., Lugol's solution): 10 drops q8hr PO

  d. Inhibition of peripheral beta-adrenergic activity

    (1) Most beta-blockers also block peripheral conversion of T_4 to T_3

    (2) Propranolol: 0.5-1.0 mg/min IV to total dose of 2-10 mg IV q 3-4 hr; may treat with 20-40 mg PO q6hr after initial control with IV administration; occasional patient has required up to 2 g PO/day due to variability of hepatic metabolism in thyrotoxic individuals

    (3) Esmolol: bolus with 0.5-1.0 mg/kg followed by infusion with 50 mcg/kg/min; if inadequate effect within 5 min, repeat bolus and increase infusion to 100 mcg/kg/min; can repeat procedure to 200-300 mcg/kg/min

    (4) Titrate beta-blockade to achieve heart rate ≤ 80 bpm

    (5) Use caution and a short-acting cardioselective agent such as esmolol if the patient has a history of reactive airway disease

    (6) Caution is also required in patients with CHF. Controlling the heart rate may be of benefit; however, these agents are negative inotropes and may worsen low output failure

    (7) If beta-blockers are contraindicated, other sympatholytic drugs may be useful as second-line agents (reserpine, a depleter of catecholamines; or guanethidine, an inhibitor of catecholamine release)

  e. Inhibition of peripheral conversion of T_4 to T_3

    (1) PTU (see above dosages)

    (2) Beta-blockade (see above)

    (3) Dexamethasone 1-2 mg IV or PO q6hr

  f. Definitive therapy may require surgery or radioactive iodine therapy after etiology is determined by RAIU

  g. Diagnose and treat underlying precipitating disorders (i.e., infection and other major stresses)

6.7   SICK EUTHYROID SYNDROME

1. Definitions

  a. Thyroid hormone alterations associated with acute nonthyroidal illness

  b. Two syndromes are described

    (1) Low T_3 syndrome

    (2) Low T_3/T_4 syndrome

  c. These syndromes are thought to represent euthyroid states by many; however, specific tissues may actually be hypothyroid

2. Review of normal thyroid hormone physiology

  a. Thyrotropin-releasing hormone (TRH) is released from the hypothalamus into the bloodstream

  b. TRH stimulates synthesis and release of thyrotropin (TSH) from the pituitary gland

  c. TSH stimulates the thyroid gland to produce and secrete T_4 and smaller amounts of T_3

  d. The thyroid gland secretes predominantly T_4 (80%), with smaller amounts of T_3 (20%)

  e. The remainder of T_3, the physiologically active form of thyroid hormone, is produced in extrathyroidal tissues (primarily the liver and kidneys) by monodeiodination of circulating T_4

f. T_3 and T_4 circulate bound to serum proteins; the free T_3 and T_4 are metabolically active

g. T_3 feeds back on the pituitary gland to inhibit production of TSH

h. Some of the circulating T_4 is metabolized to the inactive product reverse T_3

i. Both T_3 and reverse T_3 are rapidly cleared from the serum by further deiodination

j. Thyroid hormone activity begins with binding of T_3 to receptors on cell nuclei

k. Postbinding effects of T_3 are needed for normal cellular function

l. The T_3 resin uptake (T_3RU) test is commonly performed to give an approximation of binding proteins, primarily thyroxin-binding globulin

3. Pathophysiology
   a. In acute nonthyroidal illness, peripheral thyroid hormone metabolism is altered
   b. Exact mechanism of decreased T_3 production is unknown

4. Etiology
   a. Systemic illness (sepsis, cardiac or respiratory failure, neoplastic processes, stroke)
   b. Surgery
   c. Caloric deprivation
   d. Drug-induced (glucocorticoids, iodides, amiodarone, propylthiouracil)

5. Symptoms
   No specific symptoms are associated with thyroidal hormone alterations

6. Laboratory evaluation
   a. Serum T_3 is low (see Table 6-3)
   b. Serum T_4 is low or normal
   c. Reverse T_3 is elevated, usually this is the most useful discriminator between sick euthyroid syndrome and hypothyroidism
   d. Serum TSH is normal

7. Therapy
   a. Attempt to distinguish sick euthyroid syndrome from hypothyroidism
   b. Currently, there is no proven benefit in treating sick euthyroid patients with thyroid hormone
   c. Indeed, some believe that the sick euthyroid state may be protective by conserving energy under stress

6.8 HYPOGLYCEMIA

1. Definition
   Plasma glucose <40-50 mg/dL. This definition does not include the presence of associated symptoms since critically ill patients may not reliably demonstrate classic symptomatology

2. Pathophysiology
   a. Clinical situations that result in increased insulin, the inability of the liver to generate glucose from its glycogen stores, or problems with the counter-regulatory system may lead to hypoglycemia

b. Insulin suppresses hepatic glucose production and stimulates glucose utilization by peripheral tissues (e.g., muscle)

c. Insulin secretion lowers plasma glucose concentration

d. In response to onset of hypoglycemia, the major counter-regulatory hormones glucagon and epinephrine increase and cause an acceleration of glycogenolysis

e. Catecholamines are glucose counter-regulatory hormones but do not play essential roles as long as the secretion of glucagon is initiated; however, in the presence of glucagon deficiency (long-standing DM or patients with total pancreatectomy), catecholamines become major counter-regulatory hormones

f. Patients treated with nonselective beta-adrenergic blocking agents may have severe impairment of counter-regulation mechanisms

g. Patients with long-standing DM (10-15 years) may lose the ability to secrete epinephrine in response to hypoglycemia, becoming virtually defenseless against even moderate degrees of hyperinsulinemia

3. Etiology
See Box below

Causes of Hypoglycemia

1. Hyperinsulin states
   a. Exogenous insulin administration*
   b. Endogenous insulin excess (e.g., insulinomas)
2. Ethanol-induced (after ingestion in otherwise healthy patients or chronic alcoholics)*
3. Drug-induced (e.g., sulfonylureas, quinine, propranolol, pentamidine)*
4. System disorders*
   a. Hepatic disease (e.g., cirrhosis, fulminant viral hepatitis)
   b. Renal disease (e.g., chronic renal disease associated with liver disease, CHF, sepsis)
   c. Sepsis (e.g., gram-negative sepsis, empyema of gallbladder)
   d. AIDS
5. Extensive thermal burns*
6. Total parenteral nutrition*
7. Insulin treatment of hyperkalemia*
8. Factitious (insulin injection or sulfonylurea ingestion)*
9. Endocrine causes (hypopituitarism, hypoadrenalism, hypothyroidism)
10. Autoimmune causes (insulin antireceptor antibodies, antiinsulin autoantibodies)
11. Starvation (severe caloric restriction)
12. Alimentary following gastric surgery (e.g., gastrectomy)
13. Idiopathic (functional): typically postprandial; this is a diagnosis of exclusion and is usually not seen in the critically ill patient

---

*Designates causes likely to be seen in the critically ill.

4. Symptoms
   a. Adrenergic activation
      (1) Palpitations
      (2) Tremor
      (3) Diaphoresis
      (4) Pallor
      (5) Anxiety
   b. Neuroglycopenia
      (1) Fatigue
      (2) Faintness
      (3) Dizziness
      (4) Hunger
      (5) Inappropriate behavior
      (6) Visual symptoms
      (7) Focal neurologic symptoms
      (8) Seizures
      (9) Coma
5. Diagnostic evaluation
   a. History
      (1) Check for history of DM
         (a) Recent insulin or oral hypoglycemic therapy
         (b) If DM is long-standing, the patient may also have glucagon deficiency. Thus, there may be a higher risk for hypoglycemia since the counter-regulatory mechanisms may be ineffective
      (2) Check for history of alcohol ingestion
   b. Physical examination
      (1) Tachycardia
      (2) Pupillary dilation
      (3) Cold, moist skin
      (4) Changes in body temperature (hypothermia, hyperthermia)
      (5) Examination may be normal between hypoglycemic episodes
   c. Laboratory evaluation
      (1) Plasma glucose level <40-50 mg/dL. Whole blood glucose is usually about 15% less than the corresponding plasma glucose level
      (2) May have changes in blood counts
         (a) Acute lymphocytosis followed by neutrophilia
         (b) May have increased hemoglobin, total red blood cell (RBC) count, or packed RBC volume
      (3) ECG changes (ST depression, flat T waves, Q-T interval prolongation)
      (4) EEG changes (diminished frequency of alpha waves, increased delta waves)
      (5) Artifactictious hypoglycemia must be ruled out, especially if the laboratory result indicates hypoglycemia with no apparent cause
         (a) Samples in serum separator tubes left at room temperature for extended periods of time; blood glucose levels may decrease by 10-20 mg/dL/hr due to ongoing blood cell metabolism
         (b) Patients with increased numbers of blood cells (polycythemia vera, leukemia, leukemoid reactions) may have low measured plasma glucose levels secondary to increased metabolism

(c) Avoid these problems by collecting blood in tubes containing oxalate and fluoride (gray tubes) since the fluoride acts as a glycolytic enzyme poison

d. Diagnostic approach

   (1) Measure simultaneous blood glucose and plasma insulin levels during an episode of hypoglycemia. This is the best way to demonstrate insulin secretion inappropriate to the prevailing blood glucose concentration

      (a) Relative hyperinsulinemia can be demonstrated by the simultaneous determination of blood glucose and plasma insulin levels after an overnight fast or during a 24- to 72-hr fast

      (b) Diagnosis of hyperinsulinism can be further supported by elevated levels of plasma C peptide and proinsulin concentrations

      (c) Insulinomas can be localized by ultrasonography, CT scanning, magnetic resonance imaging (MRI), arteriography, transhepatic percutaneous venous sampling, and intraoperative high-frequency sonography

   (2) Factitious hypoglycemia resulting from administration of insulin or sulfonylurea agents is typically characterized by inappropriately high plasma insulin levels similar to insulinomas

      (a) C-peptide levels remain low in insulin-induced factitious hypoglycemia; presence of insulin antibodies in patients who have no reason to take insulin injections also suggests this etiology

      (b) C-peptide levels are elevated in sulfonylurea-induced factitious hypoglycemia, similar to insulinomas; screening for plasma or urine sulfonylureas may confirm diagnosis

      (c) Rule out alcohol ingestion as a cause in spontaneous hypoglycemia. Alcohol levels may not be helpful since hypoglycemia may not occur for as long as 36 hr after ingestion

      (d) Rule out associated systemic disorders must be ruled out as appropriate for each patient (evaluate for liver, renal, or endocrine dysfunction, or sepsis)

6. Therapy

a. If the patient is comatose, administer glucose intravenously (25-50 mL of 50% dextrose followed by infusion of 10% dextrose) until persistent or mild hyperglycemia is present

b. Treatment with dextrose should cause rapid resolution of symptoms unless organic changes have occurred in the brain

c. Some patients may require additional IV boluses of 50% dextrose with continuous infusion of 10% dextrose

d. In drug-induced hypoglycemia, especially secondary to chlorpropamide, prolonged treatment with IV dextrose may be required to keep the blood glucose levels in the 200 mg/dL range; if this does not maintain the blood glucose level >200 mg/dL, one of the following should be added

   (1) 100 mg hydrocortisone and 1 mg glucagon per L of 10% dextrose. Continue until blood glucose levels are maintained >200 mg/dL

  (2) An additional infusion of 300 mg diazoxide in 5% dextrose given over a 30-min period and repeated q4hr until blood glucose levels are maintained >200 mg/dL

  (3) When the blood glucose levels rise, stop the hydrocortisone, glucagon, and diazoxide and decrease the rate of infusion of 10% dextrose

  (4) Persistent hyperglycemia maintained on 5% dextrose is a sign to discontinue the infusion gradually over a 24-hr period

e. Insulin-induced hypoglycemia in diabetic patients may be effectively treated with 0.5-1.0 mg glucagon IV, IM, or SQ; the patient should also ingest 20-40 g of carbohydrate since the glucagon effect lasts only 1-1.5 hr

f. Insulinomas may be surgically cured with resection

g. Medical management of insulinomas is indicated for malignant insulinoma, in patients with major contraindications to surgery, and in rare patients whom surgery fails

  (1) Diazoxide (3-8 mg/kg/day PO in 2-3 divided doses) is the drug of choice as it inhibits insulin secretion

  (2) Thiazide diuretics, diphenylhydantoin, propranolol, or calcium channel blockers may also be useful

  (3) Combination chemotherapy with streptozotocin and 5-fluorouracil has been reported to achieve partial or complete remission in 60% of patients with malignant insulinomas

h. Treat the underlying cause if related to systemic disorders

7. Complications
   Prompt recognition and treatment of hypoglycemia is required to prevent long-term neurologic sequelae or death

6.9 PHEOCHROMOCYTOMA

1. Definition and epidemiology
   a. Catecholamine-producing tumor of the adrenergic system (chromaffin cells); ~ 90% are adrenomedullary
   b. Nonadrenal tumors (~ 10%) arising from the sympathetic nervous system are designated extraadrenal pheochromocytomas or functioning paragangliomas; they most commonly occur in the abdomen, chest, and neck
   c. Pheochromocytomas are rare, occurring in only 1-2/100,000 adults

2. Pathophysiology
   Symptoms are secondary to catecholamines secreted by the tumor:
   a. Alpha-1 adrenergic stimulation results in vasoconstriction
   b. Alpha-2 adrenergic stimulation results in decreased insulin secretion
   c. Beta-1 adrenergic stimulation results in cardiac inotropy/chronotropy
   d. Beta-2 adrenergic stimulation results in bronchodilation and vasodilation
   e. Dopa-1 receptor stimulation results in renal and mesenteric vasodilation
   f. Excessive levels of catecholamines are toxic to the myocardium and cardiomyopathy may result

g. Symptoms may be episodic in nature; paroxysms may last from <1 min to several hr and may occur from only once every few months to as frequently as multiple times per day

3. Symptoms
   a. Hypertension (paroxysmal or persistent)
   b. Headache
   c. Pallor
   d. Hyperhidrosis
   e. Anxiety
   f. Tachycardia
   g. Palpitations
   h. Angina
   i. Hyperglycemia
   j. Weight loss
   k. Paresthesias (2° vasoconstriction)
   l. Visual disturbances (2° hypertensive retinopathy)
   m. Dilated pupils

4. Diagnostic evaluation
   a. History
      (1) Check for the presence of the above symptoms
      (2) A pressor response to histamine, glucagon, droperidol, tyramine, metoclopramide, saralasin, tricyclic antidepressants, or phenothiazides suggests the possibility of a pheochromocytomá
   b. Physical examination
      (1) May be normal if performed during a symptom-free time interval
      (2) May exhibit above symptoms during a paroxysm
   c. Laboratory evaluation
      (1) Plasma or urinary catecholamine levels or urinary catecholamine metabolite (i.e., vanillylmandelic [VMA] or metanephrine) levels
      (2) Suppression tests using clonidine or provocative tests using glucagon are rarely needed
      (3) Measurement of plasma and urinary catecholamines are interfered with by
         (a) Stimulation of endogenous catecholamines (e.g., surgery, stroke)
         (b) Administration of exogenous catecholamines
         (c) Various drugs (i.e., alpha-2 agonists, methyldopa, converting enzyme inhibitors, monoamine oxidase inhibitors [MAOI], phenothiazines, tricyclic antidepressants)
   d. Tumors may be localized by a variety of scanning techniques (CT, MRI, or venous blood sampling for catecholamines)
   e. Arteriography is generally avoided because it can precipitate hypertensive crisis

5. Differential diagnosis
   a. Malignant hypertension
   b. Thyrotoxic crisis
   c. Hypertensive response (to stress, surgery, anesthesic)
   d. Cushing's syndrome

6. Therapy
   a. Surgical excision is the definitive treatment
   b. Preoperative management is important in determining surgical outcome
   c. Preoperative goals
      (1) Control BP
      (2) Provide adequate intravascular volume
      (3) Treat tachyarrhythmias
      (4) Treat heart failure
      (5) Treat glucose intolerance
   d. Alpha-adrenergic blockade is the basis of hypertensive therapy. Patients are generally treated 1-2 weeks prior to surgery with phenoxybenzamine, labetalol, or prazosin, which are tapered to produce 10-15 mm Hg orthostatic BP decrease; 1-2 weeks of pretreatment allows for repletion of intravascular volume (diminished by excess endogenous catecholamines)
   e. Tachycardia may occur from unopposed beta-adrenergic receptor activation and, if the heart rate is >110 bpm, a beta-blocker should be added; beta-blockers should *not* be used prior to institution of alpha-adrenergic blockade. Elimination of the vasodilative effects of beta-receptors results in unopposed alpha-adrenergic vasoconstriction and may provoke hypertensive crisis. The negative inotropic effects of beta-blockers may precipitate heart failure in the face of hypertension
   f. Reflex tachycardia is lessened with prazosin or labetalol
   g. Alpha-methylparatyrosine—an inhibitor of tyrosine hydroxylase, the rate limiting enzyme in catecholamine production—may be used in patients who cannot tolerate alpha-adrenergic blockade due to postural hypotension. This can be especially useful in patients with cardiomyopathy; phenoxybenzamine and alpha-methylparatyrosine in combination result in less tachycardia and less postoperative hypotension
   h. Treat dysrhythmias with standard antidysrhythmic agents (e.g., lidocaine)
   i. Blood should be available for transfusion in the perioperative period since pheochromocytomas are vascular tumors and bleeding is frequent
   j. Use diuretics sparingly since intravascular volume is already constricted by catecholamines; conversely, over administration of fluids can worsen heart failure
   k. Perioperatively, avoid drugs that cause catecholamine release or potentiate catecholamine action (e.g., morphine can cause histamine-induced catecholamine release)
   l. Monitor cardiovascular and metabolic functions in postoperative patients
   m. Hypoglycemia may occur following tumor removal, which causes a loss of catecholamine-induced hyperglycemia
   n. Pain is best treated with meperidine; benzodiazepines are useful for sedation
   o. Recurrent hypertension suggests the possibility of residual tumor

Selected readings

1. Arieff AI: Hyponatremia, convulsions, respiratory arrest, and permanent brain damage after elective surgery in healthy women. *N Engl J Med* 1986; 314:1529-35.
2. Arieff AI, Ayus JC: Pathogenesis of hyponatremic encephalopathy: current concepts. *Chest* 1993; 103:607-10.
3. Bartter FC, Schwartz WB: The syndrome of inappropriate secretion of antidiuretic hormone. *Am J Med* 1967; 42:790-806.
4. Benua RS, Becker DV: *Thyroid storm.* In Bardin CW, editor: *Current therapy in endocrinology and metabolism,* ed 4, Philadelphia, 1991, BC Decker.
5. Burch HB, Wartofsky L: *Hyperthyroidism.* In Bardin CW, editor: *Current therapy in endocrinology and metabolism,* ed 4, Philadelphia, 1991, BC Decker.
6. Cefalu WT: *Diabetic ketoacidosis.* In Zaloga GP, editor: *Critical care clinics—endocrine crises,* Philadelphia, 1991, WB Saunders.
7. Chernow B, Burman KD, Johnson DL, et al: T_3 may be a better agent than T_4 in the critically ill hypothyroid patient: evaluation of transport across the blood-brain barrier in a primate model. *Crit Care Med* 1983; 11:99-104.
8. Chin R: *Adrenal crisis.* In Zaloga GP, editor: *Critical care clinics—endocrine crises,* Philadelphia, 1991, WB Saunders.
9. Chin R Jr, Zekan JM: *Adrenal insufficiency.* In Zaloga GP, editor: *Problems in critical care—endocrine emergencies,* Philadelphia, 1990, JB Lippincott.
10. Czernichow P, Robinson AG, editors: *Diabetes insipidus in man, frontiers of hormone research,* New York, 1985, S Karger.
11. Field JB: Hypoglycemia: definition, clinical presentations, classifications and laboratory tests. *Endocrinol Metab Clin North Am* 1989; 18:27-43.
12. Fischer KF, Lees JA, Newman JH: Hypoglycemia in hospitalized patients: causes and outcomes. *N Engl J Med* 1986; 315:1245-50.
13. Foster DW, McGarry JD: The metabolic derangements and treatment of diabetic ketoacidosis. *N Engl J Med* 1986; 309:159-69.
14. Hall J, Robertson G: *Diabetes insipidus.* In Zaloga GP, editor: *Problems in critical care—endocrine emergencies,* Philadelphia, 1990, JB Lippincott.
15. Khaleeli A: Myxoedema coma: a review. *Pahlavi Med J* 1978; 9:126-51.
16. Kovacs L, Robertson GL: Syndrome of inappropriate antidiuresis. *Endocrinol Metab Clin North Am* 1992; 21:859-75.
17. Kreisberg RA: Diabetic ketoacidosis: new concepts and trends in pathogenesis and treatment. *Ann Intern Med* 1978; 88:681-95.
18. Malouf R, Brust JC: Hypoglycemia: causes, neurological manifestations, and outcome. *Ann Neurol* 1985; 17:421-30.
19. Morris LR, Murphy MB, Kitabchi AE: Bicarbonate therapy in severe diabetic ketoacidosis. *Ann Intern Med* 1986; 105:836-40.
20. Mueller GL: *Pheochromocytoma.* In Zaloga GP, editor: *Problems in critical care—endocrine emergencies,* Philadelphia, 1990, JB Lippincott.
21. Myers L, Hays J: *Myxedema coma.* In Zaloga GP, editor: *Critical care clinics—endocrine crises,* Philadelphia, 1991, WB Saunders.
22. Nouel O, Bernuau J, Rueff B, et al: Hypoglycemia: a common complication of septicemia in cirrhosis. *Arch Intern Med* 1981; 141:1477-8.
23. Ober KP: *Diabetes insipidus.* In Zaloga GP, editor: *Critical care clinics—endocrine crises,* Philadelphia, 1991, WB Saunders.
24. Rao RH, Vagnucci AH, Amico JA: Bilateral massive adrenal hemorrhage: early recognition and treatment. *Ann Intern Med* 1989; 110:227-35.
25. Raum WJ: *Pheochromocytoma.* In Bardin CW, editor: *Current therapy in endocrinology and metabolism,* ed 4, Philadelphia, 1991, BC Decker.
26. Reasner CA II, Isley WL: *Thyrotoxicosis in the critically ill.* In Zaloga GP, editor: *Critical care clinics—endocrine crises,* Philadelphia, 1991, WB Saunders.
27. Robinson AG: Disorders of antidiuretic hormone secretion. *Clin Endocrinol Metab* 1985; 14:55-88.

28. Shakir KM, Amin RM: *Hypoglycemia.* In Zaloga GP, editor: *Critical care clinics—endocrine crises,* Philadelphia, 1991, WB Saunders.
29. Shapiro B, Gross MD: *Pheochromocytoma.* In Zaloga GP, editor: *Critical care clinics—endocrine crises,* Philadelphia, 1991, WB Saunders.
30. Silverberg JD, Kreisberg RA: *Hyperglycemic disorders.* In Zaloga GP, editor: *Problems in critical care—endocrine emergencies,* Philadelphia, 1990, JB Lippincott.
31. Sterns RH: *The management of hyponatremic emergencies.* In Zaloga GP, editor: *critical care clinics—endocrine crises,* Philadelphia, 1991, WB Saunders.
32. Sterns RH, Riggs JE, Schochet SS Jr: Osmotic demyelination syndrome following correction of hyponatremia. *N Engl J Med* 1986; 314:1535-42.
33. Zaloga GP, Chernow B, Smallridge RC, et al: A longitudinal evaluation of thyroid function in critically ill surgical patients. *Ann Surg* 1985; 201:456-64.
34. Zaloga GP, Smallridge RC: Thyroidal alterations in acute illness. *Semin Respir Med* 1985; 7:95-107.

Environmental Disorders

7

George L. Sternbach and Joseph Varon

7.1 BURNS

It is estimated that two million people are burned annually in the United States. Although most of these burns are minor, approximately 3%-5% of burn injuries are life-threatening.

Pathophysiology

1. Partial-thickness burns involve heat damage to the epidermis or to a portion of the dermis. The dermis contains sensory nerve endings, vascular supply, hair follicles, and sweat glands
2. Full-thickness burns involve injury to tissue deep in the dermis containing the sweat glands and hair follicles. The presence of thrombosed blood vessels or charring is characteristic of full-thickness burns. However, final determination of burn depth may not be possible for several days following the injury
3. Shock may develop due to transudation and sequestration of fluid in the burned areas and elsewhere in the body. Cardiac output may drop in major burns due to myocardial dysfunction

Risk factors

1. Burn injury is the second leading cause of death among children under the age of 12 years
2. Children are more likely than adults to suffer burns. Because children do not have the ability to recognize or react to hazardous situations, they have a greater vulnerability to accidents. Half of all victims of hot-water burns are children under the age of 5 years

Clinical presentation

1. Partial-thickness burns
   a. First-degree burn: involves only the epidermis; there is blanching erythema but no bulla formation
   b. Second-degree burn: involves a portion of the dermis; produces edema and fluid exudation. Bulla formation is characteristic and these develop quickly after a burn injury. Consider infection if bulla appear 18 hr or more after a burn occurs

2. Full-thickness burns
   a. Third-degree burn: surface is dry and inelastic. Skin surface may become white or gray. This burn will not regenerate from unburned edges
   b. Fourth-degree burn: extends beyond the depth of the skin to involve underlying muscle, tendons, vascular structures, periosteum, or bone
3. Survival depends on the extent and depth of the burn, the age of the patient, and associated injuries
4. Vascular effects in burned skin are immediate vasoconstriction followed by increased capillary permeability and plasma extravasation. Burned skin also permits increased insensible water loss

Complications

1. Coagulation necrosis at the burn site produces an advantageous setting for bacterial growth. Infection is one of the most important causes of death in severe burn injury
2. Gastric dilatation and adynamic ileus occur in major burns
3. Acute hemolysis may occur due to heat damage of red blood cells (RBC)
4. Acute renal failure may occur as a result of shock
5. Hypertension may be present, especially in children
6. Multiorgan failure is the leading cause of death in patients with burns
7. Manipulation of burn wounds has been shown to result in bacteremia in 20% of cases

Treatment

1. Evaluate airway (see the section on smoke inhalation later in this chapter) and perform endotracheal intubation if indicated by upper airway edema or deterioration of arterial blood gases (ABGs). Endotracheal intubation is appropriate for any patient with acute burn injury who displays respiratory distress
2. Establish intravenous (IV) access
3. Evaluate burned areas under sterile technique
4. Assess for the presence of other injuries, especially in the case of burns associated with explosions
5. Insert nasogastric tube (to treat ileus) and urinary catheter (to monitor urine output)
6. Obtain baseline laboratory values: complete blood cell count (CBC), electrolytes, blood urea nitrogen (BUN), creatinine, glucose, ABGs, and carboxyhemoglobin level

Estimating the extent of the burned area

1. Rule of nines for body surface area (BSA)
   a. Adults: arms 9% each; legs 18% each; head 9%; trunk 18% anterior, 18% posterior; genitalia 1%
   b. Children: arms 9% each; legs 16% each; head 13%; trunk 18% anterior, 18% posterior; genitalia 1%
   c. Infants: arms 9% each; legs 14% each; head 18%; trunk 18% anterior, 18% posterior; genitalia 1%
2. Lund and Browder chart
   a. More accurate in children
   b. See Fig. 7-1

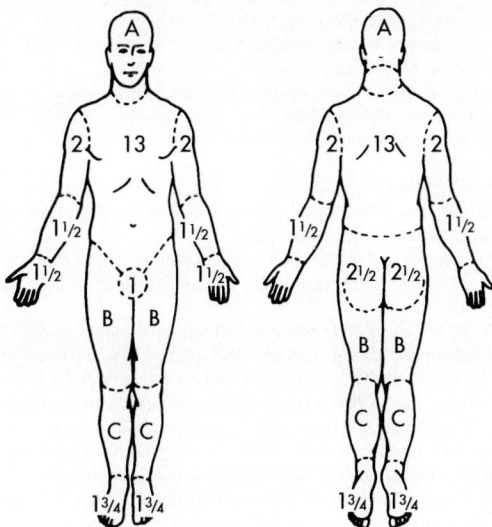

Relative percentages of areas affected by growth
(age in years)

	0	1	5	10	15	Adult
A: half of head	$9^{1/2}$	$8^{1/2}$	$6^{1/2}$	$5^{1/2}$	$4^{1/2}$	$3^{1/2}$
B: half of thigh	$2^{3/4}$	$3^{1/4}$	4	$4^{1/4}$	$4^{1/2}$	$4^{3/4}$
C: half of leg	$2^{1/2}$	$2^{1/2}$	$2^{3/4}$	3	$3^{1/4}$	$3^{1/2}$

Second degree _____ and Third degree _____ =

Total percent burned ____

Figure 7-1
Lund and Browder chart for estimation of burn extent. (From Artz CP and Yarbrough DR III: *Burns: including cold, chemical, and electrical injuries.* In Sabiston CC, Jr, editor: *Textbook of surgery: the biological basis of modern surgical practice,* ed 11, Philadelphia, 1977, WB Saunders.)

Classifying the severity of burns

1. Major burns
   a. Partial-thickness burns of >20% BSA in children or the elderly and >25% BSA in adults
   b. Full-thickness burns >10% BSA
   c. Burns involving the face, hands, feet, or perineum that may produce functional or cosmetic impairment
   d. Caustic chemical burns

    e. High-voltage electrical injury (see below)

    f. Burns complicated by inhalation injury (see below) or major trauma

2. Moderate burns

    a. Partial-thickness burns of 10%-20% BSA in children or the elderly and 15-25% BSA in adults

    b. Full thickness burns <10% BSA

Fluid resuscitation

1. Within the first 24 hr, administer isotonic balanced crystalloid solution according to recommended formula

    a. Multiple formulas for fluid administration exist that recommend 1-4 ml/kg per percentage of burn be administered within the first 24 hr

    b. The Parkland formula recommends administering 4 ml/kg of crystalloid solution per the percent BSA in the first 24 hr of treatment. Administer ½ this quantity within first the 8 hr following the burn, ¼ during the second 8 hr, and the remaining ¼ in the last 8 hr

2. Colloid-containing solutions may be administered as needed after 24 hr, at least 12.5 g of albumin for every L of crystalloid administered

3. Monitor urine output. The adult patient should have at least 50 ml/hr (or 1 ml/kg ideal body weight/hr); the child should have 1 ml/kg/hr

4. Inhalation injury may significantly increase fluid requirements

5. Some protocols (including the Parkland formula) do not account for evaporative or other water losses. Evaporative water loss is calculated as follows: (25 + % BSA) × TBSA (Total body surface area)

Topical care

1. Initially cover burned areas with dry sterile sheets

2. Clean burned areas with water and mild soap (Dial or Ivory) and remove particulate matter from the burn

3. Debride any overtly necrotic skin

4. Apply topical agents such as silver sulfadiazine or mafenide acetate

5. Use biologic dressings and synthetic skin substitutes to achieve temporary wound closure

Nutrition

1. Early enteral feeding may attenuate the hypermetabolic response by preserving the intestinal mucosal barrier (see Chapter 12)

2. High-protein diets appear preferable to conventional diets

Escharotomy

1. Circumferential burns producing a constricting eschar may result in respiratory (thorax) or circulatory (extremities) impairment

2. Escharotomy may be necessary

    a. Chest: diminished respiratory excursion, hypoxemia, diminished tidal volume (V_T)

    b. Extremities: diminished pulse and deterioration of circulation distal to the burn

3. Fasciotomy may be necessary with high-voltage electrical burns or with associated crush injury

| 7.2 | DECOMPRESSION ILLNESS (DCS) AND AIR EMBOLISM

The occurrence of DCS has paralleled the increased popularity of sport diving and can also occur in commercial divers and tunnel workers

Pathophysiology

1. DCS occurs when gas dissolved in body fluids separates to form bubbles as ambient pressure decreases. Nitrogen accumulates in tissue during a dive; the amount is dependent on the dive's depth and duration. When a diver ascends too rapidly and ambient pressure decreases, there is insufficient time for nitrogen to equilibrate, and gas bubbles form in tissue and in the venous circulation. Symptoms of DCS then occur
2. Flying shortly after diving increases the risk of DCS as decreased ambient pressure at high altitude promotes gas bubble formation

Risk factors

1. Patients who are older or obese have a higher incidence of DCS
2. Prior joint injury predisposes to the development of DCS in that joint
3. Air embolism tends to occur more frequently in less experienced divers

Clinical presentation

1. The vast majority of patients exhibit symptoms immediately following diving, though the onset may be delayed 12-36 hr
2. Clinical manifestations of DCS can be divided into two major groups
   a. Type I DCS: pain only, usually involving the joints
   b. Type II DCS: involvement of the central nervous system (CNS). This type accounts for 10-25% of instances of DCS in the United States
3. Most frequent presentation (66%-75% of cases) involves joint pain
   a. Knees, shoulders, and elbows are most commonly involved
   b. There may be slight tenderness or edema, but the severity of pain is out of proportion to objective clinical findings
4. Cutaneous DCS produces pruritus, erythematous eruption, or mottling
5. Pulmonary involvement
   a. Symptoms include pleuritic substernal chest pain, dyspnea, and cough
   b. Physical examination is usually unremarkable
6. Circulatory collapse and death may result from serious DCS
7. Spinal cord DCS produces back pain, paresthesias, weakness, or paralysis due to obstruction of epidural vertebral veins
8. Cerebral DCS may present with headache, confusion, hallucinations, delirium, seizures, visual disturbance, or cranial nerve involvement (especially, for unknown reasons, cranial nerve eight, producing vomiting, vertigo, tinnitus, and nystagmus)

Air embolism

1. Cerebral air embolism is an important cause of death in divers
2. Focal neurologic deficits occurring within 15-20 min of ascent is the most common presentation. Consider air embolism if immediate loss of consciousness occurs upon ascent

3. Mediastinal emphysema, subcutaneous emphysema, or pneumothorax may be associated with cerebral air embolism
4. Coronary embolization can produce acute myocardial infarction or cardiac arrest

Complications

1. Persistent neurologic defect may result from CNS DCS
2. Osteonecrosis may be a late consequence of bone involvement, but is not seen now as commonly as it once was

Treatment

1. Maintain left lateral decubitus Trendelenburg position when the patient has an air embolism
2. Apply 100% oxygen by mask
3. Administer normal saline intravenously as required
4. Treat seizures and cardiac dysrhythmias in standard fashion
5. Treat all patients with DCS and air embolism with recompression in a hyperbaric chamber. Recompression may be beneficial for DCS even if treatment is delayed several days. Major complications of hyperbaric oxygen therapy
   a. Barotrauma (e.g., pneumothorax, sinus trauma)
   b. Oxygen toxicity
   c. Psychiatric (e.g., claustrophobia)
6. For location of closest hyperbaric chamber, contact the Diving Accident Network of Duke University at (919) 694-2948 or (919) 684-5514

7.3   NEAR-DROWNING

Definition
    Drowning acounts for 6,000-8,000 deaths each year in the United States; children under the age of 4 comprise 40% of these fatalities. Peak incidence is during warm weather months. *Drowning* is defined as suffocation in a liquid medium. *Near-drowning* is defined as at least temporary survival from such submersion.

Pathophysiology

1. Near-drowning may be accompanied by aspiration of fluids or may be primarily the consequence of asphyxia due to laryngospasm. Aspiration of large quantities of seawater produces hypovolemia and concentration of extracellular electrolytes, whereas substantial fresh-water aspiration produces acute hypervolemia with dilution of extracellular electrolytes
    Although early medical literature emphasizes pathophysiologic differences between fresh- and salt-water drowning, aspiration of significant quantities of fluid required to produce hemodilution or electrolyte changes does not occur in most human survivors. At least 85% of survivors of drowning are thought to aspirate <22 ml of H_2O/kg of body weight
2. Adverse respiratory effects of near-drowning include
   a. Intrapulmonary shunting (both true and relative shunts)
   b. Ventilation-perfusion mismatch
   c. Decreased compliance

d. Intraalveolar influx of fluid due to capillary-alveolar leak
e. Hypoxemia resulting from any of the above
3. Hypothermia associated with immersion may predispose to cardiac dysrhythmias and exhaustion

Risk factors

1. Age distribution peaks of near-drowning victims
   a. Children under the age of 4 years
   b. Males aged 14-24 years
2. Alcohol intoxication is related to a large proportion of adult drownings

Clinical presentation

1. Respiratory findings usually predominate and include shortness of breath, air hunger, and tachypnea
   a. Auscultatory findings may include rales, rhonchi, or wheezes
   b. Respiratory deterioration may occur insidiously
2. Changes in mental status may be due to cerebral hypoxemia or head injury
3. Cardiac dysrhythmias (premature beats, bradycardia, atrial fibrillation, asystole, ventricular fibrillation) result from hypoxemia or hypothermia
4. Consider presence of hypothermia or trauma, especially cervical spine injury in appropriate settings

Complications

1. Cerebral end-organ damage due to hypoxemia mediated through cerebral edema and increased intracerebral pressure
2. Renal failure may be produced by acute tubular necrosis, hemoglobinuria, or myoglobinuria
3. Bronchial hyperreactivity may follow near-drowning
4. Hypoglycemia is common

Admission criteria for the ICU

1. Need for assisted ventilation
2. Coma or obtundation
3. Cardiac arrest or dysrhythmias
4. Hypothermia

Treatment

1. Clear airway and assure adequate respirations
   a. Apply 100% oxygen by mask to patients with spontaneous respirations
   b. Perform endotracheal intubation and mechanical ventilation in apnea and as directed by hypoxemia, hypercapnia, or for protection of airway in coma
   c. Initiate positive end-expiratory pressure (PEEP) at 3-5 cm H_2O in mechanically ventilated patients. Increase as required to maintain Po_2 ≥65 torr
   d. Monitor ABGs in all patients
   e. Administer bronchodilators in standard fashion in patients with wheezing

2. Treat cardiac dysrhythmias as indicated. Obtain an ECG on all patients with near-drowning
3. Monitor body temperature with core probe and treat hypothermia if present (see below)
4. Obtain chest x-ray (CXR) at presentation and repeat at least q6hr during the first several days
5. If circulatory shock is present, monitor with Swan-Ganz catheter
6. Consider bronchoscopy in patients who have aspirated particulate matter or contaminated water

Prognosis

1. Classification of the victim's neurologic status allows systematic assessment of prognosis
   a. Category A: awake, fully conscious
   b. Category B: stuporous but arousable
   c. Category C: comatose
2. Eighty percent of near-drowning victims recover without sequelae, 2%-9% survive with brain damage, and 12% die

7.4   ELECTRICAL INJURIES

Approximately 3% of burn injuries that require hospital admission are the result of electrical injury. Of these, approximately 40% are fatal.

Pathophysiology

1. Injuries are classified as *high voltage* (>1000 volts) or *low voltage* (<1000 volts). High voltage injuries are generally more severe, but the degree of injury also depends on tissue resistance and type of current
2. Lightning produces a current with many millions of volts but exposure may be extremely brief
3. Electrical energy causes injury through the release of heat within the tissues
4. The severity of tissue damage is directly related to the duration of contact

Risk factors

1. There is a high incidence of electrical injury among children younger than 6 years; most are related to injury by electrical outlets and cords
2. Two-thirds of injuries among adults (mostly males) involve electrical and construction workers

Clinical presentation

1. Wounds occurring at sites where electricity enters and exits the body are typically small areas of full-thickness burn. There may be considerable underlying tissue damage that is poorly reflected by the extent of visible skin damage
2. Musculoskeletal injury results from tetanic contraction of skeletal muscle during exposure. Fractures or dislocations may occur. Heat injury may produce bony or periosteal destruction
3. Electrical injury may produce vascular endothelial disruption, hemorrhage, arterial or venous thrombosis, or peripheral ischemia

4. Cardiac dysrhythmias are a frequent cause of immediate death. Dysrhythmias may continue to appear within 24 hr of injury
   a. Sinus tachycardia, supraventricular tachycardia, ventricular tachycardia, atrial fibrillation, AV block, and intraventricular conduction delay may occur
   b. Myocardial injury resulting from high-voltage injury is uncommon but may occur
   c. The most common ECG alterations are nonspecific ST-T wave changes and sinus tachycardia
5. Gastrointestinal (GI) tract injuries include intestinal perforation and stress ulcer formation with GI hemorrhage
6. Signs of CNS injury include coma, confusion, disorientation, and seizures. Central respiratory center depression may occur

Complications

1. Renal failure may result from rhabdomyolysis
2. Delayed or long-term motor paralysis may be caused by injury to the central or peripheral nervous system. Other long-term neural deficits include personality changes, memory or concentration impairment, and depression
3. Cataracts may develop 6-12 months following electrical injury to the head. Other ophthalmic sequelae include corneal ulceration, and retinal or optic nerve damage

Admission criteria

ICU admission criteria include
1. Thermal injury ≥20% BSA
2. Suspicion of inhalation injury
3. History of loss of consciousness
4. Cardiac dysrhythmias
5. Cardiopulmonary arrest
6. Rhabdomyolysis

Treatment

1. Clear the airway and support respiration if necessary
2. Administer intravenous (IV) fluids as required to maintain a urine output of at least 50-100 ml/hr or 1 ml/kg ideal body weight/hr. Traditional burn formulas for fluid replacement are not applicable to electrical burns
3. Monitor cardiac rhythm
4. Obtain CBC, electrolytes, BUN, creatinine, prothrombin time (PT), partial thromboplastin time (PTT), myoglobin, creatine kinase (CK), urinalysis (U/A), 12-lead ECG
5. If myoglobinuria appears, treat with mannitol and sodium bicarbonate (see Chapter 16)
6. Obtain surgical consultation as necessary for debridement of deep tissue. Technetium scanning may identify areas of muscular injury
7. Observe for development of sepsis, especially with *Pseudomonas* or *Clostridium* (in instances of myonecrosis). Antibiotics should be given prophylactically, as should tetanus prophylaxis

HEAT EXHAUSTION AND HEATSTROKE

There are approximately 4000 deaths annually in the United States from heat-related illness. The mortality rate of heatstroke may be 30%-80%. Heat exhaustion and heatstroke do not represent distinct pathophysiologic entities, but rather constitute heat-induced illnesses of varying severity.

Pathophysiology

Radiation of heat from the body accounts for approximately 65% of cooling, providing that the air temperature is lower than the body temperature. This mechanism becomes less effective as ambient temperature approaches 35° C. Sweating with evaporation produces approximately 30% of cooling. As ambient temperature rises, this becomes the primary method of cooling. When air temperature exceeds body temperature, heat gain by radiation is possible. As relative humidity rises, evaporative heat loss diminishes. Heat illness is exacerbated by excessive fluid loss and electrolyte depletion

Physiologic responses to increased body heat:
1. Cutaneous vasodilatation
2. Increased cardiac output to maintain blood pressure (BP)
3. Splanchnic vasoconstriction
4. Increased sweat volume

Risk factors

1. All neonates, who have poor thermoregulatory capability
2. The elderly, especially those with cardiac disease
3. Obese individuals
4. Those with underlying illnesses: congestive heart failure, coronary artery disease, hyperthyroidism, dermatologic disorders, and major burns
5. Medications and drugs: beta-adrenergic blockers, phenothiazines, lithium, cyclic antidepressants, antihistamines, amphetamines, cocaine, and phencyclidine

Clinical presentation

Heat exhaustion

1. Temperature elevation but generally less than 39° C
2. Symptoms: nausea, vomiting, headache, light-headedness, malaise, and muscular cramping
3. Diaphoresis, tachycardia, hypotension, or orthostatic hypotension
4. Mental status is unimpaired

Heatstroke

1. Temperature generally >40.5° C
2. Signs: tachypnea (respiratory rate as high as 60/min), tachycardia, and hypotension
3. Dry, hot skin is classic, but not necessary to make the diagnosis. Lack of sweating may be a late finding and diaphoretic skin is seen in about half of all cases
4. Major diagnostic point: CNS dysfunction (confusion, bizarre behavior, delirium, obtundation, coma, seizures). Ataxia may result from cerebel-

lar involvement. Most CNS deficits are reversible with treatment, but may become fixed

Complications

Heatstroke

1. Muscular injury causing rhabdomyolysis
2. Hypoglycemia
3. Hypocalcemia (does not usually require specific treatment)
4. Renal failure resulting from acute tubular necrosis or rhabdomyolysis (see Chapter 16)
5. Hepatocellular injury producing elevation of liver enzymes
6. Diffuse intravascular coagulation (DIC) may occur 1-3 days following the onset of heatstroke
7. Adult respiratory distress syndrome (ARDS) (see Chapter 15)
8. Neurologic: ataxia, dementia, cerebral edema, and brain death

Treatment

Heat exhaustion

1. Place patient in a cool environment
2. Replace fluid with normal saline or half-normal saline with the amount to be guided by vital signs. Invasive cardiovascular monitoring may be required, especially in older patients

Heatstroke

1. Maintain airway and breathing. Administer IV fluids as directed by vital signs
2. Maintain continuous monitoring of core temperature with rectal or esophageal probe
3. Initiate immediate vigorous cooling by one or more of the following measures
   a. Evaporative technique: spray patient with warm water (15° C) and cool with a fan. This method prevents cutaneous vasoconstriction and does not induce shivering. Requires low-humidity environment
   b. Ice packs to neck, axilla, and groin. This produces cooling in the area of major vessels and is useful as an adjunct to other techniques
   c. Ice-water bath. May cause cutaneous vasoconstriction. It is also difficult to monitor an immersed patient
   d. Iced gastric lavage
   e. Cool (6°-10° C) peritoneal lavage
   f. Intermittent positive pressure breathing (IPPB) with cold inhaled air
   g. Cardiopulmonary bypass (this method produces the most rapid cooling)
4. Do not administer antipyretics (e.g., salicylates or acetaminophen)
5. Administer D5%/half-normal saline to replace fluid loss
6. Monitor central venous pressure, urine output, and urine for myoglobin
7. Follow ABGs and CXR to determine the development of ARDS, coagulation studies for DIC, liver enzymes, creatine kinase (CK), BUN, and creatinine

8. May require paralysis and mechanical ventilation (especially if associated with amphetamine use)
9. If shivering occurs with cooling, chlorpromazine (25-50 mg IV) may be administered. However, this must be done with care, as chlorpromazine may produce cardiac dysrhythmias, hypotension, or neuroleptic malignant syndrome, which in itself produces hyperthermia
10. Dantrolene may be used, 1 mg/kg IV (may be increased to as high as 10 mg/kg). The mechanism appears to involve calcium release inhibition in skeletal muscle. Muscular weakness may be produced. Further research into the use of this agent in heatstroke is required

7.6 HYPOTHERMIA

1. Normal core temperature is 36°-37.5° C. Thermoregulation is controlled in the hypothalamus. Shivering is initiated in the anterior hypothalamus and is the body's most effective method to raise temperature
2. Hypothermia may be divided into mild (body temperature 33°-35° C), moderate (27°-32° C), and severe (<27° C) forms. It is seen in a variety of circumstances
3. *Primary* (accidental) *hypothermia* is caused by exposure to low environmental temperature. *Secondary hypothermia* occurs when heat conservation mechanisms are abnormal due to underlying disease. *Induced hypothermia* is used as a therapeutic measure in certain neurosurgical and cardiovascular surgical procedures

Pathophysiology

In secondary hypothermia, there may be interference with the hypothalamic temperature regulating center, or an inability to shiver, redistribute blood flow, or move from a cold environment

Risk factors

1. Infants and the elderly are the most susceptible
   a. Infants: large surface area to mass ratio and the inability to protect themselves from a cool environment
   b. Elderly: decreased sensory temperature appreciation, deficient centrally-mediated response to cold, failure to shiver, limited ability to vasoconstrict peripheral vessels
2. Drug use and intoxication
   a. Agents that depress the level of consciousness (especially ethanol) are often involved in exposure-related hypothermia
   b. Barbiturates depress core temperature by central effect
   c. Phenothiazines inhibit response to cold by alpha-adrenergic blocking activity and by direct suppression of the thermoregulatory center
3. Preexisting illness: on facing page

Clinical presentation

1. Initial sympathetic response (producing peripheral vasoconstriction and tachycardia) causes transient elevation of BP and cardiac output
   a. Increased renal perfusion produces increased urine production (cold diuresis), and may lead to hypovolemia, hemoconcentration, and increased blood viscosity

Illness Predisposing to Hypothermia

Pathologic Reduction of Metabolic Rate

Hypothyroidism
Hypopituitarism
Hypoadrenalism

Alteration of Hypothalamic Function

Anorexia nervosa
Hypothalamic tumors
Head trauma
Cerebrovascular accident
Wernicke's encephalopathy
Sarcoidosis (involving the hypothalamus)

Other Mechanisms

Hypoglycemia
Spinal cord transection
Extensive body surface burns
Exfoliative erythrodermas
Sepsis
Severe protein malnutrition

From Varon J, Sadovnikoff N, Sternbach GL: Hypothermia. saving patients from the big chill. *Postgrad Med* 1992; 92:47-59.

  b. Response is ablated <30° C
2. Clouding of sensorium regularly occurs at 30°-32° C
3. Mild hypothermia: tachypnea, tachycardia, shivering, amnesia, ataxia, and dysarthria
4. Moderate hypothermia: decreased level of consciousness, mydriasis, atrial fibrillation, and bradycardia
5. Severe hypothermia: absent reflexes and response to pain, coma, and hypotension
6. Cardiac complications
  a. Dysrhythmias: atrial fibrillation is common
  b. Patients are increasingly susceptible to ventricular fibrillation with diminishing temperature. Below 28° C, even minor procedures such as moving or repositioning the patient may initiate ventricular fibrillation
  c. Ventricular fibrillation is resistant to pharmacologic treatment or electrical defibrillation until the temperature has increased
  d. Susceptibility to ventricular dysrhythmias may persist for several days, even after normal body temperature has been restored
  e. ECG changes include PR, QT, and QRS prolongation, and J-point elevation (Osborne wave).

Complications

1. Morbidity and mortality are related to the degree and duration of hypothermia, as well as to appropriate therapy

2. Bronchorrhea and depressed cough reflexes lead to bronchopneumonia and aspiration pneumonitis
3. Punctate hemorrhages may occur in the GI tract but significant bleeding is rare
4. Pancreatitis is common
5. Fatal disseminated intravascular coagulation may occur

Treatment

Cardiovascular

1. Employ basic life-support protocols to support ventilation and circulation
2. Use endotracheal intubation and mechanical ventilation as indicated
3. Initiate CPR if cardiac arrest is present. Continue until the core temperature of 32° C is reached or response is achieved
4. Ventricular fibrillation may be resistant to defibrillation in severe hypothermia. Attempt single defibrillation; if this is not successful, continue rewarming until the temperature >30° and administer bretylium 5-10 mg/kg IV over 5-10 min, then infusion of 2 mg/min

Rewarming

1. For mild and moderate hypothermia (including most cases of secondary hypothermia) passive rewarming is indicated
   a. Remove patient from the cold environment
   b. Apply dry, unheated blankets
2. For some cases of moderate hypothermia, use active surface rewarming
   a. Heating blankets, hot water bottles, heat cradles, heat-fluidized beds, and warm-water immersion
   b. May be associated with afterdrop of core temperature as peripheral vasoconstriction is reversed, producing hypovolemic shock and ventricular fibrillation
3. For severe hypothermia, active core rewarming is indicated. Use one or more of the following
   a. Infusion of warmed IV fluids (temperature not to exceed 40° C)
   b. Intubation and ventilation with warmed, humidified oxygen. Keep airway temperature <45° C
   c. Peritoneal dialysis (usually requires 6-8 exchanges of potassium-free dialysate heated to 43° C)
   d. Gastric irrigation with warmed fluids and with introduction of intragastric balloon. May provoke dysrhythmias
   e. Mediastinal irrigation (operative technique)
   f. Extracorporeal blood rewarming with a heat exchanger at 40° C
4. If patient does not respond to rewarming consider cerebral edema

| 7.7 | SMOKE INHALATION AND CARBON MONOXIDE (CO) POISONING

CO intoxication is the leading cause of death by poisoning in the United States, accounting for 3800 accidental and suicidal deaths annually. It is also the most common cause of death in combustion-related inhalation injury. Many nonlethal exposures may, however, go undetected.

Pathophysiology

CO poisoning

1. CO combines preferentially with hemoglobin (Hg) to produce carboxy-hemoglobin (COHb). This displaces oxygen and reduces systemic arterial content
2. CO binds reversibly to Hg with an affinity over $200 \times$ that of oxygen, so a relatively minute concentration of CO in the environment can lead to toxic concentrations in blood
3. Mechanisms of toxicity
   a. Decreased oxygen-carrying capacity of the blood
   b. Alteration of dissociation characteristics of oxyhemoglobin; shifts oxyhemoglobin dissociation curve to the left
   c. Decreased cellular respiration due to binding with cytochrome c oxidase
   d. Binding to myoglobin, producing myocardial and skeletal muscle dysfunction
4. Half-life of COHb in room air is 320 min; on 100% O_2 at 1 atmosphere it is 60 min, and on 100% O_2 at 3 atmospheres, it is 23 min

Smoke inhalation

1. Smoke contains carbon particles and various gases (including nitrogen oxide, chlorine, phosgene, ammonia, and hydrogen cyanide)
2. These gases adhere to the respiratory mucosa and produce compounds that are locally and systemically toxic

Risk factors

1. The most common sources of CO are listed in the Box below
2. Smoke inhalation from fires accounts for the vast majority of cases
3. Vapor of methylene chloride (contained in many paint removers) is readily absorbed through the lungs and is converted to CO by the liver

---

Exogenous Sources of Carbon Monoxide

Smoke from all types of fires
Paint-remover containing methylene chloride
Furnaces
Gasoline-powered engines
Swimming pool heaters
Sterno fuel
Tobacco smoke
Vehicular exhaust fumes
Water heaters

From Sadovnikoff N, Varon J, Sternbach GL: Carbon monoxide poisoning: an occult epidemic. *Postgrad Med* 1992; 92:86-96.

Clinical presentation

CO poisoning

1. Symptoms and signs in acute CO poisoning depend on the COHb level (see Table 7-1)
   a. Patients with COHb levels <10% are usually asymptomatic
   b. Patients with levels >25% should be considered for hospital admission
   c. Those with levels >50% commonly have coma and seizures resulting from cerebral edema
   d. Death is likely if levels >60%
   e. Determination of treatment based only on the COHb level is inappropriate, though, because the level alone is a poor predictor of the degree of injury. Therefore, clinical assessment is vital to planning treatment
2. Chronic or subacute poisoning may present with less characteristic symptoms

Smoke inhalation

Suspect if
1. Exposure occurred in a closed space
2. There are facial or pharyngeal burns, or burned nasal vibrissae
3. There is carbonaceous sputum or hoarseness

Complications

1. Neuropsychiatric problems such as memory loss, personality changes, mutism, and parkinsonism may occur as long-term sequelae to CO poisoning
2. Indicators of a poor prognosis include an altered level of consciousness, advanced age, metabolic acidosis, and structural abnormalities on computed tomography (CT) or magnetic resonance (MR) scanning

Treatment

CO poisoning

1. Obtain COHb levels in all patients suspected of having CO exposure (e.g., all victims at a fire scene)

Table 7-1   Acute carbon monoxide poisoning

COHb Level (%)	Symptoms
10	Headache
20	Dizziness, nausea, and dyspnea
30	Visual disturbances
40	Confusion and syncope
50	Seizures and coma
>60	Cardiopulmonary failure and death

From Sadovnikoff N, Varon J, Sternbach GL: Carbon monoxide poisoning: an occult epidemic. *Postgrad Med* 1992; 92:86-96.

2. Apply supplemental oxygen 100% by mask while awaiting results
   a. The goal is to improve blood oxygen content by maximizing the fraction dissolved in plasma
   b. Monitor with serial COHb levels. Continue 100% oxygen until COHb level is <5%. Continue to monitor the level thereafter to guard against the undetected release of CO from tissue sites
3. Obtain an ECG and monitor with serial CK levels if ECG suggestive of ischemia
4. Consider treatment with hyperbaric oxygen (HBO) in
   a. Patients with serious CO poisoning (e.g, coma, neurologic deficit, cardiac or hemodynamic instability, history of loss of consciousness)
   b. Pregnant women
   c. Patients with underlying heart disease or an abnormal ECG
5. Whether HBO alters outcome is still controversial
6. If HBO treatment is unavailable, consider intubation and mechanical ventilation with administration of 100% oxygen if clinical findings merit
7. Consider transfusion with packed red blood cells in severe poisoning

Smoke inhalation

1. If findings of smoke inhalation are present, evaluate the airway with fiberoptic bronchoscopy
2. Obtain ABGs and CXR
3. Administer humidified oxygen
4. Perform early endotracheal intubation in the presence of upper airway edema

---

7.8 SCORPION ENVENOMATION

Scorpions are arachnids that typically inhabit temperate climates. The only dangerous species of scorpion in the United States is the *Centruroides* genus, which is found primarily in the southwestern states (Arizona, California, New Mexico, Texas).

Pathophysiology

The venom is complex, containing a number of proteins, polypeptides, enzymes (e.g., hyaluronidases, phospholipases), and neurotoxins. The venom affects sodium channels to prolong action potentials and produce spontaneous neural depolarizations of the sympathetic and parasympathetic systems.

Risk factors

Most serious envenomations occur in children.

Clinical presentation

1. The most common finding is severe local pain at the site of the sting. In most cases, this resolves within several hrs. There is severe tenderness to palpation or percussion over the site
2. May be accompanied by wheal and flare reaction and paresthesias at the site of the sting
3. Significant envenomation produces tachycardia, hypertension, restlessness, hyperexcitability, diaphoresis, piloerection, nystagmus, diplopia, opisthotonos, muscular fasciculations, or hypersalivation

Table 7-2   Severity of *Centruroides* scorpion envenomation

Grade	Signs and Symptoms
I	Local pain or paresthesias at site; tenderness to touch or percussion
II	Local findings; pain and paresthesias remote from sting site
III	Symptomatic skeletal neuromuscular dysfunction (muscular jerking or shaking) or cranial nerve dysfunction (e.g., blurred vision, difficulty swallowing, hypersalivation, slurred speech, tongue fasciculations)
IV	Somatic skeletal *and* cranial nerve dysfunction

From Curry SC, Vance MV, Ryan PJ, et al: Envenomation by the scorpion *Centruroides sculpturatus.* J Toxicol Clin Toxicol 1983-84; 21:417-49.

4. The most severe cases produce seizures, pulmonary edema, muscular paralysis, respiratory arrest, cardiovascular collapse, and death

Complications

These include disseminated intravascular coagulation, pancreatitis, jaundice, and renal failure

Treatment

1. Maintain airway and assist ventilations if necessary
2. Clean the wound and administer tetanus prophylaxis if indicated. Do not cool or incise wound
3. Classify *Centruroides* sting by severity of involvement according to Table 7-2
   a. Grades I and II envenomation: wound care as above and provide oral analgesics
   b. Grades III and IV: an antivenin has been produced but is not generally available. Contact the regional poison control center or Central Arizona Regional Poison Management at (602) 253-3334. Sedate and provide supportive care. High doses of phenobarbital have been recommended, but care must be taken to prevent respiratory failure
   c. Treat severe tachycardia with labetalol 10-20 mg IV

Prognosis

1. Though deaths may occur, none has been reported in the United States since 1968
2. If untreated, the sting may be lethal in 1% of adults and as many as 25% of children under the age of 5 years

7.9   SNAKEBITE

Approximately 8000 instances of poisonous snakebites occur annually in the United States, with 9-15 deaths resulting. Most bites occur in the southern and southwestern states, with a peak incidence during the summer months

There are four venomous species in the United States: rattlesnakes (genus *Crotalus* and *Sistruris*), copperheads *(Agkistrodon contortrix),* and cottonmouths *(Agkistrodon piscivorus)* all are pit vipers; or coral snakes (genus *Micrurus*). Rattlesnakes account for 65% of reported venomous snakebites.

Pathophysiology

Snake venoms are complex mixtures of toxins that have cytotoxic, hemotoxic, and neurotoxic components. Cytotoxic effects produce tissue necrosis. Hemotoxic venoms interfere with the coagulation system. Rattlesnakes are classically considered to have cytotoxic and hemotoxic venom, but neurotoxic activity may also be present. Coral snake venom has largely neurotoxic activity.

Snakes are capable of controlling the quantity of venom administered and approximately 25%-30% of bites by poisonous snakes do not result in envenomation.

Predisposition

1. The majority of victims are males younger than the age of 20
2. Severity of a bite depends on
   a. Size and species of snake
   b. Location of bite
   c. Grade of envenomation (see below)
   d. Age and medical condition of the patient

Clinical presentation

Pit vipers

1. The most important findings of pit viper envenomation are fang punctures at the bite site (usually on the extremities), local pain, and adjacent erythema and edema
   a. Edema and erythema are characteristic and usually develop within 30 min of envenomation
   b. This may spread for the following 24 hr and develop hemorrhagic bullae
   c. If there is no erythema or edema development within 4 hr of the bite, it is unlikely that envenomation has occurred
2. Grade the severity of the bite according to criteria in Table 7-3
3. Swelling resulting from edema and capillary rupture may produce increased fascial compartment pressure
4. Severe envenomation produces hypotension due to hemorrhage and third-space fluid loss, shock, paresthesias, muscular fasciculations. Nausea, vomiting, giddiness, and elevation or depression of temperature may be produced. Coma, convulsions, and death may result
5. Hematologic sequelae of severe envenomation include anemia due to hemolysis, hypothrombinemia, thrombocytopenia, hypofibrinogenemia, and hypercoagulability. GI tract, urinary tract, or intracerebral hemorrhage may result
6. CNS effects include seizures, coma, and respiratory paralysis

Table 7-3   Severity of pit viper envenomation

Grade	Envenomation	Findings
0	None	Fang marks; minimal pain; <2.5 cm circumferential edema
I	Minimal	2.5-12.5 cm edema and erythema in first 12 hr
II	Moderate	15-36 cm edema and erythema in first 12 hr
III	Severe	Edema >36 cm in 24 hr; systemic symptoms present (including coagulation defects)
IV	Very severe	Systemic symptoms; rapid development of edema, erythema; ecchymoses, bullae; coagulation defects

From Parrish HM: Influence of treated snakebites in the United States. *Publ Health Rep* 1966; 81:269-76.

Table 7-4   Severity of coral snake envenomation

Grade	Envenomation	Findings within 36 hr of Bite
0	None	Minimal local swelling; no systemic symptoms
I	Moderate	Systemic symptoms but no respiratory paralysis
II	Severe	Complete respiratory paralysis

From Parrish HM, Kahn MS: Bites by coral snakes: report of 11 representative cases. *Am J Med Sci* 1967; 253:561-568.

Coral snakes

1. Coral snakebites do not produce prominent swelling or other local findings
2. Neurotoxic venom may cause ptosis, diplopia, dysphagia, dysarthria, salivation, paresthesias, muscular fasciculations, loss of deep tendon reflexes, muscular weakness, and respiratory paralysis
3. Onset of symptoms may be delayed 1-5 hr following the bite
4. Grade severity of the bite according to the criteria in Table 7-4. Repeat evaluation every 15 min for the first 4 hr following the bite

Complications

1. Renal failure may result from disseminated intravascular coagulation or acute tubular necrosis
2. Anaphylaxis and serum sickness are potential complications of treatment with antivenin

Treatment

Pit viper

1. Wound care
   a. Do not apply ice to bite

    b. Use of tourniquets, incision, and suction is traditional but controversial

    c. Measure the circumference of the bitten extremity and repeat the measurement qhr. With massive swelling, measurement of intrafascial pressure may be indicated

2. Obtain CBC, platelet count, prothrombin time (PT), partial thromboplastin time (PTT), thrombin time, fibrinogen level, fibrin split products, electrolytes, BUN, and creatinine. These values should be repeated q4hr

3. Type and crossmatch for 4 U packed red blood cells

4. Administer IV normal saline as indicated by hypotension. Institute Swan-Ganz catheter monitoring in hemodynamically unstable patients

5. Antivenin
    a. Perform skin or eye test for horse serum hypersensitivity. If negative, proceed with antivenin administration. If positive, consider the risk of envenomation against the possibility of anaphylactic reaction. In severe envenomation, antivenin infusion may be preceded with 250 mg methylprednisolone IV. Be prepared to treat anaphylaxis (see Chapter 20)
    b. No universally accepted standard recommendations exist for antivenin administration
    c. No antivenin is required for grades 0 or I pit viper bites
    d. Administer to grades II-IV bites. Test dose: 2-0.5 ml IV over 5 min; if no adverse effect, administer remainder over 30 min to 2 hr. Individualize dosage to severity and rate of progression. Grade II: up to 5 vials. Grade III: 5-15 vials. Grade IV: 15-20 vials
    e. Observe for 3-5 hr after initial administration; administer an additional vial q 1-2 hr if pain persists or swelling progresses

6. Use of fasciotomy in severe envenomation with increased intrafascial pressure is controversial. This may be necessary if intrafascial pressure >30 torr. Obtain surgical consultation as required in instances of massive edema

Coral snakes

1. An antivenin is available for bites of Eastern coral snakes. Administer antivenin to all bite victims of this snake, even prior to the appearance of symptoms. Dosage is 3-6 vials in 300-500 ml normal saline

2. There is no antivenin available for bites of the Arizona coral snake

3. Perform endotracheal intubation if there are any signs of bulbar paralysis such as diplopia or dysphagia

4. Institute respiratory support with mechanical ventilation as required. Antivenin may not completely reverse respiratory depression

| 7.10 | **SPIDER BITE**

Black widow spider

The black widow spider is a member of the *Latrodectus* genus, and is found throughout the United States. The female, larger and more dangerous than the male, is black or brown with a characteristic red hourglass marking on the ventral abdomen.

Pathophysiology

Black widow venom is extremely potent. The major activity of the venom lies in provoking the release of catecholamines at adrenergic synaptic terminals and depletion of acetylcholine from motor nerve endings.

Risk factors

There is high risk for mortality among the following patients:

1. Patients younger than 16 or older than 65 years
2. Those with hypertension or cardiovascular disease (envenomation may cause heart failure, cerebrovascular accident, or myocardial ischemia)

Clinical presentation

1. Pain at the bite site may be minimal, but severe pain may develop in the extremity, along with painful lymphadenopathy, erythema, swelling, and piloerection 20-60 min following the bite
2. Cramping and painful muscular contractions in the back, thigh, abdomen, and chest produces abdominal rigidity, tonic contractions, and tremor
3. There may be restlessness, weakness, dizziness, urinary retention, diaphoresis, salivation, nausea, vomiting, priapism, and hypertension
4. Distinction must be made from the acute abdomen (the onset of severe pain within the abdominal cavity): despite rigidity, there is minimal tenderness and no rebound tenderness

Complications

1. Hypertensive crisis
2. Paralysis and respiratory arrest, especially in children
3. Severe envenomation may produce shock and/or coma

Treatment

1. Clean wound and apply cool compresses (not ice) to the bite site
2. Administer diazepam (5-10 mg IV q3hr as needed) and methocarbamol (1000 mg IV no faster than 100 mg/min and 1000 mg additionally as IV infusion) for symptomatic treatment of muscular spasm
3. Calcium gluconate 10% (1-2 ml/kg IV over 20 min, maximum 10 ml) may also provide relief of muscular spasm, but this is transient, lasting <30 min
4. Treat elevated BP if diastolic BP >130 torr (see Chapter 5)
5. Antivenin
   a. Administration is recommended for symptomatic patients <16 or >65 years old; those with preexisting hypertension or cardiovascular disease; and those displaying respiratory distress, pronounced hypertension, or persistent severe muscular symptoms despite above treatment
   b. Prior to administration, test the skin for horse serum sensitivity (included with antivenin)
   c. Administer 1 vial diluted in 50 ml normal saline over 15-30 min. A second vial will be required only in severe cases

Prognosis

1. Prognosis for recovery with treatment is good and deaths are rare
2. There is a 0.5% incidence of anaphylaxis and a 2% incidence of serum sickness associated with antivenin use

Brown recluse spider

This spider is of the *Loxosceles* species and is present throughout the southern United States. It is tan or brown with a violin-shaped mark on the dorsum of the cephalothorax.

Pathophysiology

The venom contains a variety of enzymes including hyaluronidase, protease, collagenase, and sphingomyelinase D, which are thought to be responsible for dermal necrosis and hemolysis.

Risk factors

Most severe envenomations occur in children.

Clinical presentation

1. Local pain and burning, bulla formation at the site of the bite, becoming necrotic over hrs to days
2. Systemic signs and symptoms: fever, chills, petechiae, nausea, vomiting, and weakness
3. Severe cases may produce hemolysis, disseminated intravascular coagulation, thrombocytopenia, jaundice, or shock

Complications

1. Severe hemolysis may result in death
2. Renal failure may result from hemoglobinuria or myoglobinuria

Treatment

1. There is no commercially available antivenin in the United States
2. Begin IV infusion with normal saline
3. Obtain CBC, platelet count, electrolytes, BUN, creatinine, PT, PTT, and U/A
4. Clean the wound and administer tetanus prophylaxis if indicated. Do not cool or incise wound
5. Some recommend the use of dapsone (50-200 mg/day), a leukocyte inhibitor that relieves pain, and reduces erythema and induration. Do not administer to children
6. Obtain surgical consultation for wound care

Selected readings

Christensen JA, Sherman RT, Balis GA, et al: Delayed neurological injury secondary to high voltage current with recovery. *J Trauma* 1980; 20:166-8.

Craig SR: When lightning strikes: pathophysiology and treatment of lightning injuries. *Postgrad Med* 1986; 79:109-24.

Curley G, Irwin RS: Disorders of temperature control: part I. Hyperthermia. *Intensive Care Med* 1986; 1:5-14.

Curry SC, Vance MV, Ryan PJ, et al: Envenomation by the scorpion *Centruroides sculpturatus*. *J Toxicol Clin Toxicol* 1983-84; 21:417-49.

Deming RH: Burns. *N Engl J Med* 1985; 313:1389-98.

Dick APK, Massey EW: Neurologic presentation of decompression sickness and air embolism in sport scuba divers. *Neurology* 1985; 35:667-71.

Dietch EA: The management of burns. *New Engl J Med* 1990; 323:1249-53.

Hunt JL, Mason AD, Masterson TS, et al: The pathophysiology of acute electrical injury. *J Trauma* 1976; 16:335-40.

Knochel JP: Heatstroke and related heat stress disorders. *DM* 1989; 35:301-78.

Kobernick M: Electrical injuries: pathophysiology and emergency management. *Ann Emerg Med* 1982; 11:633-8.

Lavelle JM, Shaw KN: Near-drowning: is emergency department cardiopulmonary resuscitation or intensive care unit cerebral resuscitation indicated? *Crit Care Med* 1993; 21:368-73.

Levin DL: Near-drowning. *Crit Care Med* 1980; 8:590-95.

Modell JH: Drowning. *New Engl J Med* 1993; 328:253-6.

Modell JH: Drowning vs near drowning: a discussion of definitions. *Crit Care Med* 1981; 9:351-2.

Modell JH, Graves SA, Kuck EJ: Near-drowning: correlation of level of consciousness and survival. *Can Anesth Soc J* 1980; 27:211-5.

Myers R, Bray P: Delayed treatment of serious decompression illness. *Ann Emerg Med* 1985; 14:254-7.

Parrish HM: Influence of treated snakebites in the United States. *Publ Health Rep* 1966; 81:269-76.

Parrish HM, Kahn MS: Bites by coral snakes: report of 11 representative cases. *Am J Med Sci* 1967; 253:561-8.

Paton BC: Accidental hypothermia. *Pharmacol Ther* 1983; 22:331-77.

Robinson L, Miller RH: Smoke inhalation injuries. *Am J Otolaryngol* 1986; 7:628-32.

Russell FE: *Snake venom poisoning,* Philadelphia, 1980, JB Lippincott.

Sadovnikoff N, Varon J, Sternbach GL: Carbon monoxide poisoning: an occult epidemic. *Postgrad Med* 1992; 92:86-96.

Snyder CC, Knowles RP: Snakebites: guidelines for practical management. *Postgrad Med* 1988; 83:53-75.

Spyker DA: Submersion injury: epidemiology, prevention and management. *Pediatr Clin North Am* 1985; 32:113-25.

Strauss R: Diving medicine. *Am Rev Respir Dis* 1979; 119:1001-23.

Varon J, Sadovnikoff N, Sternbach GL: Hypothermia: saving patients from the big chill. *Postgrad Med* 1992; 92:47-59.

Wingert WA, Chan L: Rattlesnake bites in Southern California and rationale for recommended treatment. *West J Med* 1988; 148:37-44.

Gastrointestinal
Disorders

8

Alex E. Lechin and Joseph Varon

8.1 GASTROINTESTINAL BLEEDING

1. Classification
   a. Upper: above the ligament of Treitz
   b. Lower: below the ligament of Treitz
2. Etiology
   The most common causes of acute gastrointestinal (GI) bleeding that require admission to the intensive care unit (ICU) are depicted in Table 8-1. The most common source of GI bleeding in the ICU is gastroduodenal stress ulcerations.
3. Diagnostic evaluation
   a. History: Although the history and physical examination in a critically-ill patient with acute GI bleeding may be limited by the patient's clinical condition, the following need to be investigated
      (1) History of hematemesis or melena
      (2) Time of onset
      (3) Amount of blood
      (4) Color and character
      (5) Drug or alcohol use (i.e., nonsteroidal antiinflammatory drugs [NSAID], prednisone, sodium warfarin)
      (6) Past medical history (e.g., cirrhosis, peptic ulcer disease [PUD], inflammatory bowel disease [IBD])
   b. Physical examination: The precise cause of acute GI bleeding is unlikely to be evident from physical examination alone, except in chronic liver disease, Osler-Weber-Rendu disease, or hemorrhoids
      (1) General appearance may vary from the patient who is not in acute distress to the patient who is in hypovolemic shock
      (2) Vital signs: itachycardia and postural hypotension. An increase in heart rate (HR) of 10-20 beats/min (bpm) and a drop in blood pressure (BP) of >20 mm Hg upon assumption of an upright position are generally indicative of significant, acute volume (blood) loss
      (3) Other signs of hypovolemia: altered mental status and low urine output

Table 8-1 Etiology of acute GI bleeding

Upper	Lower
Esophagus	Small intestine
Mucosal tear	A-V malformations
Esophageal rupture	Inflammatory bowel disease
Esophagitis	Ischemia
Neoplasms	Meckel's diverticulum
Varices	Neoplasms
Stomach	Large intestine
A-V (arteriovenous)	Diverticulosis
malformations	Hemorrhoids
Gastritis (any etiology)	Inflammatory bowel disease
Neoplasms	Infections
Peptic ulcer disease	Ischemia
Stress ulcers	Neoplasms
Duodenum	
A-V malformations	
Neoplasms (rare)	
Peptic ulcer disease	

Table 8-2 Advantages and disadvantages of NG tubes in acute GI bleeding

Advantages	Disadvantages
Documents the presence or absence of blood	Causes patient discomfort
Monitors the rate of bleeding	Irritates esophageal and/or gastric mucosa
Lavages and decompresses the stomach	Increases the incidence of sinusitis
	Possibly causes esophageal or gastric perforation

    (4) Associated findings: petechiae, jaundice, hepatomegaly, and splenomegaly

    (5) Rectum: look for hemorrhoids, fissures, etc. Examine stools for blood even if the patient has an upper GI source

  c. Place a nasogastric (NG) tube in *all* patients with acute GI bleeding. The major advantages and disadvantages of NG tubes are depicted in Table 8-2

  d. Laboratory evaluation: all patients admitted to the ICU with GI bleeding should undergo the laboratory tests depicted in the Box on p. 151.

  e. Radiologic evaluation: All patients should undergo chest radiograph and abdominal x-rays. These may show evidence of perforation, obstruction, and may indicate ischemic changes. Contrast studies have a low diagnostic yield and may be hazardous for the critically ill patient. They may also interfere with other diagnostic studies (i.e., endoscopy, angiography).

Initial Laboratory Evaluation in GI Bleeding

- Complete blood count (CBC): Repeat hemoglobin/hematocrit (H/H) q4 hr until the patient is stable or bleeding has been controlled
- Blood urea nitrogen (BUN), creatinine, and electrolytes
- Prothrombin time (PT) and partial thromboplastin time (PTT)
- Type and crossmatch for 2-8 U of packed red blood cells (PRCBs), FFP
- Other tests are ordered according to suspected or known underlying disease (e.g., liver function tests [LFTs] and CR)

Special tests may be required in the evaluation of acute GI bleeding. These include:
   (1) Selective angiography may be used as a tool for both diagnosis and therapy (e.g., embolization). A bleeding rate ≥ 0.5 ml/min is needed at the time of the procedure for diagnosis
   (2) Radionuclide scans: sensitive in detecting lesions with lower bleeding rates
   f. Endoscopy is indicated in the vast majority of patients requiring ICU admission for GI bleeding:
   (1) Perform an upper endoscopy when blood is obtained from the NG tube or frank hematemesis is present
   (2) Perform a flexible sigmoidoscopy initially if lower GI bleeding is suspected. If this is not diagnostic, consider colonoscopy
4. Initial ICU management
   a. As in any critically ill patient, the management of acute GI bleeding starts with assessment of the airway, breathing, and circulation (ABCs). A low threshold for endotracheal intubation is recommended in the event of clouding of consciousness or overt shock to prevent aspiration
   b. Insert at least 2 large-bore (16-gauge) IV catheters
   c. Infuse blood, plasma expanders, and/or normal saline to maintain a mean arterial pressure ≥ 65 mm Hg
   d. Some authors recommend NG placement in all patients with GI bleed and lavage of the stomach until the return is clear
   e. Correct pre-existing coagulopathy (e.g., FFP and vitamin K)
   f. Histamine$_2$ (H$_2$)-receptor blockers may prevent further hemorrhage. Continuous infusions are preferred (i.e., ranitidine 150-300 mg/24 hr IV infusion if renal function is normal)
   g. Once the patient's condition is stable, endoscopic and/or angiographic verification of the source of bleeding will allow more definitive therapy
5. Specific management of selected conditions
   a. Variceal hemorrhage
   (1) Vasopressin infusion: start at 0.2-0.4 U/min (up to 1 U/min). Some of the major complications of vasopressin (e.g., myocardial ischemia) can be prevented by the co-administration of low doses of nitroglycerin

(2) Sclerotherapy is indicated at the time of diagnostic endoscopy. Two or three treatments are usually done within a 10-day period

(3) Balloon tamponade: temporizing measure only. It is usually reserved for hemorrhage that fails to stop after therapy with vasopressin and sclerotherapy. Use Sengstaken-Blakemore or Minnesota tubes

(4) Surgical therapy: every patient with a major esophageal bleed should receive surgical consultation in case an emergent intervention is needed. Indications for surgical therapy include
   (a) Child's classification A or B: patients in whom vital signs cannot be stabilized medically
   (b) Continuous bleed for ≥48 hr despite sclerotherapy and balloon tamponade
   (c) Third acute episode of esophageal bleed in spite of previous sclerotherapy

b. Hemorrhage from ulcers and erosive lesions
   (1) Endoscopy therapy with sclerosing agents, laser coagulation, or heater probe
   (2) Surgical intervention is indicated in cases of
      (a) Visible vascular pedicle on endoscopy
      (b) Transfusion of ≥6 U blood in 24 hr
      (c) Arterial spurting

c. Active lower GI bleed
   (1) If a lesion is reachable with sigmoidoscopy or colonoscopy, local therapy may be attempted (e.g., laser coagulation)
   (2) Arterial embolization is indicated if the above fails
   (3) Surgical consultation is necessary for all patients with active lower GI bleeding in case an emergent intervention is needed

8.2 ACUTE MESENTERIC ISCHEMIA (AMI)

1. Definition
Acute reduction in blood flow to the intestine leading to inadequate perfusion. AMI may be a reflection of generalized poor perfusion or may result from local pathology

2. Epidemiology
The incidence of AMI has increased over the past few decades. Rising incidence may be attributable to advances in medical technology and new therapies that extend the life of critically ill patients who are prone to develop AMI (e.g., elderly). The mortality rate in AMI is 55%-100%.

3. Etiology
   a. Occlusive
      (1) Atherosclerotic narrowing of the mesenteric bed
      (2) Systemic emboli from any source (e.g., endocarditis)
      (3) Vasculitis
   b. Nonocclusive
      (1) Splanchnic vasoconstriction
         (a) Hypovolemia
         (b) Hypotension

      (c) Low cardiac output

      (d) Use of vasopressor agents

4. Risk factors

    The most common predisposing conditions are depicted in the Box below.

5. Diagnostic evaluation

    a. History and physical examination

      The classic complaint of severe abdominal pain that is out of proportion to the findings of physical examination, in the authors' experience, is rarely seen. If peritoneal signs are present (e.g., rebound tenderness), intestinal infarction is likely to have occurred. Abdominal distention, emesis, and other signs of intestinal obstruction may occur in patients with AMI *in situ*. Lower GI bleeding may occur.

    b. Laboratory studies reveal

      (1) Leukocytosis in 75% of patients

      (2) Metabolic acidosis

      (3) Elevated amylase, CK (6-12 hr after infarction has occurred), lactate, and phosphate

    c. Radiologic evaluation

      (1) Plain abdominal x-rays

        (a) Useful in excluding other causes of abdominal pain (e.g., mechanical obstruction, perforation)

        (b) Seventy percent of patients will show at least one of the following

          (i) Ileus

          (ii) Ascites

          (iii) Small bowel dilation

          (iv) Separation of small bowel loops

          (v) Thickening of valvulae conniventes

          (vi) Thumbprinting

      (2) Barium studies are *contraindicated* in these patients as they may interfere with arteriography

      (3) Arteriography: For an adequate study the patient needs to be hemodynamically stable. Early use of this test is the key to diagnosis. It provides a "road map" for the surgeon

6. Therapy

    a. As in any critically ill patient, the management of AMI starts with assessment of the ABCs

Risk Factors for the Development of Acute Mesenteric Ischemia

- Age $\geq$50 years
- Atherosclerotic heart disease
- Congestive heart failure
- Recent myocardial infarction
- Valvular heart disease

    b. Ensure adequate hydration and place Swan-Ganz catheter if necessary to maximize cardiac output, oxygen delivery, and volume status

    c. Patients with suspected embolic or thrombotic occlusion should undergo *urgent* laparotomy for possible resection. Heparin and broad-spectrum antibiotics are indicated prior to surgery. Most patients will undergo a "second-look" operation within 24 hr of the initial laparotomy

    d. In those cases with nonocclusive AMI, intraarterial infusions of vasodilators (e.g., papaverine 30-60 mg/hr) are advocated by some

| 8.3 | FULMINANT HEPATIC FAILURE AND ENCEPHALOPATHY |

1. Definition
   a. Acute fulminant hepatic failure (FHF) is defined as acute liver failure associated with the development of hepatic encephalopathy within 8 weeks of the onset of symptoms attributable to hepatocellular dysfunction. This definition assumes that there is no preexisting liver disease
   b. Hepatic encephalopathy (HE) is a complex neuropsychiatric syndrome precipitated by abnormal liver function. This syndrome is a feature of acute and/or chronic hepatocellular failure
2. Etiology
   Common causes of FHF and HE are depicted in the Box below.
3. Diagnostic evaluation
   a. History: Detailed history should be obtained from family members. The following points need to be investigated
      (1) History of preexisting liver disease
      (2) Drug or alcohol use
      (3) Toxin exposure or ingestion

Causes of Acute Liver Failure

Viral hepatitis (i.e., A,B,C)
Drugs or toxins
  Acetaminophen
  Acute alcohol intoxication
  Carbon tetrachloride
  Halothane
  Isoniazid
  Monoamine oxidase inhibitors (MAOI)
  Mushroom poisoning
Fatty liver of pregnancy
Shock of any etiology
Massive liver infiltration (e.g., leukemia)
Decompensation of chronic liver failure

b. Physical examination: This may vary from the patient who is not in distress to the patient in overt shock
   (1) Vital signs: tachycardia and hypotension
   (2) Associated findings: petechiae, jaundice, hepatomegaly, and splenomegaly
   (3) Encephalopathy may begin with confusion, disorientation, and irrational behavior. Coma may develop rapidly. (See Table 8-3)
c. Laboratory and radiologic evaluation: All patients with HE and/or FHF should undergo the following tests:
   (1) Chest x-ray (CXR), abdominal X-rays
   (2) Blood glucose (may reveal hypoglycemia)
   (3) Serum bilirubin (a value >23 mg/dL is the best predictor of nonsurvival)
   (4) Aspartate aminotransferase (AST), alanine aminotransferase (ALT): little prognostic value because levels tend to fall as the patient's condition worsens
   (5) Serum albumin decrease reflects poor outcome
   (6) Serum electrolytes
   (7) CBC
   (8) Head computed tomography (CT) scan to rule out a structural lesion (e.g., hemorrhage)
   (9) Lumbar puncture (LP) needs to be considered and performed if meningitis is suspected
   (10) If the etiology of FHF is unknown, order the following
       (a) Acetaminophen level
       (b) Hepatitis profile
           (i) Viral hepatitis A (HAV) is diagnosed by detection of HAV-IgM in patient's serum
           (ii) Viral hepatitis B (HBV) is diagnosed by
               • Detection of HBV surface antigen (HB_sAg)
               • Anti-HBV core antigen (HB_c) IgM
           (iii) Viral hepatitis C (HCV): detection of anti-HCV
           (iv) Viral hepatitis D (HDV): detection of anti-HDV in a patient co-infected with HBV
       (c) Alkaline phosphatase
       (d) Amylase

Table 8-3   Clinical stages of hepatic encephalopathy

Stage	Neurologic Findings
I	Confusion, mild changes in personality, and psychometric defects
II	Drowsiness to lethargy
III	Somnolent but arousable
IV	Coma

       (e) Serum ammonia level

       (f) Electroencephalogram (EEG) to assess clinical response and prognosis in patients with HE

4. Complications of FHF

In acute liver failure all organ systems are involved to some extent.

  a. Central nervous system (CNS): hepatic encephalopathy and cerebral edema

  b. Cardiovascular: dysrhythmias (particularly in patients with advanced FHF) and hypotension

  c. Pulmonary: hypoxemia advancing to acute respiratory distress syndrome (ARDS)

  d. Renal: development of renal failure with FHF carries a poor prognosis

     (1) In most instances the renal failure is related to prerenal causes

     (2) Hepatorenal syndrome is a diagnosis of exclusion. It is associated with a normal urine sediment, a urinary sodium concentration of <20 mmol/L, and resolution if liver function improves

  e. Hematologic: thrombocytopenia and diminished clotting factors with episodes of severe bleeding

  f. Infection: susceptibility to infection is increased in patients with FHF

  g. Metabolic: hypoglycemia, metabolic acidosis, hypokalemia, and hyponatremia

5. Management

  a. Supportive therapy

     (1) As in any critically ill patient, the management of AMI starts with assessment of the ABCs

     (2) The usual indications for endotracheal intubation and assisted mechanical ventilation apply to these patients

  b. The use of corticosteroids for patients with FHF has not been proven to improve survival and indeed may worsen the clinical picture

  c. Some authors suggest avoiding parenteral nutrition because protein and amino acids may worsen the clinical picture. However, new total parenteral nutrition (TPN) solutions with "branched-chain" amino acids are probably efficacious and help to maintain a positive nitrogen balance

  d. The management of FHF-associated cerebral edema is no different from that for non–hepatic-related causes (see Chapter 11)

  e. There is some preliminary evidence showing that the benzodiazepine antagonist flumazenil may have some role in improving the signs and symptoms of HE

  f. Investigational data has shown some improvement in hemodynamics of patients with FHF treated with acetylcysteine

  g. Liver transplantation may be an alternative form of therapy (in a few specialized transplant centers) for some patients with no known contraindication to the procedure

  h. Liver "dialysis": a few specialized centers are currently exploring this form of therapy

8.4 PANCREATITIS

1. Definition
   Acute pancreatitis is an inflammatory process of the pancreas with a wide range of clinical severity from self-limited to a lethal disease complicated by multiple organ-system failure (10% of cases).

2. Etiology
   The most common causes of pancreatitis are:
   a. Alcoholism
   b. Gallstones
   c. Hyperlipidemia
   d. Trauma (blunt or penetrating)
   e. Infections (e.g., mumps, mycoplasma)
   f. Hypoperfusion states (e.g., shock, cardiopulmonary bypass)
   g. Hypercalcemia
   h. Drugs (e.g., sulfonamides, thiazides)

3. Diagnostic evaluation
   a. History: Ninety-five percent of patients with acute pancreatitis present with abdominal pain; 50% of those patients present with upper abdominal discomfort radiating to the back. Nausea and vomiting are also present
   b. Physical examination: Depending on the severity of the situation the patient may have overt signs of shock or be hemodynamically stable. Other findings include:
      (1) Abdominal tenderness and distention
      (2) Abdominal ileus
      (3) Low-grade fever (note: if fever is >39° C, cholangitis, peritonitis, or a pancreatic abscess is suggested)
      (4) Mild jaundice
      (5) Ascites
      (6) Pleural effusion
   c. Laboratory evaluation
      (1) CBC shows marked leukocytosis. Thrombocytopenia may be present in those cases complicated by disseminated intravascular coagulation (DIC)
      (2) Amylase is elevated initially, but may decrease after 2-3 days if necrosis of the pancreas is widespread. False-positive results may occur in perforation of the esophagus, stomach, intestine; gynecologic disorders; renal failure; severe burns; diabetic ketoacidosis (DKA); salivary gland disorders; and macroamylasemia
      (3) Lipase: hyperlipasemia persists longer than hyperamylasemia. However, if necrosis of the pancreas is widespread, these values may be normal
      (4) Serum calcium is usually low. When levels are <8 mg/dL, the prognosis is poor
      (5) Other electrolyte imbalances, as well as hyperglycemia, are usually present
      (6) Metabolic acidosis may be present

(7) Urinalysis (U/A) may reveal proteinuria, casts (25% of cases), and glycosuria

d. Radiologic evaluation: Every patient with suspected acute pancreatitis should get a CXR (e.g., to rule out free air under the diaphragm and evidence of pleural effusions and an abdominal x-ray (e.g., for signs of intestinal obstruction, ileus, gallstones, the so-called sentinel loop of pancreatitis, or the colon "cut-off" sign). When the diagnosis remains in doubt, especially in the more severely ill, the following can be obtained:

  (1) Ultrasonography (US) is the modality of choice in patients with edematous pancreatitis and suspected biliary pancreatitis. It is also used to follow up phlegmon or abscesses. Unfortunately, US cannot be accurately performed in obese patients and in those with moderate to severe ileus

  (2) CT is the most useful tool in assessing the retroperitoneum. Its use in acute pancreatitis is mainly to follow up significant complications (i.e., abscess, phlegmon, pseudoaneurysms)

4. Management

a. The management of acute pancreatitis starts with assessment of the ABCs.

b. Adequate hydration: if necessary place a Swan-Ganz catheter to maximize cardiac output, oxygen delivery, and volume status

c. Correct underlying factors

d. Control pancreatic enzyme secretion

  (1) Nasogastric suction

  (2) H_2-receptor blocking agents (e.g., ranitidine 300 mg/24 hr IV infusion if renal function is normal)

  (3) Many clinicians use the following agents in acute pancreatitis; however, clinical studies have not supported the routine use of these agents

    (a) Calcitonin (300 IU/24 hr)

    (b) Somatostatin (250 mcg IV bolus, then 250 mcg/hr as IV drip)

    (c) Glucagon

  (4) The use of intramuscular (IM) clonidine (not yet available in the United States) is of interest for patients who are hemodynamically stable with acute pancreatitis. Preliminary data show encouraging results

e. Sedation and analgesics: Patients may require substantial amounts of analgesics, usually with meperidine

f. Ensure adequate parenteral nutrition (see Chapter 12)

g. Correct hypocalcemia *only* if there is clinical evidence of tetany

5. Complications

The most common complications of acute pancreatitis are depicted in the Box on the facing page.

a. Those patients who demonstrate a fever >39° C with a white blood cell count (WBC) over 20,000/mm^3 should be evaluated for the presence of a pancreatic abscess with the use of CT. If there are any fluid collections, CT-guided, fine-needle aspiration is indicated for Gram's stain and cultures

Complications of Acute Pancreatitis

Intravascular fluid depletion
  Prerenal azotemia
  Shock
ARDS (3-7 days after onset)
Cardiac dysfunction
Pancreatic abscess
Pancreatic pseudocysts
Chronic pancreatitis
Permanent diabetes mellitus
Multiorgan-system failure

---

    b. If the suspected diagnosis is pancreatic abscess, start broad-spectrum antibiotics and obtain an emergent surgical consultation

    c. Some authors advocate necrosectomy in patients with necrotizing pancreatitis

  6. Prognosis

    a. In assessing the severity of the disease and the prognosis, several classifications have been used. The most commonly utilized is *Ranson's criteria* (initially developed for patients with alcoholic pancreatitis)

     (1) Three or more of the following criteria must be met:

       (a) Age > 55 years

       (b) WBC >16,000/mm^3

       (c) Glucose >200 mg/dL

       (d) Base deficit >4 mEq/L

       (e) Lactate dehydrogenase (LDH) >350 IU/L

       (f) AST (SGPT) >250 IU/L

     (2) Development of the following within 48 hr indicates a worsening prognosis

       (a) Hematocrit (hct) drop >10%

       (b) BUN rise >5 mg/dL

       (c) Pao$_2$ <60 torr

       (d) Calcium <8 mg/dL

       (e) Fluid sequestration >6 L

     (3) Mortality rates correlate with the number of criteria present

       • 0-2 criteria = 1% mortality

       • 3-4 criteria = 16% mortality

       • 5-6 criteria = 40% mortality

       • 7-8 criteria = 100% mortality

    b. Intensive care management and prompt surgical consultation have lowered the mortality of acute pancreatitis

Selected readings

Cello JP: Diagnosis and management of lower gastrointestinal tract hemorrhage. *West J Med* 1985;143:80-7.

Cello JP, Crass RA, Grendell JH, et al: Management of the patient with hemorrhaging esophageal varices. *JAMA* 1986;256:1480-4.

Frantizides CT, Tsiftisis D, Pissiotis C, et al: Radionuclide visualization of acute occlusive and nonocclusive intestinal ischemia. *Ann Surg* 1986;203:295-300.

Gammal SH, Jones EA: Hepatic encephalopathy. *Med Clin North Am* 1989;73:793-813.

Haddock G, Garden OJ, McKee RF, et al: Esophageal tamponade in the management of acute variceal hemorrhage. *Dig Dis Sci* 1989;34:913-8.

Harrison PM, Wendon JA, Gimson AES, et al: Improvement by acetylcysteine of hemdynamics and oxygen transport in fulminant hepatic failure. *N Engl J Med* 1991;324:1852-7.

Hunter GC, Guernsey JM: Mesenteric ischemia. *Med Clin North Am* 1988;72:1091-115.

Katelaris PH, Jones DB. Fulminant hepatic failure. *Med Clin North Am* 1989;73:955-70.

Lechin F, Ven der Dijs B, Lechin M, et al: Clonidine treatment of acute pancreatitis: report of five cases. *Acta Gastroenterol Latinoam* 1992;22:119-24.

Ottinger LW: Mesenteric ischemia. *N Engl J Med* 1982;307:535-7.

Panes J, Teres J, Bosch J, et al: Efficacy of balloon tamponade in treatment of bleeding gastric and esophageal varices: results in 151 consecutive episodes. *Dig Dis Sci* 1988;33:454-9.

Ranson JH: Acute pancreatitis: pathogenesis, outcome and treatment. *Clin Gastroenterol* 1984;13:843-63.

Ranson JH, Rifkind KM, Roses DF, et al: Prognostic signs and the role of operative management in acute pancreatitis. *Surg Gynecol Obstet* 1974;139:69-81.

Silverstein FE, Feld AD, Gilbert DA: Upper gastrointestinal tract bleeding: predisposing factors, diagnosis and therapy. *Arch Intern Med* 1981;141:322-7.

Sitzmann JV, Steinborn PA, Zinner MJ, et al: Total parenteral nutrition and alternate energy substrates in treatment of severe acute pancreatitis. *Surg Gynecol Obstet* 1989;168:311-17.

Hematologic Disorders

Alex E. Lechin

9.1 ANEMIA

1. Definition
   Absolute decrease in the circulating red blood cell (RBC) mass.
2. Etiology
   a. Decreased RBC production
      (1) Deficiency of hematinic agents (i.e., iron, vitamin B_{12}, folate)
      (2) Bone marrow failure
   b. Increased RBC destruction or loss
      (1) Hemolysis
      (2) Hemorrhage
3. Diagnostic evaluation
   The approach to the anemic patient in the ICU changes depending on whether the patient was anemic when admitted or if the anemia developed during the ICU stay.
   a. If the patient was anemic when admitted to the ICU:
      (1) The symptoms of anemia depend on the degree of anemia, the rapidity of development, cardiopulmonary reserve, and underlying disease
      (2) As a general rule hemoglobin (Hb) <7 g/dL represents severe anemia. Such patients may present with dyspnea upon exertion, lightheadedness, angina, and/or fatigue
      (3) Absence of symptoms in patients with Hb <7 g/dL suggests a gradual onset
   b. History
      Inquire about previous hematologic values, family and ethnic history (i.e., sickle-cell, thalassemia), history of splenectomy, cholelithiasis at an early age, medications, drugs, alcohol use, dietary habits, gastrectomy, and bleeding
   c. Physical examination
      (1) General appearance: nutritional status or evidence of specific nutritional deficiencies; and there may be evidence of chronic illness
      (2) Vital signs: tachycardia, postural hypotension, other signs of hypoperfusion (i.e., decreased mental status, low urine output), petechiae, and/or purpura

161

(3) Associated findings: jaundice, glossitis (i.e., pernicious anemia, iron deficiency), and/or neurologic abnormalities (i.e., vitamin B_{12}, folate deficiency). Lymphadenopathy, hepatomegaly, and splenomegaly (i.e., hemolysis, neoplasms, infiltrative disorders). Heart: listen for flow murmurs and/or prosthetic valves sounds (i.e., increased RBC destruction). Rectal: examine stools for blood

d. Laboratory evaluation

This usually provides a diagnosis and should always be done stepwise unless the patient's condition requires emergent transfusion. In this case, before transfusion, obtain a blood sample for red cell indices, peripheral blood smear, as well as iron, folate, and vitamin B_{12} studies

(1) Hb and hematocrit (hct) estimate RBC mass and severity of anemia and should be monitored serially in the patient suspected to have active bleeding. Acute blood loss does not immediately influence hct.

(2) Mean corpuscular volume (MCV) is a measure of the average size of RBC. Classification of the anemia according to the MCV is helpful in generating a differential diagnosis and workup. Examine the smear to determine whether multiple cell populations are present

   (a) Low MCV (<80) generally limits the diagnosis to a few disorders: iron deficiency, thalassemia, sideroblastic anemia, other hemoglobinopathies, and some cases of anemia of chronic disease

   (b) High MCV (>100): megaloblastic anemia, liver disease, alcoholism, drugs (i.e., methotrexate, zidovudine [AZT]), and myelodysplastic syndrome

   (c) Normal MCV: acute blood loss, hemolytic anemia, pituitary or thyroid failure, aplastic anemia, myelofibrosis, and anemia of chronic disease

(3) Reticulocyte count is also essential in the evaluation of the anemic patient; it reflects the rate of production of RBCs by the bone marrow. According to the reticulocyte count anemia can be classified into

   (a) Increased RBC destruction (i.e., bleeding, hemolysis) reflected in a high reticulocyte count

   (b) Decreased RBC production (i.e., iron deficiency, anemia of chronic disease) reflected in an abnormally low reticulocyte count

e. Bleeding is the first concern in patients who develop anemia while in the ICU. Common sites of bleeding are the gastrointestinal (GI) tract, venipunctures, pulmonary tree, genitourinary tract, and the retroperitoneum. Development of anemia in the ICU should prompt additional investigation (i.e., gastric aspiration to look for blood, stools to check for gross or occult blood, prothrombin time [PT], partial thromboplastin time [PTT], and platelet count)

4. Therapy

   Patients who are acutely bleeding

   a. General measures

    (1) Airway management: assess the need for intubation to prevent aspiration, especially in upper GI bleeding

    (2) Obtain adequate venous access. Large-bore peripheral catheters allow greater volume administration rates than long central lines

    (3) Obtain blood for type and crossmatch, as well as diagnostic laboratory evaluation as discussed above

    (4) Fluid resuscitation: start with colloids or crystalloids; continue with whole blood or packed RBC as required

       (a) Healthy adult patients can tolerate blood losses up to 20-30% of blood volume if adequate replacement with crystalloid is provided

       (b) Patients with impaired cardiac reserve, coronary artery disease, or advanced age can develop symptoms with a decrease of approximately 10% of blood volume

    (5) Identify the source of bleeding

    (6) Monitor end points. There are two goals when monitoring ICU patients with acute bleeding

       (a) Adequate blood volume replacement (e.g., reflected in vital signs, urine output, mental status, central venous pressure [CVP], pulmonary capillary wedge pressure [PCWP])

       (b) Control of bleeding: follow serial Hb, hct, and monitor the bleeding site (e.g., GI and genitourinary tracts)

  b. Specific measures depend on the cause of the bleeding

    Patients who are not acutely bleeding

       (a) Therapy for anemia depends on its etiology

       (b) Do not use specific Hb concentration as the only parameter to decide on the need for transfusion. Transfusion of red cells is usually not necessary in patients with either chronic stable anemia or anemia of acute blood loss unless the patient is symptomatic. Patients with chronic anemia with Hb levels >7 g/dL rarely require blood transfusion unless cardiopulmonary or cerebrovascular disease is present

       (c) Patients in the ICU who are receiving mechanical ventilation and have Hb values <9.0-10 g/dL are commonly transfused to this level to improve oxygen delivery (DO_2)

9.2   LEUKOPENIA

1. Definitions

Blood leukocyte count below the normal range (in the authors' laboratories <3800/μl). *Neutropenia* is defined as absolute neutrophil count <2000/μl for Caucasians, and <1500/μl for blacks and Yemenite Jews. *Lymphopenia* is defined as absolute lymphocyte count <1500/μl.

2. Etiology

  a. Neutropenia: see Table 9-1

  b. Lymphocytopenia: see Table 9-2

3. Diagnostic evaluation

  a. History

    (1) Ethnic background: black or Yemenite Jew

    (2) Family history: congenital or hereditary defect

Table 9-1 Etiology of neutropenia

False Decrease in WBC	Decreased Production	Increased Neutrophil Destruction, Utilization, Sequestration	Combination (Increased Destruction and Decreased Production)
Counts done long after blood has been drawn	Bone marrow injury due to ionizing radiation or drugs	Hypersplenism	Sepsis
Disintegration of fragile cells (i.e., blasts, immature WBCs)	Bone marrow replacement or destruction by tumor or infection	Autoimmune	Antineutrophil antibodies
Presence of paraproteins (i.e., monoclonal gammopathies), which can produce WBC clumping	Nutritional deficiencies: vitamin B_{12}, folate	Sepsis	Drugs
	Congenital stem-cell defects		Felty's syndrome

Table 9-2   Etiology of lymphocytopenia

Decreased Production	Increased Destruction, Utilization, Loss	Unknown Mechanisms
Primary immuno-deficiency diseases (i.e., HIV)	Collagen vascular diseases Acute infections or stress Ionizing radiation Cytotoxic drugs	Malignancies Chronic infection

    (3) Medications (e.g., chemotherapeutic agents and antibiotics)
    (4) Alcohol and dietary history
    (5) Diet habits: nutritional deficiency (i.e., B_{12}, folate)
    (6) Underlying illness: malignancies, human immunodefiency virus (HIV)
  b. Physical examination
    (1) General appearance: acute distress, mental status, changes and/or evidence of chronic illness
    (2) Vital signs: fever, hypotension, tachycardia, tachypnea, low urine output (e.g., sepsis)
    (3) Associated findings: e.g., hepatomegaly or splenomegaly, lymph-adenopathy, abdominal masses, oral thrush, skin rash, purpura, and/or jaundice
  c. Laboratory evaluation
    (1) Complete blood count (CBC) and differential to assess the degree and type of leukopenia
    (2) Bone marrow aspiration and biopsy are pivotal in the evaluation of the leukopenic patient without obvious cause. Analysis of the bone marrow:
      (a) Will classify the leukopenia by revealing the degree of bone marrow cellularity: decreased production, decreased survival, or a combined defect
      (b) May indicate the etiology of the leukopenia such as aplastic anemia, bone marrow infiltration (e.g., leukemia), and/or infection
    (3) Other laboratory tests that may help in identifying the cause of leukopenia are blood and tissue cultures, vitamin levels, and autoantibodies
  d. Therapy
    The mainstay of therapy for the leukopenic patient is to treat the underlying disease. For example, discontinue offending medications in patients with suspected drug-induced leukopenia. Also treat vitamin deficiency when suspected
    (1) Granulocyte-colony stimulating factors ([G-CSF] and granulocyte-macrophage colony stimulating factor [GM-CSF]) represent a new line of therapy for the treatment of leukopenia secondary to a decrease in bone marrow production. Currently they are indicated for chemotherapy-induced severe leukopenia. Other indications for these agents are not well defined

    (2) Transfusions of WBC concentrates have not been proven to be of benefit in many controlled trials

    (3) Supportive therapy for the leukopenic patient requires special consideration, particularly in the ICU environment where there is a higher risk for nosocomial infections

        (a) Granulocyte counts $<1000/\mu l$ result in severe immunocompromise

        (b) Patients who are immunocompromised should not receive rectal manipulations. Enforce strict hand washing for caregivers. Avoid intramuscular (IM) or subcutaneous (SQ) routes

        (c) If the temperature rises $>38.5°$ C, the patient should be fully examined, pancultured, and started on broad-spectrum antibiotics

9.3 THROMBOCYTOPENIA

1. Definition
   Platelet count $<150,000/\mu l$.
2. Etiology
   See Table 9-3.
3. Diagnostic evaluation
   a. History
      Inquire about bleeding, thrombotic events, mental status changes, alcohol use, drugs and medications, and associated illness
   b. Physical examination
      (1) Vital signs: fever, tachycardia, hypotension, tachypnea, and oliguria (i.e., sepsis)
      (2) Purpura, hematomas, gingival bleeding, lymphadenopathy, hepatomegaly or splenomegaly, and abdominal masses
   c. Laboratory evaluation
      (1) CBC and platelet count
         (a) Platelet counts $>50,000/\mu l$ are not associated with significant bleeding problems. Severe spontaneous bleeding is unusual in patients with counts $>20,000/\mu l$ in the absence of coagulation factor abnormalities
         (b) Thrombocytopenia associated with anemia suggests thrombotic thrombocytopenic purpura (TTP), hemolytic-uremic syndrome (HUS), disseminated intravascular coagulation (DIC), or other microangiopathic processes
         (c) Pancytopenia suggests leukemia, aplastic anemia, or other bone marrow disorders
      (2) Peripheral blood smear: note platelet size and other abnormalities (i.e., fragmented RBC may indicate TTP or DIC, increased platelet size suggests accelerated destruction)
      (3) Coagulation evaluation: PT, PTT, D-dimer, and fibrin degradation products may indicate the presence of consumption coagulopathy (e.g., DIC)
      (4) Bone marrow aspiration and biopsy (not always necessary) to assess the number of megakaryocytes and the presence of bone marrow disorders (i.e., leukemia, aplastic anemia, tumor infiltration)

Table 9-3   Etiology of thrombocytopenia

Decreased Survival or Sequestration	Decreased Production	Developed while in ICU
Autoimmune primary (ITP); secondary (collagen vascular disease [SLE]); viral infections; drug-induced (heparin, quinidine, sulfas); post-transfusion	Primary bone marrow disorders (e.g. aplastic anemia, primary thrombocytopenia)	Drug-induced (e.g. heparin, H_2-blockers, diuretics)
Hypersplenism (portal hypertension, infiltrative disorders)	Bone marrow infiltration (e.g., tumor, infection)	Disseminated intravascular coagulation
Thrombotic thrombocytopenic purpura (TTP), hemolytic-uremic syndrome (HUS)	Drug-induced (e.g. alcohol, thiazides, alkylating agents)	Sepsis
Disseminated intravascular coagulation	Infection	Post-transfusion
Sepsis		

4. Therapy

Detailed treatment for the various causes of thrombocytopenia is beyond the scope of this chapter. The following concentrates on relevant topics for the acute management of patients in ICU setting

a. As hemostasis approaches normal at platelet counts >50,000/μl, transfuse patients with active bleeding (6-10 U) to attempt to achieve levels >50,000/μl

b. Lumbar puncture (LP) and organ needle-biopsies, (e.g., lung, liver, and kidneys) are more hazardous than thoracentesis, paracentesis, and bone marrow biopsy. Transfusion to 50,000/μl prior to such procedures is indicated

c. Patients with a platelet count <20,000/μl are at higher risks for hemorrhage; however, there is no real threshold for prophylactic platelet transfusion

d. Discontinue all nonessential medications including heparin. Consider changing H_2-blockers to coating agents or antacids. Avoid agents known to inhibit platelet function (e.g., nonsteroidal antiinflammatory drugs [NSAIDs] and ticarcillin)

e. Avoid trauma (e.g., IM and SQ injections, rectal manipulations, hard toothbrushes, razors) in thrombocytopenic patients

f. TTP/HUS deserve special consideration because their management differs

(1) TTP is a syndrome characterized by microangiopathic hemolytic anemia, fever, fluctuating neurologic deficits, and renal insufficiency. HUS is felt to be a variant of this syndrome in which renal failure is the predominant feature. TTP/HUS should be considered a medical emergency

(2) Do not give platelet transfusions to patients with TTP/HUS unless life-threatening bleeding occurs

(3) Therapy for TTP/HUS includes plasma exchange by plasmapheresis if available; otherwise, by fresh frozen plasma transfusions. IV steroids can be used and, in unresponsive cases, vincristine has been recommended

| 9.4 | ANTICOAGULATION AND FIBRINOLYSIS

Anticoagulants and thrombolytic agents are potentially life-saving when used prophylactically or therapeutically in critically ill patients.

1. Anticoagulation

a. Heparin

(1) Mechanism of action

Heparin acts by potentiating the activity of the plasma protease-inhibitor antithrombin III, which rapidly inhibits the activity of factors XII_a, XI_a, X_a, IX_a, and thrombin (factor II)

(2) Heparin prolongs thrombin time (TT), bleeding time, PTT, and to a lesser extent, PT

(3) Heparin half-life is 1-3 hr, but in patients with pulmonary embolism clearance it is accelerated 20%-40% compared to normals

(4) Indications

(a) Prophylaxis of deep venous thrombosis (DVT) and pulmonary embolism (PE): All patients in the ICU should be on some form of DVT prophylaxis (commonly heparin 5000 U SQ q12hr). Heparin has proved to be an effective agent in DVT prophylaxis except after major orthopedic procedures (particularly hip and knee replacement) and prostate surgery

(b) Full anticoagulation (PTT approximately 2 × normal) in pulmonary embolism or DVT, arterial thrombosis, and other disorders: 5000-10,000 U IV bolus is commonly used with infusion rates of 1000 U/hr (12-25 U/kg/hr)

(5) Monitoring of anticoagulation

(a) Not required for prophylactic doses

(b) For full anticoagulation adjust the heparin dosage to maintain the PTT at 1.5-2 × control. To avoid the tendency to under-anticoagulate patients on heparin therapy, a standardized dosage regimen has been developed (see Table 9-4)

(6) Complications

(a) Bleeding occurs in 7%-20% of patients during the full dosage heparinization. Hemorrhage typically occurs from the GI tract, urinary tract, or surgical incisions. Less common sites include intracranial, retroperitoneal, soft tissue, nasal, and pleural space. Bleeding is associated with the intensity of the anticoagulation, (e.g., when the PTT is >3 × normal, the risk of hemorrhage is substantially higher)

(b) Thrombocytopenia: heparin use is associated with thrombocytopenia in 5-30% of patients and its incidence is higher with the use of bovine-lung heparin

(i) If thrombocytopenia is mild (>100,000/µl) and is not associated with bleeding or thrombotic events, heparin therapy can be continued

(ii) Severe thrombocytopenia rarely occurs. It may be associated with bleeding or paradoxic thrombotic events. Di-

Table 9-4   Standardized protocol for dosing of intravenous heparin

PTT*	Dosage Adjustment†	Repeat PTT
<50	5000 U bolus, increase infusion by 2400 U/24 hr	6 hr
50-59	Increase infusion by 2400 U/24 hr	6 hr
60-85	Therapeutic range, no change	Next morning
86-95	High therapeutic range, decrease infusion by 1920 U/24 hr	Next morning
96-120	Stop infusion for 30 min, decrease infusion by 1920 U/24 hr	6 hr
>120	Stop infusion for 60 min, decrease infusion by 3840 U/24 hr	6 hr

*Normal PTT range is 27-35 seconds.

†Dosage protocol is based on an initial IV bolus of 5000-10,000 U followed by continuous infusion of 24,000 U/24 hr. The first PTT should be obtained 6 hr after the bolus of heparin.

agnosis is made by detection of heparin-dependent IgG. Treatment is to discontinue *all* heparin and *avoid* platelet transfusion
      (c) Osteoporosis may be seen with long-term use of heparin
      (d) Hypoaldosteronism is seen rarely
      (e) Antidote: heparin is generally undetectable in the patient's plasma within 3 hr after discontinuation of therapy. In the rare instance that anticoagulation must be reversed more rapidly, protamine sulfate can be used
  b. Warfarin
  Warfarin is the most frequently used oral anticoagulant in the United States. Sometimes the transition to chronic oral therapy is begun before the patient leaves the ICU. Sometimes oral therapy must be initiated because of heparin-induced thrombocytopenia or, in certain cases, as DVT prophylaxis. The clinician caring for the critically ill can also encounter patients who have accidentally or purposely overdosed with warfarin
    (1) Mechanism of action
      Warfarin interferes with the hepatic vitamin K-dependent carboxylation of factors II, VII, IX, and X. It also inhibits the synthesis of the anticoagulant factors protein C and protein S; thus it may be thrombogenic. The antithrombotic effects of warfarin occur only after several days of treatment. In patients on IV anticoagulation therapy who require chronic oral anticoagulation, overlap heparin and warfarin for at least 48 hr
    (2) Indications
      (a) Prophylaxis of DVT and PE, especially in those patients for whom heparin has not been effective
      (b) For chronic anticoagulation therapy
    (3) Dosage
      (a) Loading dosage: 10-15 mg PO qd for 3 days
      (b) Maintenance dosage: 2-15 mg PO qd to keep PT value 1.2-1.5 × control or INR 2.0-3.0
    (4) Complications
      (a) Bleeding occurs in 2.4%-8.1% of patients who are chronically anticoagulated. The risk is dose-related and proportional to the prolongation of the PT. Treatment consists of fresh frozen plasma (FFP) transfusions. Vitamin K replacement is recommended only for warfarin overdose because its onset of action is delayed and it complicates reinstitution of warfarin therapy
      (b) Warfarin skin necrosis secondary to a paradoxical hypercoagulable state due to the warfarin-induced protein C reduction
2. Fibrinolysis
  a. Fibrinolytic therapy has an expanding role in the treatment of many thromboembolic disorders. Four fibrinolytic drugs are currently marketed: streptokinase (SK), anisoylated plasminogen/streptokinase activator complex (APSAC), urokinase (UK), and recombinant tissue plasminogen activator (rt-PA). All four drugs activate the fibrinolytic

system by converting plasminogen to the active enzyme plasmin. Plasmin degrades fibrin and dissolves the thrombus

b. Indications
(1) Acute myocardial infarction (MI): thrombolytic therapy for acute MI is discussed in Chapter 5
(2) PE—the effectiveness and role of thrombolytic agents in acute MIs are firmly established. However, the use of these agents in pulmonary thromboembolism remains infrequent and controversial mainly because of the fear of a negative benefit:risk ratio. SK and UK have both been shown to be more effective than heparin alone in accelerating clot lysis and improving pulmonary tissue perfusion. Current recommendations for the use of fibrinolysis in PE apply to patients with massive pulmonary embolism, persistent systemic hypotension, and in whom rapid resolution of pulmonary obstruction is desired
(3) DVT: even more debated is the use of thrombolytic agents in the treatment of DVT. Potential advantages of fibrinolysis over anticoagulation include the prevention of PE by lysing the source of thrombus *in situ,* rapid restoration of normal venous circulation with a prompt resolution of symptoms, and prevention of valve damage, that would otherwise result in chronic venous insufficiency. Risks include a much higher incidence of bleeding

c. Dosage
Selected thrombolytic regimens
(1) PE
UK: 4400 U/kg bolus, followed by 4400 U/kg/hr for 24 hr
UK: 15,000 U/kg bolus over 10 min
SK: 250,000 U over 30 min, followed by 100,000 U/hr for 24 hr
rt-PA: 100 mg as continuous peripheral infusion over 2 hr
(2) DVT
SK: 250,000 U over 30 min, followed by 100,000 U/hr for 48-72 hr
rt-PA: 0.5 mg/kg over 4-8 hr
rt-PA: 0.05 mg/kg/hr for 24 hr
(3) MI (see Chapter 5)

d. Monitoring
(1) Clinical monitoring should include serial neurologic examinations to detect central nervous system (CNS) hemorrhage and frequent vital signs to detect bleeding. Frequently examine all puncture sites
(2) Laboratory monitoring should include Hb/hct, platelet, fibrinogen, PT, and PTT

e. Complications
(1) Bleeding is the greatest limitation of the thrombolytic drugs and the factor that has limited their acceptance for the treatment of DVT and PE
(2) Allergic reactions including skin rashes, fever, and hypotension are rare and usually associated with the use of SK and APSAC. The induction of antibodies against streptococcal antigens can occur after the administration of SK or APSAC, or after streptococcal infection that may neutralize the fibrinolytic activity of SK

| BLOOD AND BLOOD PRODUCT TRANSFUSIONS

Transfusion therapy may be associated with several immediate and delayed adverse effects. Therefore, carefully weigh the risks and benefits before administering any blood product. The use of blood components should be guided by a rational diagnostic and therapeutic approach.

1. Whole blood
   Whole blood stored more than 24 hr contains few viable platelets or granulocytes; factors V and VIII are decreased, but stable clotting factors are maintained. One U is 450 ml and, transfused to an average-sized adult, increases the Hb by 1 g/dl and the hct by 3%.
   a. Indications: symptomatic anemia with or without massive hemorrhage
   b. Risks
      (1) Allergic reactions
      (2) Infectious diseases (i.e., HIV and hepatitis B [HBV])
      (3) Febrile reactions
      (4) Volume overload
      (5) Noncardiogenic pulmonary edema
2. Packed red blood cells (PRBC)
   Removal of 200-250 ml of plasma from whole blood results in packed RBC. Transfusion of 1 U of PRBC will increase the Hb and hct by the same amount as 1 U of whole blood. 1 U is 250-300 ml.
   a. Indications: symptomatic anemia
   b. Risks: same as for whole blood (see above)
3. Leukocyte-poor PRBC
   Most of the WBC are removed from the packed RBC by saline washing.
   a. Indications
      (1) Symptomatic anemia and allergic or febrile reaction from leukocyte antibodies
      (2) Paroxysmal nocturnal hemoglobinuria
   b. Risks: same as for whole blood (see above)
4. FFP
   Separated from freshly drawn whole blood and then frozen. Volume 200-250 ml. Rich in all coagulation factors; 1 ml supplies approximately 1 U of coagulation activity. FFP should be compatible with ABO. Crossmatching is not required
   a. Indications
      (1) Bleeding due to coagulation factor deficiency
      (2) Treatment of TTP/HUS
      (3) Rapid reversal of vitamin K deficiency or warfarin overdose
   b. Risks
      (1) Same as for whole blood (see above)
5. Cryoprecipitate
   Made by thawing 1 U of FFP at 4° C. A white precipitate forms; most of supernatant plasma is removed and refrozen. Volume 10 ml. A pack of cryoprecipitate contains von Willebrand's factor, lesser amounts of factor VIII, fibrinogen, factor XIII, and fibronectin. ABO compatibility is preferred.
   a. Indications
      (1) von Willebrand's disease

      (2) Mild to moderate hemophilia A

      (3) Factor XIII deficiency

      (4) Fibrinogen deficiency

  b. Risks

      (1) Infectious diseases

      (2) Hyperfibrinogenemia

      (3) Allergic reactions

6. Platelets

  Platelet packs are obtained from whole blood and 1 U contains at least 5.5×10^{10} platelets in approximately 50 ml volume. In a normal 70 kg adult, 1 U of platelets should increase the platelet count by 5000-10,000/mm^3.

  a. Indications

      (1) To correct bleeding secondary to thrombocytopenia or abnormal platelet function

      (2) Prophylactically (e.g., in patients with chemotherapy-induced thrombocytopenia the threshold is somewhat controversial—10,000-20,000/mm^3) and prior to invasive procedures (target counts of 50,000/mm^3)

  b. Risks

      (1) Infectious diseases

      (2) Allergic reactions

      (3) Alloimmunization

7. Complications of transfusion therapy

  a. Disease transmission: HIV, hepatitis, cytomegalovirus (CMV), Epstein-Barr virus (EBV), Chagas' disease, and malaria

  b. Allergic reactions characterized by fever, chills, urticaria, and respiratory distress. These events are secondary to antileukocyte antibodies or antibodies against antigenic proteins in donor plasma. Therapy is symptomatic (acetaminophen, antihistamines, and, rarely, epinephrine or glucocorticoids are needed)

  c. Related to red cell transfusion

      (1) Acute hemolytic reactions: fever, chills, back pain, nausea, vomiting, hypotension, dark urine, and chest pain. Acute renal failure with hemoglobinuria and DIC may occur. If suspected

        (a) Inform the blood bank

        (b) Stop the transfusion

        (c) Replace all IV tubing

        (d) Send clotted and edetate (ETDA)-treated blood samples from the patient's blood along with the remainder of the U of blood to the blood bank for crossmatch

        (e) Send blood samples for DIC screen, bilirubin, and free Hb

      (2) Management

        (a) Intravascular volume expansion plus mannitol to keep urine output >100 ml/hr or 1 cc/kg/hr

        (b) Alkalinization of urine with IV bicarbonate to keep urine pH >7 to avoid Hg tubular precipitation

        (c) Treatment of DIC

      (3) Delayed hemolytic transfusion reactions: 24 hr to 25 days post-transfusion. These are secondary to an amnestic (1-3 days) or pri-

mary (7-25 days) antibody response to RBC antigens. Patients usually develop a drop in the Hb and hct with an increase in bilirubin. Coombs' test is positive
   (4) Noncardiogenic pulmonary edema (ARDS) caused by antileukocytic antibodies
   (5) Coagulopathy associated with a large volume of PRBC transfusions, secondary to dilution of platelet and coagulation factors. Treatment consists of FFP and platelet transfusions
   (6) Citrate intoxication is also seen with large volume transfusion of PRBC. Patients present with hypocalcemia, hypotension, and drop in cardiac output. Treatment: IV calcium
 d. Volume overload, especially in patients with congestive heart failure (CHF). Diuretics may be needed post-transfusion
 e. Platelet alloimmunization develops in patients who have received multiple transfusions. Approximately 75% of patients receiving platelets on a regular basis will become alloimmunized to platelet antigens. Increments <20% of expectation generally indicate alloimmunization. Patients may respond to single-donor platelets, but human leukocyte antigens (HLA) matched platelets may be needed

9.6 | DISSEMINATED INTRAVASCULAR COAGULATION (DIC)

1. Definition
   DIC is a dynamic pathologic process triggered by activation of the clotting cascade with resultant generation of excess thrombin within the vascular system. Most consider DIC to be a systemic hemorrhagic syndrome; however, this is only because hemorrhage is obvious and often impressive. What is less commonly appreciated is the significant amount of microvascular thrombosis and, in some instances, the large-vessel thrombosis that occurs. This thrombosis is usually the more life-threatening insult.
2. Etiology
   See Table 9-5
3. Diagnostic evaluation
   Since DIC is associated with an underlying disease state, the clinical evaluation is directed toward identifying the primary illness, the status of the coagulation system, and the focal and systemic consequences of the DIC-associated hemorrhage and/or thrombosis.

Table 9-5   Etiology of disseminated intravascular coagulation (DIC)

Obstetric accidents (amniotic fluid embolism, abruptio placentae)
Intravascular hemolysis
Sepsis
Malignancy
Trauma
Vascular disorders

a. Clinical findings associated with the primary illness will vary according to the precipitating event (e.g., obstetric accident, infection, malignancy)
b. Clinical findings associated with the coagulation status
 (1) Bleeding (e.g., from venipuncture sites, mucous membranes, hemorrhagic bullae, hematuria, GI)
 (2) Purpura, petechiae, and subcutaneous hematomas
c. Clinical findings associated with end-organ thrombosis and hemorrhage
 (1) Lungs: respiratory distress, hypoxia, and ARDS
 (2) Kidneys: proteinuria and renal insufficiency
 (3) Liver: Budd-Chiari syndrome, hepatitis, and hepatic failure
 (4) Skin: necrosis and acrocyanosis
 (5) CNS: mental status changes and neurologic deficits
d. Laboratory evaluation
 (1) Peripheral blood smear will show fragmented RBC and thrombocytopenia with large platelets
 (2) Prolonged PT and PTT
 (3) Thrombocytopenia usually around 60,000/μl, but values ranging from 3000-100,000/μl may be seen
 (4) Decreased fibrin level
 (5) Decreased antithrombin III level
 (6) Elevated levels of fibrin degradation products (FDP)
 (7) There is an elevation of D-dimer neoantigens: specific test for degradation products of fibrin, whereas nonspecific FDP may be derived from either fibrinogen or fibrin

4. Therapy
The treatment of DIC is confusing and controversial. Therapy must be individualized according to the cause of DIC, severity of hemorrhage, severity of thrombosis, hemodynamic status, and age.
a. The most important and effective treatment for DIC is the removal of the triggering disease process (i.e., evacuate the uterus, control shock, control infection, remove tumors, consider chemotherapy, radiotherapy, or other indicated therapy)
b. Anticoagulation is rarely needed in cases of obstetric complications. Evacuation of the uterus usually stops the intravascular clotting process
c. If the patient continues to bleed or clot significantly after 6 hr of initiating therapy directed to stop or blunt the triggering event, anticoagulation therapy may be indicated. There is general agreement on the need for anticoagulation in acute promyelocytic leukemia and perhaps DIC with solid tumors. The authors favor the use of low-dose, subcutaneous heparin at dosages of 80-100 U/kg q6hr. Other anticoagulant modalities available are IV heparin and antithrombin III concentrates
d. If the patient continues to bleed after reasonable attempts to treat the triggering event of the DIC and if anticoagulation therapy has been initiated, clotting factor depletion is the most probable cause of bleeding and replacement therapy should be considered

| 9.7 | HEMOLYTIC SYNDROMES

1. Definition
Premature destruction of RBC. This process may occur either because of abnormal factors in the intravascular environment or because of defective RBC.
2. Etiology: see Table 9-6
3. Diagnostic evaluation
   a. History and physical examination
   Clinical manifestations will depend on the underlying disorder, the severity of the anemia, and whether the hemolysis is intravascular or extravascular
      (1) Intravascular hemolysis can present as an acute event with back pain, dyspnea, chills, fever, tachycardia, dark urine, hypotension, and renal failure
      (2) Extravascular hemolysis is usually less dramatic and may be accompanied only by jaundice and splenomegaly
   b. Laboratory evaluation
      (1) Elevated reticulocyte count
      (2) Peripheral blood smear can provide a diagnosis in cases of spherocytosis; microangiopathic disorders will show the presence of fragmented RBC; Heinz bodies suggest enzymatic defects; the presence of anisocytosis or sickle cells is consistent with hemoglobinopathies
      (3) Other laboratory data suggestive of hemolysis are
         (a) Hemoglobinuria (indicative of intravascular hemolysis)
         (b) Hemoglobinemia (indicative of intravascular hemolysis)

Table 9-6 Etiology of hemolytic syndromes

Acquired Hemolytic Disorders	Hereditary Hemolytic Disorders
Autoimmune hemolytic anemia	
Warm-reactive antibody (idiopathic, neoplasia, collagen vascular disorder, drugs)	Membrane defects (spherocytosis, elliptocytosis)
Cold-reactive antibody (idiopathic, mycoplasma infection, lymphoproliferative disorder, paroxysmal cold hemoglobinuria)	Enzymatic defects (glucose-6-phosphate dehydrogenase [G6PD] deficiency)
Microangiopathic hemolytic anemia (TTP, DIC, eclampsia)	Thalassemias
Direct toxic effect (malaria, clostridial infection)	Hemoglobinopathies
Splenomegaly	
Membrane defects	
Paroxysmal nocturnal hemoglobinuria	
Spur-cell anemia	

(c) Low levels of haptoglobin

(d) Elevated lactate dehydrogenase (LDH)

(e) Positive Coombs' test

4. Sickle-cell disease

Definition

A heterogenous group of defects of hemoglobin synthesis that can all cause clinically significant illness due to sickling of red cells. Sickle-cell Hb (Hb S) is less soluble when deoxygenated. It forms polymers that precipitate inside the RBC, leading to membrane abnormalities, decreased deformability, and increased blood viscosity

a. Clinical manifestations

Secondary to vasoocclusive phenomena, which may lead to microinfarcts with resultant painful crises and, eventually, chronic organ damage

b. Diagnosis

Demonstration of sickling under reduced oxygen tension. Perform Hg electrophoresis to discriminate homozygous (SS) from heterozygous (AS) and to determine the presence of other abnormal Hg

c. Treatment

The treatment of sickle-cell disease is supportive and limited to the management of acute and chronic complications. Frequently these patients need to be admitted to the ICU due to the severity and life-threatening dimensions of their acute attacks

(1) Treat with antibiotics at the first evidence of infection. Pneumococcal sepsis is a leading cause of mortality. Other prevalent pathogens include *E. coli, Haemophilus influenzae, Salmonella, Shigella,* and *Mycoplasma pneumoniae*

(2) Painful crises: initiate IV hydration; adequate analgesic (usually a regular schedule of opioids is necessary); administer oxygen when hypoxemia is present; correct acidosis

(3) Look for precipitating events (i.e., infections, surgery, dehydration, trauma, cold temperatures, alcohol ingestion). When abdominal pain is one of the manifestations, rule out other causes of abdominal pain (i.e., acute abdomen, hepatobiliary disease)

(4) Acute chest syndrome is characterized by pleuritic chest pain, fever, cough, hypoxia, and pulmonary infiltrates. Lung scans and pulmonary angiograms are usually of no help. In addition, the latter test is associated with added risk because of possible induction of sickling by the hypertonic contrast media. Differentiation between pneumonia and infarction is often difficult. Features favoring infarction include painful bone crisis, clear chest radiograph at onset, lower lobe disease, and negative blood cultures. Treatment includes oxygen therapy, mechanical ventilation when indicated, empiric antibiotic therapy, and correction of acidosis

(5) Sickle-cell crisis associated with cerebrovascular accidents or repeated venoocclusive crisis may benefit from transfusion or exchange transfusion to keep the Hb S levels <39%

5. Autoimmune hemolytic anemia (AIHA)

a. Warm-reactive antibody AIHA

Is usually extravascular and IgG-mediated. This type of hemolytic anemia can be seen in the ICU not only in patients admitted with collagen vascular diseases or lymphomas, but also in drug-induced hemolytic anemias

(1) Diagnosis is made by signs of hemolysis and positive direct Coombs' test
(2) Treatment
    (a) If the suspected mechanism is drug-induced, discontinue all nonessential medications
    (b) 60% of cases respond to steroid therapy (e.g., prednisone 1-1.5 mg/kg PO qd)
    (c) Splenectomy increases the success rate to ≈ 80%-90%
    (d) Reserve cytotoxic drugs for patients who fail to respond to steroid plus splenectomy
    (e) Transfusions are indicated only in severe cases of anemia. In emergency situations most patients can be managed with careful transfusion (ABO and Rh-compatible blood); administer slowly and watch for reactions

b. Microangiopathic hemolytic anemia (MAHA)

This is a syndrome caused by traumatic intravascular hemolysis. Intraluminal deposition of fibrin strands in small vessels is presumed to be responsible for the red cell destruction

(1) Etiology includes DIC, TTP, HUS, malignant hypertension, vasculitis, and eclampsia
(2) Diagnosis
    (a) Evidence of hemolysis (e.g., reticulocytosis, elevated LDH, decreased haptoglobin)
    (b) Fragmented RBC in the peripheral blood smear
(3) Treatment
    Therapy is directed toward the underlying disorder. Management of TTP, HUS, and DIC is discussed elsewhere. Transfusion is rarely indicated

c. Glucose-6-phosphate dehydrogenase (G6PD) deficiency

Hereditary deficiency of the enzyme G6PD in the red cells. This is a sex-linked disorder that affects men and, rarely, women of Mediterranean, African, or Chinese ancestry. The disease is associated with episodic hemolysis

(1) Clinical manifestations
    (a) Hemolytic episodes are sometimes triggered by infections and the ingestion of some drugs (e.g., sulfonamides, antimalarials, nitrofurantoin, nalidixic acid)
    (b) Patients present with acute intravascular hemolysis associated with hemoglobinemia, hemoglobinuria, decreased haptoglobin, and jaundice
    (c) Peripheral vascular collapse can occur in severe cases
    (d) Hemolysis is usually self-limited even if the exposure to the oxidant agent continues, since only the older G6PD-depleted population of RBC is affected
(2) Diagnosis
    Definitive diagnosis requires the measurement of levels of the enzyme. This must be made several weeks after the episode because

enzyme levels can be normal during the hemolytic event. This is due to the presence of high numbers of young red cells that are relatively rich in G6PD

   (3) Therapy

      (a) Transfusion therapy as indicated

      (b) Protect renal function during hemolytic episodes: IV hydration to maintain a good urine output and alkalinization of urine (to keep urine pH >7)

      (c) Prevent hemolytic episodes by identifying deficient individuals, treating infections promptly, and avoiding exposure to oxidant agents

Selected readings

Angelli G, Parise P: Bolus thrombolysis in venous thromboembolism. *Chest* 1992; 101(suppl):172-82.

Bick RL: Disseminated intravascular coagulation. *Hematol Oncol Clin North Am* 1992; 6:1259-85.

Cruickshank MK, Levine MN, Hirsh J: A standardized heparin nomogram for the management of heparin therapy. *Arch Intern Med* 1991; 151:333-7.

Dale DC: *Neutropenia and neutrophilia*. In Williams WJ, Beutler E, Erslev AJ, Lichtman MA, et al, editors: *Hematology*, New York, 1990, McGraw-Hill.

Deykin D: Warfarin therapy. *N Engl J Med* 1970; 283:691-7.

Elliott CG: Thrombolysis in cardiopulmonary disease. *Chest* 1992; 101(suppl):163-71.

Feinstein DI: Treatment of disseminated intravascular coagulation. *Semin Thromb Hemost* 1988; 14:351-63.

Goldhaber SZ: Evolving concepts in thrombolytic therapy for pulmonary embolism. *Chest* 1992; 101(suppl):183-5.

Gore JM: Prevention of severe neurologic events in the thrombolytic era. *Chest* 1992: 101(suppl):124-30.

Haire WD: Pharmacology of fibrinolysis. *Chest* 1992; 101(suppl):91-7.

Murphy S: Guidelines for platelet transfusion. *JAMA* 1988; 259:2453-4.

Schmidt GA: *Anticoagulants and thrombolytic agents*. In Hall JH, Schmidt GA, Wood LD, editors: *Principles of critical care*, New York, 1992, McGraw-Hill.

Wessler S, Gitel SN. Heparin: new concepts relevant to clinical use. *Semin Hematol* 1979; 53:525-31

Wheby MS: Anemia. *Med Clin North Am* 1992; 76:549-745.

10

Infections in the Intensive Care Unit

Victor Fainstein

The number of infectious complications encountered in the intensive care unit (ICU) continues to increase. Patients who would not have survived in the past now improve due to new technology. However, the length of stay and the many devices employed to improve care also predispose patients to difficult and often fatal infections. Thus, the clinical characteristics of ICU patients have changed. Immunocompromised and post-transplant patients, as well as the geriatric population, are now regularly treated in the ICU with the consequent increase in morbidity, mortality, and cost.

The management of infectious diseases requires a specific approach to the critically ill patient who is admitted to the ICU. The clinician must first differentiate the patient transferred from another location within the hospital from the patient directly admitted to the ICU from the community. This differentiation is paramount in categorizing the etiologic agents, understanding the pathophysiology of their processes, and most important, in deciding which therapeutic antimicrobial interventions are needed.

10.1 PNEUMONIA (NOSOCOMIAL)

1. For the patient who has been transferred to the ICU after several days in the hospital, emphasis should be placed on the nosocomial aspects of infection and on the following important facts:
   a. Nosocomial infections have a 20%-60% mortality rate
   b. 15% of all hospital deaths are the result of nosocomial infections
   c. Successful treatment depends on the underlying disease, specific causative organisms, and timely institution of therapy
2. Risk factors
   a. Intubation
   b. Admission to the ICU, especially for the patient who is receiving sedation
   c. Antibiotics: broad-spectrum agents rapidly change normal flora in the mouth and gastrointestinal (GI) tract
   d. Surgery, especially thoracic, abdominal, or neurosurgery (which increases the risk of aspiration)
   e. Chronic lung disease
   f. Advanced age

180

g. Immunosuppression
3. Etiologic agents
    a. Common
        (1) *Klebsiella* sp
        (2) *E. coli*
        (3) *Pseudomonas aeruginosa*
        (4) *Staphylococcus aureus*
        (5) *Enterobacter* sp
        (6) *Acinetobacter* sp
    b. Less common
        (1) Anaerobic mouth flora (e.g., *Streptococcus*)
        (2) Other gram-negative bacilli (e.g., *Serratia* sp, *Xanthomonas* sp)
        (3) *Haemophilus influenzae*
        (4) *Legionella* sp
        (5) *Candida* sp
        (6) *Aspergillus* sp
        (7) Influenza virus
        (8) *Streptococcus pneumoniae*
        (9) Tuberculosis (typical and atypical)
        (10) Miscellaneous, according to prevalent organisms in each hospital
4. Clinical manifestations
    Patients in the ICU, especially those who are intubated or sedated, do not
    manifest the usual symptoms of pneumonia (like cough, chest pain, or
    dyspnea). Patients who are neutropenic are unable to mount an inflamma-
    tory response and therefore, the sputum does not show purulent material.
    Subtle changes in oxygenation, fever, and clinical deterioration are clues
    to the diagnosis of pneumonia in intubated patients. Leukocytosis or leu-
    kopenia can be the first manifestation of occult pneumonia. In some in-
    stances, e.g., *Pneumocystis* pneumonia, the presence of spontaneous
    pneumothorax can be the first indication of pulmonary involvement.
    Thick, foul-smelling sputum is characteristic of anaerobic and aspiration
    pneumonia.
5. Diagnostic studies
    a. Obtain sputum for Gram's stain *immediately* for every patient
    b. Obtain other stains (i.e., acid-fast bacilli [AFB], Giemsa, wet prep)
    c. Chest x-ray (CXR): look for new or changing infiltrates
    d. Order serologic tests if appropriate (i.e., *Legionella*, fungal, cryptococ-
        cal antigen, counter immunoelectrophoresis [CIE])
    e. Differentiate between the concept of colonization and true infection;
        this distinction is sometimes very difficult
    f. Remember the microbiologic pattern of your hospital
    g. Be aggressive in trying to obtain a diagnosis (i.e., bronchoalveolar la-
        vage). Transtracheal aspirates are not commonly employed
6. Treatment
    a. Empiric treatment is the most commonly utilized in the ICU
    b. Common regimens
        (1) Beta-lactam plus aminoglycoside (i.e., piperacillin and gentami-
            cin)
        (2) Cephalosporin plus aminoglycoside (i.e., ceftazidime and gen-
            tamicin)

- (3) Clindamycin plus gentamicin
- (4) Clindamycin plus quinolone (i.e., ciprofloxacin)
- (5) Imipenem-cilastatin plus aminoglycoside
- (6) Add trimethoprim/sulfamethoxazole (TMP-SMX) if *Pneumocystis carinii* pneumonia is suspected
- (7) Add erythromycin if *Legionella* is suspected
- c. Proven gram-negative infection
  - (1) Continued double therapy as described above is preferred (i.e., piperacillin 4 g IV 4-6 hr; gentamicin 2-3 mg/kg q8hr or q12hr)
  - (2) Continue single-agent therapy (i.e., ceftazidime 2 g IV q8hr; ciprofloxacin 400 mg IV q 8-12 hr; imipenem-cilastatin 500 mg-1 g IV q6hr or ticarcillin and clavulanic acid 3.1 g IV q 4-6 hr)
- d. Aspiration pneumonia
  - (1) Penicillin G 12-24 million U IV/day
  - (2) Clindamycin 600-900 mg IV q8hr
  - (3) Ticarcillin and clavulanic acid 3.1 g IV q6hr
  - (4) Imipenem-cilastatin 0.5-1 g IV q6hr
    Controversy exists in this regard. Some authors recommend no therapy as in many cases aspiration only gives a chemical pneumonitis
- e. Proven gram-positive infection (depending on the microorganism)
  - (1) Nafcillin 1-2 g IV q 4-6 hr
  - (2) Vancomycin 0.5-1 g IV q 8-12 hr
  - (3) Clindamycin 900 mg IV q8hr
  - (4) Penicillin G 12-24 million U IV/day
- f. Atypical
  - (1) Erythromycin 0.5-1 g IV q6hr
  - (2) TMP-SMX 15-20 mg/kg/day
  - (3) Doxycycline 100 mg IV q12hr
  - (4) Rifampin 300 mg IV q12hr
  - (5) Amphotericin B 0.6-1 mg/kg/day

The duration of therapy is not well defined but most authors agree on treating gram-negative and anaerobic pneumonia for 2-3 weeks. Gram-positive processes are usually treated from 10-14 days and atypical pneumonias receive 2 weeks of antimicrobial therapy. *Candida* pneumonia requires prolonged treatment with up to 1.5 g of amphotericin B as a total dose.

7. Prevention
  - a. Preoperative and postoperative measures for prevention of pneumonia
    - (1) Identify high-risk patients
    - (2) Treat respiratory infections and remove respiratory secretions
    - (3) Initiate instruction and therapy to expand the patient's lungs (i.e., chest physiotherapy, incentive spirometry)
  - b. Ensure proper hand-washing
  - c. Appropriate maintenance of in-use respiratory therapy equipment
    - (1) Use sterile fluids in nebulizers
    - (2) Properly use single-dose and multidose medications for respiratory therapy
  - d. Properly sterilize and disinfect reusable respiratory equipment
  - e. Properly suction the respiratory tract
  - f. Protect patients from other infected patients or staff

10.2   PNEUMONIA (COMMUNITY-ACQUIRED)

Etiologic agents

1. Common organisms
   a. *Streptococcus pneumoniae*
   b. *Staphylococcus aureus*
   c. *Branhamella catarrhalis*
   d. *Haemophilus influenzae*
   e. *Klebsiella* sp
   f. Influenza
   g. Respiratory syncytial virus
   h. *Chlamydia pneumoniae*
   i. *Legionella* sp
   j. *Mycoplasma* sp
2. Less common
   a. *Pneumocystis carinii*
   b. *Mycobacterium tuberculosis*
   c. *Cryptococcus* sp
   d. *Chlamydia psittaci*
   e. *Coxiella burnetii*
   f. *Histoplasma* sp
   g. *Nocardia* sp
   h. *Strongyloides stercoralis*
3. Common manifestations
   a. Fever, cough, dyspnea, and sputum production (usually purulent)
   b. Hypoxemia is common
   c. Anxiety
   d. Leukocytosis and, in severe infections, leukopenia
4. Uncommon presentations occur in patients who are
   a. Elderly
   b. Immunocompromised (especially neutropenic)
   c. Post-transplant
   d. infected with atypical organisms
5. Clinical clues for diagnosis
   a. *Acute onset:* bacterial, viral, aspiration, tularemia, *Pneumocystis*
   b. *Subacute onset:* viral, *Legionella*, *Hemophilus* sp, mycoplasma, Q fever, psittacosis, *Chlamydia, Pneumocystis*
   c. *Aerogenic route:* any segment
   d. *Hematogenous:* most commonly in both lung bases as blood flow is preferential to these areas
6. Associations
   a. Psittacosis: birds
   b. Typhoid: turtles
   c. *Pasteurella multocida:* dogs
   d. Q fever: cattle
   e. Tularemia: rabbits
   f. *Legionella:* air conditioners
   g. Anthrax: hides
   h. *Echinococcus* and paragonomiasis: foreign travel
   i. *Neisseria meningitidis,* group A streptococci: barracks

7. Treatment

Empiric treatment is usually dictated by geographic background, clinical presentation, and host status. Penicillin or a second- or third-generation cephalosporin, in addition to erythromycin, is the preferred initial choice.

a. *Streptococcus pneumoniae*
   (1) Penicillin (resistance can be seen)
   (2) Erythromycin
   (3) Vancomycin
b. *Haemophilus influenzae*
   (1) Second-generation cephalosporin (i.e., cefuroxime 1.5 g IV q8hr)
   (2) Third-generation cephalosporin (i.e., ceftriaxone 2 g IV q24hr)
c. *Staphylococcus aureus*
   (1) Oxacillin (3 g IV q4hr)
   (2) Cefazolin (2 g IV q8hr)
   (3) Clindamycin (900 mg IV q8hr)
   (4) Vancomycin (1 g IV q12hr)
d. *Legionella* sp
   (1) Erythromycin (0.5-1 g IV q6hr)
   (2) Rifampin (300 mg IV PO q12hr)
   (3) Ciprofloxacin (400 mg IV q12hr)
e. *Branhamella catarrhalis*
   (1) Beta-lactamase stable antibiotic (i.e., cefuroxime 1.5 g IV q8hr)
   (2) Penicillin or cephalosporin
f. *C. pneumoniae:* tetracycline (500 mg to 1 g IV q6hr for 2 weeks)
g. *Mycoplasma* sp: erythromycin (preferred) or tetracycline (in adults)
h. Influenza
   (1) Amantadine (100 mg PO q12hr)
   (2) Ribavirin requires a special device for medication delivery
8. Complications after 72 hr
a. Persistent fever
b. Empyema
c. Obstruction
d. Lung abscess
e. Resistant organism
f. Focus of infection

10.3 SEPSIS

1. More than 400,000 cases of sepsis are estimated to occur in the U.S. annually with an associated mortality of 20%-60%. Despite improvements in antimicrobial therapy and supportive care, the incidence and mortality rate associated with sepsis have not declined. This is partly a consequence of an array of medical advances that can place patients at increased risk for development of infection and, potentially, sepsis.
2. Sepsis and related disorders
a. New definitions
   (1) Bacteremia: positive blood cultures (may be transient)
   (2) Sepsis: clinical evidence suggestive of infection *plus* signs of a systemic response to the infection including all of the following

    (a) Tachypnea: respiration >20 bpm (if patient is mechanically ventilated, min volume 10 L/min)

    (b) Tachycardia (heart rate [HR] >90 bpm)

    (c) Hyperthermia or hypothermia (core or rectal temperature >38.4° C or <35.6° C)

  (3) Sepsis syndrome (may also be considered *incipient septic shock* in patients who later become hypotensive): clinical diagnosis of sepsis outlined above *plus* evidence of altered organ perfusion (one or more of the following):

    (a) Pao_2/FIo_2 <280 (in the absence of other pulmonary or cardiovascular disease)

    (b) Lactate level above the upper limit of normal

    (c) Oliguria (documented urine output <0.5 ml/kg body weight for at least 1 hr in patients with urinary catheters in place)

    (d) Acute alteration in mental status

    (e) Positive blood cultures are not required

  (4) Early septic shock: clinical diagnosis of sepsis syndrome as outlined above *plus* hypotension (systolic blood pressure [BP] <90 mm Hg or a 40 mm Hg decrease below baseline systolic BP) that lasts <1 hr and is responsive to conventional therapy (IV fluid administration and/or pharmacologic intervention)

  (5) Refractory septic shock: clinical diagnosis of the sepsis syndrome outlined above *plus* hypotension (systolic BP <90 mm Hg or a 40 mm Hg decrease below baseline systolic BP) that lasts for >1 hr despite adequate volume resuscitation and that requires vasopressors

3. Pathophysiology

Cell walls of gram-negative bacteria contain proteins, lipids, and lipopolysaccharides. Endotoxin (lipopolysaccharide) has three components: an O-specific polysaccharide, the R-core, and lipid A. Lipid A may be the major culprit in initiating the endotoxic symptoms. It is this component of endotoxin that stimulates the release of tissue necrosis factor (TNF) and can also activate the complement pathway. The sepsis syndrome is caused by endothelial damage following endotoxin-stimulated activation of neutrophils, coagulation, complement, and macrophages. Macrophages are stimulated to release TNF, interleukins, leukotrienes, thromboxane, and other cardioactive substances. Endotoxemia markedly increases the risk of myocardial depression and multiorgan failure. Of those patients with positive blood cultures, those with severe endotoxemia have five times the mortality rate of those who do not have endotoxemia.

4. Priorities in the treatment of sepsis

  (1) Early recognition

  (2) Cardiovascular/pulmonary support

  (3) Fluid resuscitation

  (4) Vasopressor agents

  (5) Empiric antibiotic therapy

  (6) Monoclonal antibodies (not yet proven to be effective)

  (7) Other immunotherapeutic agents (investigational)

  (8) Corticosteroids are *not* effective

  (9) Drainage of any foci of infection

5. Prognosis

Mortality in sepsis is a function of the severity of physiologic derangements, the duration of illness, and the number of organ system failures. These organ systems include (but are not limited to) the lungs, kidneys, and liver. When the pulmonary system becomes dysfunctional, the resultant clinical entity is known as the adult respiratory distress syndrome (ARDS). The sequence has been termed the multiple organ dysfunction syndrome (MODS). MODS is the most common cause of demise in patients who experience uncontrolled inflammation and infection.

10.4   TOXIC SHOCK SYNDROME

1. Clinical case definition (see Box below)
    a. Severe febrile illness (>38.9 °C) with rash (erythroderma followed by desquamation), hypotension or syncope, and multiorgan system involvement including at least four of following: mucous membrane, GI muscular, central nervous system (CNS), renal, hepatic, hematologic, cardiopulmonary, and metabolic
    b. Hypotension, probably due to small-vessel and capillary leakage with extravascular accumulation of fluid (edema)
    c. Blood cultures are usually negative
    d. Acute episode followed by desquamation
    e. No evidence of other causes (e.g., streptococcal, scarlet fever, Kawasaki's disease, Rocky Mountain spotted fever)
2. Epidemiology and other clinical features
    a. Affects mostly young menstruating women. Tampon use, especially continuous use, and Rely brand in some studies. *S. aureus* coloniza-

---

Toxic Shock Syndrome

Criteria for Diagnosis

Temperature <38.9° C
Systolic BP <90 mm Hg
Rash with subsequent desquamation (especially on palms and soles)
Involvement of ≥3 of the following organ systems:
    GI: vomiting or severe diarrhea
    Muscular: severe myalgias or five-fold increase in creatine kinase (CK)
    Mucous membranes: frank hyperemia
    Renal insufficiency: blood urea nitrogen (BUN), creatinine double of normal
    Liver: enzymes twice the upper limits of normal
    Blood: thrombocytopenia <100,000/mm^3
    CNS: disorientation without focal findings
    Negative tests for leptospirosis, Rocky Mountain spotted fever, and measles

tion of the vagina. Recurrence rate of 30%. Decrease in the number of reported cases

b. Also occurs in nonmenstruating women, men, and children (colonization or focal infection with *S. aureus,* including postoperative infections). Common occurrence after surgery. The fatality rate is 5%-10%

3. Etiology

Exotoxin(s) of *S. aureus* appear to cause the disease. Streptococci have been shown recently to cause the same syndrome.

4. Differential diagnosis

Kawasaki disease, scarlet fever, leptospirosis, Rocky Mountain spotted fever, and measles.

5. Treatment

Most important are volume expansion and correction of hypotension; removal of tampon, if present, in menstruating women; debridement of wounds, etc; antistaphylococcal antibiotics (after cultures are obtained). Steroids have not been proven to be effective or to alter outcome.

10.5 MENINGITIS

1. Acute meningitis is a medical emergency that requires early recognition, rapid diagnosis, precise antimicrobial therapy, and aggressive ICU support.

a. Etiologic agents

(1) *Streptococcus pneumoniae* is the most common cause in adults

(2) *Neisseria meningitis* is common among young people and children

(3) *Haemophilus influenzae* is common in children up to 12 years of age

(4) *Staphylococcus aureus* and *S. epidermidis* are seen in the elderly and in postoperative patients

(5) *Listeria monocytogenes* are usually mistaken for diphtheroids as contaminants

(6) Streptococci (other than *Streptococcus pneumoniae,* especially group B, in neonatal disease),

(7) Gram-negative bacilli after surgery or trauma

(8) *Mycobacterium tuberculosis* is increasing in frequency

(9) *Cryptococcus* usually occurs in immunosuppressed patients (e.g., AIDS, impaired cell-mediated immunity)

(10) Syphilis presentation is variable

(11) Herpes simplex

(12) *Toxoplasma* can present as meningoencephalitis or brain abscess

(13) *Naegleria:* epidemiologic history is paramount

(14) Other viruses (e.g., echovirus, St. Louis, equine, and western encephalitis)

b. Associations: epidemiology and organisms

(1) Coxsackie virus or echovirus, *Leptospira:* summer and fall

(2) *S. pneumoniae:* previous meningitis

(3) *S. pneumoniae:* alcoholism

(4) *N. meningitidis:* young adults

(5) *S. pneumoniae, Listeria,* gram-negative bacilli: the elderly

(6) *Cryptococcus* sp: lymphoma
(7) *N. meningitidis,* echovirus
(8) *H. influenzae, S. pneumoniae,* anaerobic bacteria: sinusitis
(9) Aerobic, gram-positive cocci: cellulitis
(10) Mixed flora: brain abscess
(11) Amoebas: swimming in fresh water
(12) *N. meningitidis:* other family members with meningitis
(13) *Leptospira:* water contact
(14) Gram-negative bacilli, *Staphylococcus, Candida:* hospital-acquired
(15) Head trauma
    (a) Close fracture: *S. pneumoniae,* gram-negative bacilli
    (b) Craniotomy: gram-negative bacilli, *Staphylococcus*
    (c) Cerebrospinal fluid (CSF) rhinorrhea: *S. pneumoniae*
c. CSF findings are depicted in Table 10-1.
d. Diagnostic approach
    (1) Order antigen detection for *H. influenzae, S. pneumoniae,* and *N. meningitidis*
    (2) Obtain high-volume CSF for AFB concentrate and fungal cultures (20-30 ml)
    (3) If CSF is normal or viruses are suspected, repeat lumbar puncture (LP) in 24-36 hr
    (4) Upon admission, obtain serologies for viral infections (e.g., St. Louis encephalitis, California encephalitis)
    (5) Obtain serologies in serum and CSF for fungal infections
    (6) Polymerase chain reaction (PCR) will probably be helpful in the near future (especially for tuberculosis and cytomegalovirus infections)
e. Treatment
    The goal of therapy in acutely ill patients is to institute treatment before the pathologic process of inflammation can produce irreversible

Table 10-1 Cerebrospinal fluid findings according to etiology

Bacterial	Tuberculous	Viral	Chronic
Glucose >40 mg/dl (blood ratio <0.4)	30-45 mg/dl	20-40 mg/dl	30-40 mg/dl
Protein 100-500 mg/dl	100-500 mg/dl	50-100 mg/dl	100-500 mg/dl
WBC 1000-10,000/cc^3	100-400/cm^3	10-1000/cm^3	100-500/cm^3
Gram's stain (+) 60%-80% (untreated) 40%-50% (previously treated)	AFB smear (+) in up to 40%	Smears are usually negative	Special stains needed India ink capsule (+)75% AFB (+)30%

progression and/or death. Time is essential in this situation. Empiric therapy must be instituted immediately after diagnosis is made and should be based on the differentiation of a community-acquired process from a hospital and/or postoperative process. If community-acquired, the usual treatment includes a third-generation cephalosporin (cefotaxime 2 g IV q4hr or ceftriaxone 2-4 g q 12-24 hr). Add ampicillin 2 g IV q4hr if *Listeria* is suspected. In postoperative cases, especially after neurosurgical procedures, initiate ceftazidime 2 g IV q8hr and vancomycin 500 mg to 1 g IV q 6-12 hr. If an anaerobic component or brain abscesses are part of the differential diagnosis, also give metronidazole 500 mg-1 g IV q6hr

2. Pneumococcal meningitis
   a. This is still the most common cause of bacterial meningitis in adults. Underlying diseases include sickle-cell disease; splenectomy and splenic dysfunction; hypogammaglobulinemia; alcoholism; head trauma (CSF fistula); and chronic pulmonary, hepatic, or renal disease
   b. Associated infections: pneumonia, otitis, bacteremia, endocarditis, and mastoiditis
   c. Therapy: penicillin 4 million U IV q4hr. Other alternatives include ceftriaxone 2-4 g qd or cefuroxime 1.5 g IV q8hr. If in doubt, perform *in vitro* susceptibilities

3. *Haemophilus meningitis*
   a. Underlying disease (adults): alcoholism, compromised host defenses, head trauma with CSF fistula
   b. Associated infections: pneumonia, sinusitis, and otitis. Secondary cases in close contacts
   c. Therapy: ampicillin (if sensitive) 12 g/day. Other useful antibiotics include cefuroxime, cefotaxime, ceftriaxone, and chloramphenicol

4. Meningococcal meningitis
   a. Primarily seen in children, adolescents, and young adults. Secondary in close contacts. Predisposing factors include complement defects
   b. Disseminated neisserial infection (often recurrent in persons with C_5-C_8 deficiency). Waterhouse-Friderichsen syndrome is an acute, often fatal syndrome of septic shock associated with massive adrenal necrosis, that is associated with bacteremia due to this organism. It requires early recognition, antibiotic therapy, and especially aggressive ICU/hemodynamic support
   c. Early antimicrobial therapy is needed. Penicillin or cephalosporins are the agents of choice

5. *Listeria* meningitis: not always seen in compromised host. Epidemiologic history is important. Therapy with ampicillin or TMP-SMX.

6. *Staphylococcus aureus* and *Staphylococcus epidermidis* are common after neurosurgery and/or ventricular-peritoneal shunt placement, as well as Ommaya reservoir insertion.
   a. Therapy
      (1) Methicillin-sensitive: oxacillin 12 g/day
      (2) Methicillin-resistant: vancomycin 500 mg-1 g IV q 6-12 hr plus rifampin or TMP-SMX
      (3) An infected shunt may need to be removed early in the course of therapy if the patient is not responding. It is necessary to re-

peat LP at 2-3 days in order to reach this decision (persistent growth of organisms despite adequate therapy)

7. Gram-negative bacilli

This is a challenging infection to treat with high rates of morbidity and mortality. There is development of resistance while on therapy (especially with *Enterobacter* sp). Most organisms will respond to ceftriaxone, cefotaxime, or ceftazidime. For *Pseudomonas aeruginosa,* ceftazidime 2g IV q8hr is the drug of choice. Intraventricular aminoglycosides are helpful but do not penetrate the CSF and intrathecal do not reach the ventricles.

8. Complications of bacterial meningitis
   a. Brain abscess: usually follows trauma, contiguous infection, hematogenous dissemination
   b. Subdural empyema: primarily a disease of the young but, in the elderly, it may complicate neurosurgery or subdural hematoma
   c. Epidural abscess: usually accompanied by focal osteomyelitis and subdural empyema
   d. All of the above are caused by mixed bacteria; they usually require drainage and prolonged IV antibiotic therapy

9. Herpes meningitis/encephalitis

This is a devastating, necrotizing type of encephalitis. Temporal spikes on electroencephalogram (EEG) are characteristic. Recently, magnetic resonance imaging (MRI) has been shown to be of great value for diagnosis. PCR in cerebrospinal fluid is diagnostic. However, etiologic diagnosis is usually made by brain biopsy. Treatment is given with acyclovir 15 mg/kg q8hr (high dosage) for 2 weeks. Careful attention to hydration is mandatory to avoid renal insufficiency.

10.6   ACQUIRED IMMUNODEFICIENCY SYNDROME (AIDS)

Opportunistic infections are the most common causes of morbidity and mortality in patients with HIV disease. Patients with helper/inducer T cells (CD4 cells) <250 are at risk for developing severe infectious complications. Their approach is depicted in Table 10-2.

1. Summary of current therapeutic approaches
   a. Pulmonary disease
      (1) Disease due to PCP (see Table 10-3)
      (2) Disease due to *M. tuberculosis*
          (a) Start with at least 4 drugs, preferably 5: isoniazid (INH) 300 mg/day, rifampin 600 mg/day, pyrazinamide 15 mg/kg/day, ciprofloxacin 750 mg PO bid, ethambutol 15-20 mg/kg/day
          (b) If TB is sensitive to INH and/or rifampin, continue for 12-18 months (not in the ICU)
          (c) If TB is resistant to INH or rifampin (multiply drug-resistant) continue with 5-6 drugs and adjust according to sensitivities. Prognosis is very poor
          (d) Follow liver function tests (LFT) initially weekly and later monthly
          (e) If unable to use PO, give IV INH and rifampin (same dosage) and IM streptomycin (1 g qd)

Table 10-2   Approach to HIV patient with opportunistic infections

Clinical Presentation	Common Organism*	Diagnostic Procedure
Pulmonary infiltrates	*P. Carinii* (PCP); tuberculosis (TB); *Mycobacterium avium intracellulare* (MAI); *Histoplasma*, aerobic bacteria, *Legionella*	Bronchoalveolar lavage and/or lung biopsy; appropriate serologies
Seizures, headache, vertigo, facial palsy	*Toxoplasma*, *Cryptococcus*, MAI, herpes, cytomegalovirus (CMV)	MRI, head CT, LP, and appropriate serologies
Esophagitis	*Candida*, herpes, CMV, *Cryptosporidium*	Endoscopy with biopsy and washings
Diarrhea	CMV, *Cryptosporidium*, *Giardia*, MAI, *Isospora*, *C. difficile*, *Salmonella*	Stool culture (initially),† AFB stain, colonoscopy, and biopsy
Persistent fever	MAI, *Histoplasma*, TB, *Cryptococcus*	CT abdomen, bone marrow‡; blood cultures with special stains (AFB)

*Note: each of these syndromes can be caused by noninfectious processes.
†Also useful to obtain fecal leukocytes for diagnosis of colitis.
‡Performed when fever persists despite initial evolution.

Table 10-3 Recommended management for PCP

Antibiotic	Mild to Moderate	Severe (Usually in ICU)
TMP-SMX	2-3 double-strength tabs PO tid for 14-21 days	5 mg/kg IV q6hr for 3 weeks
Pentamidine	3-4 mg/kg IV-IM qd	4 mg IV qd
Trimethoprim, dapsone	Trimethoprim 100 mg PO tid; dapsone 100 mg PO qid	?
Clindamycin, primaquine	Clindamycin 600 mg PO tid; primaquine 30 mg PO qid	900 mg IV q8hr for 3 weeks
Atovaquone	750 mg PO tid	For 2-3 weeks
Trimetrexate, leucovorin	Trimetrexate 45 mg/m^2/day IV for 21 days; leucovorin 30 mg/m^2 IV q6hr for 10 days and then PO q6hr for 14 days	Same as mild to moderate
Cortocosteroids adjunctive therapy	?	Solu-Medrol 40 mg IV or (equivalent PO bid) for 5 days Wean gradually over 10 days

(3) Pulmonary disease due to *Histoplasma capsulatum*
  (a) Initiate therapy with amphotericin B at 0.8-1 mg/kg/day
  (b) Search for other sites of involvement (i.e., bone marrow biopsy, LP, CXR, barium enema, and small bowel series)
  (c) Once the patient is stable, switch to fluconazole 200 mg PO bid
(4) Pulmonary disease due to *Legionella* sp
  (a) Initiate therapy with erythromycin 3-4 g IV/day
  (b) If patient is not responding, add rifampin (600 mg/day) and/or ciprofloxacin 400 mg IV q12hr
(5) Pulmonary disease due to bacteria
  (a) Common organisms are
    (i) *Streptococcus pneumoniae*
    (ii) *Haemophilus influenzae*
    (iii) *Pseudomonas,* especially if sinusitis is present
(6) Add antibacterial therapy empirically on admission
  (a) Ticarcillin-clavulanic acid 3.1 g IV q6hr (will also cover anaerobes in the sinuses)
  (b) Cefuroxime 1.5 g IV q8hr
  (c) Adjust when cultures and sensitivities become available
(7) Pulmonary disease due to MAI
  (a) Clofazamine 100-200 mg PO/day
  (b) Rifampin 600 mg PO/day
  (c) Ethambutol 25 mg/kg PO/day
  (d) Ciprofloxacin 750 mg/PO bid or ofloxacin 500 mg/PO bid
  (e) Amikacin 7.5 mg IM or IV q12hr; or clarithromycin 1 g PO bid; or azithromycin 600-900 mg PO qd
  (f) Treatment is given for at least 6 months
b. Enteric pathogens in patients with AIDS (see Table 10-4).
c. CNS infections in AIDS
  (1) Cryptococcal meningitis

Table 10-4 Enteric pathogens commonly seen in patiens with AIDS

Organism	Antimicrobial Agent	Direction of Therapy (Days)
Giardia lamblia	Metronidazole 250 mg PO tid	5
Entamoeba histolytica	Metronidazole 750 mg tid and di-iodohydroxyquin 650 mg PO tid	10
Shigella sp.	Ampicillin 500 mg IV qid; ceftriaxone 2 g IV qd	14
C. jejunum	Ciprofloxacin 500 mg IV q12 hr	7
Isospora belli	TMP-SMX 1 double-strength PO qid	14
CMV	Ganciclovir 5 mg/kg IV q12 hr	30
Herpes simplex	Acyclovir 1200 mg/day	10
Oral thrush	Ketoconazole 200-400 mg/day PO	10
Candida esophagitis	Fluconazole 200-400 mg IV/day	7-10

        (a) Acute: Amphotericin B 0.5-0.8 mg/kg/day $\pm$ 5-fluorocytosine 100 mg/kg/day until stable or improving. Then switch to flu-conazole 400 mg/day PO for 3 months

        (b) Maintenance: fluconazole 200-400 mg/day PO

    (2) Toxoplasmosis

        (a) Pyrimethamine 200 mg PO loading dose followed by 75 mg PO qd with folinic acid 5 mg PO qd. (No IV presentation available)

        (b) Sulfadiazine 1.5 g PO q6hr; or clindamycin 900 mg IV/PO qid

    (3) CMV (including retinitis)

        (a) Ganciclovir 5-10 mg/kg IV q12hr for 14 days (initial therapy)

        (b) Foscarnet 60mg/kg IV q8hr for 14 days (initial therapy)

    (4) Herpes simplex

        (a) Acyclovir 10-15 mg/kg IV q8hr

    (5) Syphilis

        (a) Crystalline penicillin 24 million U/day for 14 days

        (b) Ceftriaxone 2-4 g IV/day for 14 days

2. Important facts to remember in treating HIV-infected patients in the ICU

   a. Patients may have more than one infection at the same time

   b. Blood precautions should be instituted *immediately* to avoid unnecessary exposure

   c. Noninfectious processes can mimic infections (e.g., tumors)

   d. Patients require a full physical examination daily including mouth, perirectal area, and eyes

   e. Superinfections are common (i.e., fungal and resistant bacteria)

   f. When fever persists, consider LP (lumbar puncture), and liver and bone marrow biopsy

   g. Obtain CD4-CD8 counts if not recently done

   h. Establish code status early

   i. Privacy and respect toward patient are essential and mandatory

10.7 INFECTIONS IN THE IMMUNOCOMPROMISED HOST

1. The number of critically ill patients admitted to the ICU with impaired host defense mechanisms has dramatically increased in recent years. Knowledge and recognition of the basic deficiency enable the physician to predict the type and site of infection and allow the institution of early empiric therapy (see Tables 10-5 and 10-6).

2. Categorize immunocompromised patients admitted to the ICU according to the time of acquisition of infection. Hospital-acquired infections have different etiologic agents from infections from the community despite having the same basic immunologic defect.

10.8 ANTIMICROBIALS (see Table 10-7).

Defect	Organism	Manifestations
Phagocytes/neutrophils (i.e., neutropenia)	Gram-positive cocci, gram-negative bacilli, *Pseudomonas aeruginosa*, *Candida* sp, *Aspergillus* sp, *Mucor* sp, *Absidia* sp, *Fusarium* sp	Bacteremia Sepsis Tissue invasion Pneumonia, rhinocerebral and cutaneous
Complement (i.e., C_5–C_8 deficiency)	*Neisseria* sp, *Streptococcus pneumoniae*, *H. influenzae*, *Pseudomonas aeruginosa*, *Brucella* sp	Fulminant sepsis Recurrent infection Pneumonia Sepsis Recurrent fever
Antibody (i.e., IgA-IgG deficiency)	Gram-positive cocci, *H. influenzae*, herpes simplex, *Giardia lamblia*	Pneumonia Otitis Meningitis Encephalitis Liver disease Diarrhea
Cell-mediated immunity (i.e., decrease in CD4 counts)	*Salmonella*, *Listeria* sp, *Mycobacterium* sp, *Nocardia* sp, *Cryptococcus neoformans*, *Histoplasma capsulatum*, *Coccidioides immitis*, herpes simplex, varicella zoster, CMV, *P. carinii*, *Strongyloides stercoralis*, *Toxoplasma gondii*	Diarrhea Sepsis Meningitis Pneumonia CNS/lungs Lungs Mucocutaneous Disseminated Pneumonia CNS Myocardium

Table 10-6 Common clinical presentations in compromised ICU patients

Reason for Admission	Common Pathogen	Initial Therapeutic Approach
Fever and neutropenia	Early: gram-negative bacilli gram-positive cocci (usually catheter-related) Late: resistant gram-negative bacilli fungi (*Candida* sp, *Aspergillus* sp, *Fusarium* sp. *Mucor* sp)	Early empiric therapy mandatory
Sepsis: postsplenectomy	Encapsulated bacterial organisms	Emergency institution of antibacterial therapy
Neurologic deterioration in a patient with cell-mediated immune deficit	Intracellular organisms	Obtain CT, LP (lumbar puncture); treat for bacteria and possibly for *Cryptococcus*
Sepsis after solid organ transplantation	Immediately after surgery: common local bacteria Not related to surgery: virus, fungus, *Nocardia* sp.	Choose antibacterials according to site Empiric therapy with extensive work-up needed
Bilateral pulmonary infiltrates	Organism depends on causative defect	Treat empirically and obtain bronchioalveolar lavage and biopsy (if possible)
Diabetic ketoacidosis	Bacterial organisms, mucormycosis, Aspergillosis	Treat for mixed bacterial infection
AIDS	Depends on sites of infection	See section on AIDS
Postoperative status and malnutrition	Antibiotic-resistant, gram-negative bacilli Group D streptococci, *Candida* sp	Utilize broad-spectrum therapy

Antibiotic regimens commonly used in the ICU

Drug	Dosage	Renal Adjustment Creatinine Clearance >80 / 50-10 / <10	Comments and Side Effects
Aminoglycosides (i.e., gentamicin)	1-2 mg/kg IV q8hr	8-12 hr 12 hr 24-48 hr	Monitor levels, renal function, and hearing
Broad-spectrum penicillin (i.e., piperacillin)	3-4 g IV q68hrs	4-6 hr 8-12 hr 12-24 hr	Monitor Na^+ and coagulation profile
Imipenem	500 mg-1 g q6hrs	6 hr 12 hr 24 hr	Seizures, twitching, facial palsies
Cephalosporins (i.e., ceftazidime)	2 g IV q8hr	6-12 hr 12 hr 24 hr	Penetrates CSF well
Aztreonam	2 g IV q8hr	6-12 hr 12 hr 24 hr	Tolerated in penicillin-allergic patients
Vancomycin	1 g IV q12 hr	6-12 hr 2-3 days weekly	Infuse in at least 1 hr
Oxacillin	6-12 g IV	4-6 hr 6-8 hr 8-12 hr	Monitor levels; interstitial nephritis

Continued.

Table 10-7 Selected antimicrobials commonly used in the ICU—cont'd

Drug	Dosage	Renal Adjustment Creatinine Clearance >80 / 50-10 / <10	Comments and Side Effects
Acyclovir	2-3 g/day IV	8 hr / 12-24 hr / 24-48 hr	Monitor WBC and renal function
Ganciclovir	5 mg/kg IV	12 hr / 12 hr / 24-48 hr	Monitor bone marrow depression
Clindamycin	600-900 mg IV	8 hr / 8 hr / 8 hr	Diarrhea
Chloramphenicol	3-4 g IV or PO	6 hr / 6 hr / 6 hr	Monitor bone marrow function
Metronidazole	30 mg/kg/day IV or PO	6 hr / 6 hr / 6 hr	Metallic taste
Amphotericin B	0.5-1 mg/kg IV/day	24 hr / 24 hr / 48 hr	Monitor renal function
Fluconazole	200-400 mg q12hr IV or PO	12 hr / 24 hr / 48 hr	Interacts with anticoagulants

Continued

Table 10-7 Selected antimicrobials commonly used in the ICU—cont'd

Drug	Dosage	Renal Adjustment Creatinine Clearance >80 / 50-10 / <10	Comments and Side Effects
Itraconazole	2-4 g PO	12-24 hr 24 hr 24 hr	
TMP-SMX	4-5 mg/kg IV (TMP) or higher	6-12 hr 12-24 hr 24-48 hr	Monitor WBC; skin rash
Doxycycline	100-200 mg IV	12-24 hr 12-24 hr 12-24 hr	Impairs neutrophil function
Erythromycin	1-4 g/day IV	6 hr 6 hr 6 hr	Preferably given through central IV line
Ribavirin	Aerosolized 190 mg/ml at 12.5 L/min over 18 hr and the rest over 6 hr. Repeat qid for 10 days	? ? ?	Requires special device for medication delivery

10.9 INFECTIOUS DISEASE "PEARLS" FOR ICU CARE

1. Hand-washing is the single most important procedure to prevent infection
2. Improving nutritional status is of great importance for the outcome of infections
3. Remove bladder catheters as soon as possible
4. Complete daily physical examination is mandatory
5. The Gram's stain is the best and least expensive test for early diagnosis of several infections (e.g., pulmonary, soft tissue, meningitis)
6. Hypothermia, especially in elderly patients, suggests sepsis
7. Change central catheters q 5-7 days
8. Change peripheral lines q 2-3 days
9. If a prolonged ICU stay is expected, early placement of subcutaneous catheters is recommended
10. Patients with high fever require special attention to fluid management
11. Antibiotics interact with many other drugs (see previous tables)
12. Drug-induced fever is not uncommon (common agents are antibiotics, H_2-antagonists, and phenytoin)
13. Fever may last for several days even when appropriate antimicrobial therapy has been instituted
14. Closely follow the clinical situation; it is more important than laboratory results

Selected readings

Bartlett MS, South JW: *Pneumocystis carinii:* an opportunist in immunocompromised patients. *Clin Microbiol Rev* 1991; 4:137-46.

Bodey GP, Fainstein V: *Systemic candidiasis.* In Bodey GP, Fainstein V, editors: *Candidiasis,* New York, 1985, Raven Press.

Bone RC: Sepsis, the sepsis syndrome, multiorgan failure: a plea for comparable definitions. *Ann Intern Med* 1991; 114:332-6.

Craven DE, Kunches LM, Kilinsky S: Risk factors for pneumonia and fatality in patients receiving continuous mechanical ventilation. *Am Rev Respir Dis* 1986; 133:792-9.

Cross PA: Epidemiology of hospital-acquired pneumonia. *Semin Respir Infect* 1987; 2:2-10.

Eisenstein BI: The polymerase chain reaction: a new method of using molecular genetics for medical diagnosis. *N Engl J Med* 1990; 322:178-183.

Fainstein V: *New antimicrobial agents in the compromised host.* In Pulvener A, editor: *Antimicrobial agents and immunity,* New York, 1985, Medicine (Baltimore).

Friedland G, Klein R: *Infectious complications of HIV: tuberculosis and other bacterial infections.* In DeVita VT Jr, Hellman S, Rosenberg SA, editors. *AIDS: etiology, diagnosis, treatment, and prevention,* ed 3, Philadelphia, 1992, JB Lippincott.

Harvey RL, Myers JP: Nosocomial fungemia in a large community teaching hospital. *Arch Intern Med* 1987; 147:2117-24.

Hughes JM: *Epidemiology and prevention of nosocomial pneumonia.* In Remington JS, Swartz MN, editors: *Current clinical topics in infectious diseases,* New York, 1988, McGraw-Hill.

McArthur JC: Neurologic manifestations of AIDS. *Medicine* (Baltimore) 1987; 66: 404-13.

Miller PJ, Wenzel RP: Etiologic organisms as independent predictors of death and morbidity associated with bloodstream infections. *J Infect Dis* 1987; 156:471-7.

Pennington JE: *Community-acquired pneumonia and acute bronchitis in respiratory infections: diagnosis and management,* New York, 1973, Raven Press.

Pizzo PA, Robichand KJ, Gill FA: Empiric antibiotic and antifungal therapy for cancer patients with prolonged fever and granulocytopenia. *Am J Med* 1982; 72:101-7.

Scheld WM: Drug delivery to the central nervous system: general principles and relevance to therapy for infections of the central nervous system. *Rev Infect Dis* 1989; 2(suppl7):1669-79.

Stratton CW: Bacterial pneumonia: an overview with emphasis on pathogenesis, diagnosis, and treatment. *Heart Lung* 1986;15:226-34.

Vane JR, Angaard EE, Botting RM: Regulatory functions of the vascular endothelium. *N Engl J Med* 1990; 322:323-8.

Ziegler EJ, McCutchan JA, Fiener J: Treatment of gram-negative bacteremia and shock with human antiserum to a mutant *Escherichia coli. N Engl J Med* 1982; 307:1225-30.

11 Neurologic Disorders

Robert E. Fromm, Jr. and Joseph Varon

11.1 **BRAIN DEATH**

1. Definition

   Traditionally, death has been defined as the absence of spontaneous respirations and spontaneous pulse. A more contemporary definition of death includes the concept of *brain death,* defined as the permanent cessation of all brain function. The evolution of this concept coincides with the increasing use of transplantation; thus, it is an important concept for the critical care practitioner to master.

2. Legal status of brain death

   In the United States, the concept of brain death and the criteria for its diagnosis have been codified in the vast majority of states. Physicians operating outside of areas with specific legislation on brain death often rely on common law for legal certification of death, but the judicial acceptance of the brain death concept is universal in the United States.

3. Determination of brain death

   Specific requirements for determination of brain death vary from institution to institution. In most institutions, specific sets of criteria are established. The recognition of irreversibility in most instances requires that the cause of the coma be established and be sufficient to account for the loss of brain function observed. For example, when drugs or toxins have been implicated, blood levels of these agents must be absent or below therapeutic levels prior to the determination of brain death by clinical examination.

   a. Clinical determination of brain death

      (1) The common checklist for the diagnosis of brain death is depicted in the Box on p. 203.

      (2) The specific brain stem functions tested vary from site to site, but every institutional protocol includes a number of simple bedside tests demonstrating the absence of brain stem function. One such example is the cold water caloric test (see Box on p. 203).

      (3) In most institutions, two clinical observers must concur with the diagnosis of brain death and so note that in the patient's chart

      (4) The final component of the clinical evaluation of brain death is usually the apnea test (see Box on p. 204).

Clinical Determination of Brain Death

1. Coma of established cause
   Temperature $\geq 32°$ C
   Absence of significant central nervous system (CNS) depressants or significant metabolic disturbances
   Patient not in shock
2. Absence of spontaneous movements, decerebrate or decorticate posturing
3. Absence of brain stem responses
   Pupils fixed
   Corneal reflex absent
   Unresponsiveness to pain in the distribution of the cranial nerves (i.e., supraorbital pressure)
   Absence of cough or gag reflex
   Absence of "doll's eyes"
   No eye movement with cold water (caloric test) bilaterally
4. Absence of respiratory activity for at least three min (see apnea test)

Cold-Water Caloric Test

1. Elevate the patient's head at a 30° angle
2. Inject 50 ml of ice water into each external ear canal using an IV catheter (after determination that the ear canal is free of cerumen). Observe the patient for several min for the presence of eye movements

(5) Ancillary tests for brain death
   Other tests used in determining brain death include
   (a) Electroencephalogram (EEG): an isoelectric EEG is not required as a criterion for brain death in most institutions; however, it may be used as a confirmatory test
   (b) Cerebral angiography: In the presence of toxic substances or sedative agents, the irreversibility of coma may not be determined clinically. The four-vessel cerebral angiogram may be used to determine the absence of brain blood flow; thus, the irreversible nature of coma, confirming the diagnosis of brain death
   (c) Cerebral radionuclide studies: ^{99m}Tc nuclear imaging studies of the cerebral circulation have been used in some centers as a corroborative test in determining brain death. This procedure is not as sensitive for cerebral blood flow as four-vessel arteriography in determination of brain death

The Apnea Test

1. Oxygenate with 100% FiO_2 for 5-10 min before the test
2. Keep O_2 at 4-8 L/min delivered through a canula in the endotracheal tube while the patient is disconnected from the ventilator.* (If hypotension and/or dysrhythmias develop, immediately reconnect to the ventilator. Consider other confirmatory tests)
3. Observe for spontaneous respirations
4. After 10 min, obtain arterial blood gases (ABG). Patient is apneic if $PCO_2 \geq 60$ torr and there are no respiratory movements

*In patients with chronic obstructive pulmonary disease (COPD), the PaO_2 must be <50 torr at the end of the apnea test.

    (6) The patient who is brain dead is *dead.* The physician *does not* require any permission of the family or other individuals to remove a dead patient from mechanical ventilation or other life-support maneuvers

11.2   COMA

1. Definition
   Coma is a term denoting neurologic unresponsiveness. It represents part of a continuum from normal functioning to the absence of neurologic functioning with intermediate states of drowsiness and stupor. Consciousness is separated into two components: level of arousal and the content of consciousness.
   a. Level of arousal depends on the interaction between the reticular activating system of the brain stem and the cerebral hemispheres bilaterally
   b. Content of consciousness exists within the cerebrum. (These two components may be affected individually.) For example, *dyskinetic mutism* is a term applied to patients who appear to be awake (with open eyes that on occasion may even track movements within the room) but have an absence of the content of consciousness. An individual who suffers basilar artery occlusion may develop the "locked-in" syndrome. In this syndrome the content of consciousness is preserved, but the ability to communicate directly with the environment is taken away
2. Etiology
   Coma is a frequent cause of hospital admission. Common causes of coma are depicted in the Box on p. 205.
3. Diagnosis
   a. Careful history and physical examination: history should include information leading up to the discovery of the comatose patient. Pertinent points in the physical examination include evidence of head trauma (e.g., hemotympanum), cerebrospinal fluid (CSF) rhinorrhea, contusions, or lacerations. A complete neurologic examination to look for focal signs should be recorded

Common Causes of Coma

- Cerebrovascular accidents
- CNS trauma
- CNS infections
- Drug intoxication
- Metabolic
- Metastatic or primary CNS neoplasias
- Systemic infection (sepsis)
- Unknown

CSF Studies in Patients with Coma of Unknown Etiology

Tube I
  Cell count with differential
Tube II
  Glucose, protein
Tube III
  Gram's stain, acid-fast bacilli (AFB) stain, routine cultures, India ink and/or cryptococcal antigen, pneumococcal antigen, Venereal Disease Research Laboratories test for syphilis (VDRL)
Tube IV
  Special studies as indicated (e.g., lactic acid, rheumatoid factor)

b. Toxic-metabolic phenomena are found eventually to be responsible for the majority of patients with coma without obvious cause; thus, seek evaluation for hypoglycemia or hyperglycemia, hyponatremia or hypernatremia, renal failure, liver dysfunction with subsequent hepatic encephalopathy, and toxin ingestions as the cause of coma

c. CT scan of the head: mass lesions (supratentorial or in the posterior fossa) may be found unexpectedly at CT scan and account for unconsciousness; thus, all patients with coma of unknown etiology should have neuroimaging studies completed

d. Lumbar puncture (LP): patients without evidence of mass lesion should undergo CSF examination primarily to rule out infection. Specific diagnostic studies are noted in the Box above.

4. Treatment

Always remember the ABCs (airway, breathing, and circulation).

a. Comatose patients with absent airway protective reflexes should undergo endotracheal intubation (with assisted mechanical ventilation in those patients with inadequate spontaneous ventilations)

    (1) Circulation; assess blood pressure (BP) and pulse rate to determine the adequacy of cardiovascular function

b. Specific management is dictated by the clinical condition of the patient

(1) The patient with an infectious source should be treated aggressively with IV antibiotics. For patients with mass lesions, consider early surgical intervention

(2) Patients with toxic-metabolic events should receive appropriate therapy with close monitoring of electrolytes and/or drug levels

(3) Many clinicians recommend empiric therapy of the comatose patient with naloxone, a narcotic antagonist (2-8 mg IV), and dextrose (50 g IV push). However, some data suggest that high levels of glucose may be deleterious to injured neurons; thus, with the advent of bedside glucose testing many advocate the determination of blood glucose prior to the administration of dextrose

(4) Flumazenil, a specific benzodiazepine antagonist, is also available; however, in the absence of specific knowledge of benzodiazepine overdose, the authors do not recommend its administration because of its potential for seizures in patients with tricyclic antidepressant overdose

c. Nonspecific management

(1) IV access for the administration of medications

(2) Consider nasogastric decompression through an NG tube

(3) Place a urinary catheter for urine monitoring and ease of nursing care for the comatose patient

(4) Administer deep venous thrombosis prophylaxis to all patients in whom no contraindications exist (i.e., heparin 5000 U SQ q12hr)

(5) Administer stress ulcer prophylaxis in every comatose patient (e.g., H_2-blockers, sucralfate)

(6) Take care and comfort measures (including lubrication of conjunctival spaces and eye taping)

(7) Ensure passive range of motion of upper and lower extremities for the prevention of contractures

(8) Ensure skin care (including frequent turning and positioning)

11.3   INTRACRANIAL HYPERTENSION

1. Physiology

a. The contents of the cranial vault include the brain, CSF, and the cerebral blood volume. These contents are constrained by the skull itself

b. The brain is a highly metabolic organ and very dependent on continued blood supply

c. Because of the closed nature of the cranial vault, cerebral blood flow is dependent on the difference between mean arterial pressure (MAP) and intracranial pressure (ICP). (See Appendix I)

2. Etiology

A large number of intracranial processes may result in a rise in ICP and impairment of cerebral blood flow (see the Box on p. 207). These specific entities may require individualized therapy and are discussed in other sections of this book.

3. Management

a. ABCs

b. Positioning of the patient: 30° head-up tilt is recommended for those patients who do not have contraindications (e.g., hypotension)

Causes of Intracranial Hypertension

- Brain tumors
- Fulminant hepatic failure
- Head injury
- Meningitis and/or encephalitis
- Subarachnoid hemorrhage
- Vasculitis
- Other

---

c. Hyperventilation: the fastest way to control ICP is hyperventilation. Acute reductions in arterial PCO_2 result in vasoconstriction and decrease in intracranial blood volume. Specific PCO_2 values of approximately 25-35 torr are commonly advocated, although to the authors' knowledge no controlled studies have demonstrated the utility of these specific target values

d. Osmotic agents: mannitol, at doses of 0.25-1 g/kg of ideal body weight intravenously over 10-20 min pulls water from the brain and results in a decrease in ICP. Maintain plasma osmolality <340 mOsm/L. Note: The initial administration of mannitol may result in paradoxical increases in ICP; thus, many authors recommend prior therapy with a loop-acting diuretic (i.e., furosemide)

e. Short-acting anesthetics may result in reduction of cerebral blood flow; thus, reductions in ICP. Pentobarbital is the most commonly used agent. The usual dose of this agent is 10 mg/kg ideal body weight as the loading dose and 100 mg/hr for maintenance

f. Corticosteroids: The only clear role in the management of intracranial hypertension is in cerebral edema secondary to certain neoplasms. Their use in trauma, cerebrovascular accidents (CVAs), and metabolic causes has not been demonstrated to improve outcome and therefore cannot be routinely recommended

g. CSF drainage: an intraventricular catheter may be placed percutaneously at the bedside and permit simultaneous monitoring and therapy of ICP. Sustained elevations of ICP >20 cm H_2O can be managed by withdrawal of CSF through the intraventricular catheter

h. Some authors have advocated *not* using positive end-expiratory pressure (PEEP); however, in conditions in which this therapy is required (i.e., low lung compliance), routinely used levels of PEEP (3-7 cm H_2O) are not expected to impair cerebral blood drainage

i. Other methods less commonly used to decrease ICP include controlled hypothermia, indomethacin, and flumazenil

11.4 CEREBRAL VASCULAR DISEASE

1. Epidemiology
   Approximately 250,000 people die in the United States each year of cerebral vascular disease. Many more develop catastrophic and lesser degrees of neurologic deficits.

2. Classification

A number of different syndromes comprise the disorders labeled cerebral vascular accidents (CVAs). These disorders can be broadly grouped into two large categories: those that produce vascular insufficiency (secondary to thrombosis, embolism, or stenosis leading to focal areas of ischemia); and those that produce ruptures of the vascular tree causing intracranial hypertension and secondary cerebral ischemia.

a. Vascular insufficiency

(1) Transient ischemic attacks (TIAs) are defined as the sudden or rapid onset of neurologic deficits secondary to cerebral ischemia that lasts from a few min to up to 24 hr without residual signs or symptoms. Atherosclerosis is the most frequent cause

(2) Stroke

(a) Definition: rapid onset of neurologic deficits involving a set vascular territory with neurologic signs and symptoms lasting >24 hrs

(b) Risk factors are similar to those for TIA. An increasing frequency of stroke related to vasospasm secondary to cocaine abuse has been noted in the last decade in the United States

(c) Classification of stroke

Both thrombosis and embolism may result in vascular insufficiency and the phenomena of stroke. Clinically, the differentiation of thrombosis and embolism is quite difficult. However, some clinical characteristics of each are noted in Table 11-1

(i) Embolic stroke: the most common causes include emboli secondary to atrial fibrillation, valvular heart disease, bacterial and nonbacterial endocarditis, trauma, emboli secondary to myocardial infarction or ventricular aneurysm, atrial myxoma, and paradoxical embolism secondary to endocardial disease

(ii) Thrombotic stroke occurs when a clot develops in a cerebral vessel. Intrinsic or extrinsic diseases of the cerebral vessels may contribute to thrombotic strokes. These include

• Arteriosclerosis
• Fibromuscular dysplasia

Table 11-1 Clinical characteristics of embolic and thrombotic strokes

	Embolism	Thrombosis
Predisposing factors	Valvular heart disease	Atherosclerosis
	Endocarditis	Diabetes
	Myocardial infarction	Hypertension
	Atrial fibrillation	Arteritits
History of prior TIA	Uncommon	Common
Onset of symptoms	Rapid onset	Progression over hours

- Extension of embolism or dissection into cerebral arteries because of arteritis (Takayasu's disease, giant cell arteritis, and other vascular diseases)
- Increased viscosity secondary to proteins or increased cellular elements (i.e., Waldenström's macroglobulinemia, leukemias with elevated blast counts, and erythrocytosis of any cause)
- TIAs are a risk factor for completed stroke with the highest risk in the first 3 months immediately following the onset of TIAs

(d) Initial evaluation and the management of cerebral ischemic syndromes
  - ABCs: Secure the airway and assist with breathing and circulation as with any patient presenting with a potentially critical illness
  - Carefully examine the patient. Emphasis should be on the neurologic examination to localize the area deficits and on other areas of the physical examination to rule in or rule out secondary causes for the ischemic syndrome
  - Laboratory evaluation
    Complete blood count, prothrombin time (PT), partial thromboplastin time (PTT), glucose, electrolytes, blood urea nitrogen (BUN), and creatinine are routinely ordered. Chest radiograph, ECG, and CT scan of the head (to rule out hemorrhage, infarction, subdural hematoma, or intracranial masses)
  - In any patient with new neurologic abnormalities, LP should be considered to rule out infectious causes and for the completion of the evaluation for subarachnoid hemorrhage (after head CT scan has ruled out increased ICP).
  - Echocardiography
    For patients with a history or a physical examination suggestive of cardiac abnormality, order echocardiography
  - Other useful studies may include duplex ultrasonography and cerebral angiography

(e) In patients with embolic CVAs with progressively worsening neurologic deficits (stroke in evolution), anticoagulation, beginning with heparin, is recommended. In addition, heparin is commonly prescribed for patients with recurrent TIAs despite antiplatelet therapy. Anticoagulation is contraindicated in patients with CT or LP evidence of hemorrhage. Anticoagulation is relatively contraindicated in patients with gastrointestinal (GI) bleeding or coagulation disorders and in patients with hypertension

(f) BP control: therapy to maintain systemic BP at approximately 150/100 mm Hg is advocated. Caution must be exercised as reductions in BP may worsen the clinical condition by producing ischemia in poorly perfused CNS regions

(g) Thrombolytic therapy; at the current time this therapy for ischemic stroke is undergoing intensive investigation. The authors cannot recommend routine administration of thrombolytic therapy for ischemic strokes

b. Rupture of the vascular tree

(1) Subarachnoid hemorrhage (SAH) accounts for about 10% of all strokes and 16%-20% of cerebral vascular deficits. Etiology of SAH includes ruptured aneurysms of cerebral vessels, bleeding from arteriovenous malformations of the CNS, and trauma

(a) Clinical manifestations

(i) Neurologic deficits may include focal neurologic signs as well as coma

(ii) Generalized excruciating headache with neck stiffness is classically described

(b) Evaluation and management

(i) ABCs as noted previously

(ii) CT scan of the head demonstrating subarachnoid blood is seen in approximately 90% of cases

(iii) Perform LP in patients whose CT scan is negative and for whom clinical suspicion is still high

(iv) Keep the patient at bed rest. Order cardiac monitoring and frequent (q1-2 hr) neurologic assessments

(v) Prescribe analgesic for headache. (Acetaminophen and codeine are commonly used)

(vi) Prescribe stool softeners and mild laxatives to prevent constipation (and thus, increased ICP)

(vii) BP control: Keep systolic BP in the range of 140-160 mm Hg (ischemia of poorly perfused regions may occur; therefore carefully follow clinical status as BP control is obtained). Calcium channel blockers (i.e., nimodipine 60 mg q4hr × 21 days) have been advocated to prevent cerebral blood vessel spasm following subarachnoid hemorrhage. Use these in patients without contraindications

(viii) Surgical management: Considerable controversy exists in the surgical management of patients with SAH and aneurysms. The propensity for bleeding from aneurysms leads to the desire to surgically obliterate any accessible lesions. The timing of the operation is debated. Many neurosurgeons prefer to wait 5-10 days after the event because of cerebral vasospasm; others advocate early surgery

(ix) Nonoperative interventions (e.g., embolization of arteriovenous [AV] malformation) are also options

(2) Intracerebral hemorrhage

Intracerebral hemorrhage commonly occurs following trauma. When it occurs spontaneously, it is frequently accompanied by hypertension. Neurologic abnormalities, as seen in other types of strokes, are usually present and the specific diagnosis requires neuroimaging studies

(a) Management

(i) ABCs as required for every critically ill patient

(ii) Control severe hypertension: as noted above, cerebral ischemia may occur with reductions in BP. However, control of hypertension may reduce cerebral edema and improve neurologic function. Short-acting intravenous agents are advocated (labetalol, trimethaphan). Reductions in BP should not exceed 20% of baseline value

(iii) Additional management of intracranial hypertension as noted above may be required

(iv) Continue supportive therapy as required for all ICU patients

(3) Surgical evacuation of the hematoma should occur in patients with accessible lesions that have progressive signs of deterioration

11.5   STATUS EPILEPTICUS

1. Definition
   Status epilepticus is defined as seizure activity continuing for 30 minutes or intermittently over a 30-minute period without the patient regaining consciousness. It is a condition that may lead to permanent neurologic damage or even death.

2. General approach
   The management of seizure disorders is based on clinical information.
   a. Most seizures stop spontaneously within 30-90 seconds
   b. The diagnosis of *status epilepticus* is straightforward and can be determined in most cases through observation of the patient
   c. Generalized seizure disorders without motor findings may lead to changes in mental status or coma and may not be clinically apparent; thus, further diagnostic testing (e.g., EEG) may be required
   d. Continued seizure disorders may result in enzyme elevation (creatine kinase [CK]), making the diagnosis of other clinical conditions more difficult (e.g., myocardial infarction [MI])

3. Specific management
   a. ABCs: as in all critically ill patients, maintain airway, breathing, and circulation. Position the patient so that motor activity cannot cause harm. Administer oxygen and ensure continuous observation of the patient
   b. Obtain blood glucose, calcium, magnesium, and other electrolytes; BUN; liver function tests; anticonvulsant levels; complete blood count; and toxicology screen
   c. Establish a normal saline infusion and administer intravenously 50 ml of 50% glucose, 100 mg of thiamine
   d. Establish ECG and BP monitoring
   e. Diazepam 5 mg over 1-2 min IV, repeated every 5-10 min; or lorazepam 2-4 q5 min can be administered in those patients continuing to have seizure activity
   f. Recurrence of seizures within 15-20 min following administration of benzodiazepines is quite frequent, and other antiepileptic agents should be instituted. Administer phenytoin 18 mg/kg IV at a rate 50 mg/min or less as a loading dose for patients not previously receiving

phenytoin. If dysrhythmias and/or hypotension ensue, stop the infusion and resume at a slower rate

g. Persistent seizures following phenytoin administration should result in administration of phenobarbital IV at rates of 50-100 mg/min until the seizure stops or until a loading dose of 20 mg/kg ideal body weight total has been given

h. Continued seizures should prompt the administration of other medications: lidocaine, 1-3 mg/kg ideal body weight as loading dose and 2-4 mg/min has been advocated; pentobarbital sodium 15 mg/kg ideal body weight as the loading dose followed by 0.5-3 mg/kg/hr; or inhalation anesthetics (e.g., isoflurane)

i. EEG monitoring is appropriate for patients receiving general anesthetic control of status epilepticus

j. Ensue review of laboratory data, additional history, and physical examination for underlying disorders that may have resulted in the status epilepticus

k. Careful physical and laboratory evaluation for underlying disease processes should ensue following control of the status epilepticus. Patients without clear etiology should undergo head CT scan and LP unless contraindicated

l. Continuous motor seizures may lead to muscle breakdown; and thus the release of myoglobin and other intracellular components into the circulation. The concern is with maintenance of adequate hydration as well as protection from pigment- induced renal failure. (See Chapter 16)

11.6 NEUROMUSCULAR DISORDERS

1. Guillain-Barré syndrome (GBS)
   a. Definition
      GBS is an acute demyelinating disorder of the peripheral nervous system that results in motor and sensory symptoms with few sensory signs. The vast majority of cases result in complete recovery; however, in up to 25% of patients, respiratory failure due to weakness of the respiratory muscles ensues and mechanical ventilation is required for a period of time. Peaks of occurrence are in the 15- to 35-year-old and the 50 to 75-year-old age groups
   b. Clinical manifestations
      GBS presents in a typical pattern. The usual history is that of a patient with a normal previous health status interrupted by a mild upper respiratory or GI illness followed by ascending weakness and numbness. Other factors include recent vaccination or surgery. Major clinical manifestations are depicted in the Box on p. 213. Atypical presentations may include a descending paralysis
   c. Diagnostic evaluation
      (1) Perform a careful physical examination attempting to rule out other causes of neuropathology (e.g., spinal cord lesions, infection, metabolic, or toxic)
      (2) LP usually reveals elevated protein. There are usually few mononuclear leukocytes in the CSF with <10 lymphocytes/cm^3
      (3) Eighty percent of all patients show slow nerve conduction

Major Clinical Manifestations of Guillain-Barré Syndrome

- Distal paresthesias (initially lower extremities)
- Rapidly progressive motor weakness (ascending neuropathy)
- Symmetry is seldom absolute
- Facial weakness is common (33% of cases)
- Recovery usually begins 2-4 weeks after progression stops
- Sinus tachycardia and labile BP are common
- CSF protein elevation (after the first week)
- Nerve conduction abnormalities are detectable

    d. Management
       (1) ABCs
       (2) Supportive measures: close monitoring of respiratory function with frequent measurements of the vital capacity and/or negative inspiratory force (NIF) are indicated
       (3) A vital capacity of <10 ml/kg is an indication to consider intubation and assisted mechanical ventilatory support
       (4) Perform active and passive range of motion of lower and upper extremities to prevent the formation of contractures
       (5) Institute decubitus ulcer prevention and care
       (6) Prevent thromboembolism with appropriate therapy (i.e., heparin 5000 U SQ q12hr in patients without contraindications)
       (7) Plasma exchange presumably removes or dilutes circulating factors implicated in the pathogenesis of GBS. It has been shown to decrease ventilatory dependence in GBS
       (8) Corticosteroids have not been proven to be of value in this syndrome

2. Other chronic neurologic disorders
    a. A number of chronic progressive neurologic disorders may result in patient admission to the ICU for physiologic support. These include amyotrophic lateral sclerosis, multiple sclerosis, severe Parkinson's disease, and others. Many of these patients are admitted because of the need for aggressive tracheobronchial toilet or mechanical ventilation
    b. The decision to institute aggressive therapy is a major concern in managing these patients. It is preferable that this decision be addressed with the patient and family prior to the need for these services so that unwanted supportive measures are not forced upon them

11.7 | DELIRIUM IN THE ICU

1. Epidemiology
Ten percent of medical and surgical patients become delirious during their hospitalization. These patients are at risk for harm to themselves (e.g., by the discontinuation of an IV line, arterial line, nasogastric tubes) and

others. Patients who develop delirium are at greater risk of mortality. Patients at high risk for the development of delirium are:

    a. Those at the extremes of age (the elderly and children)
    b. Those with preexisting brain injury
    c. The drug-dependent
    d. Those who are postcardiotomy
    e. Those with HIV disease

2. Clinical features
    a. A prodromal state manifested by restlessness, irritability, anxiety, or sleep difficulty
    b. A rapidly fluctuating course. Patients are intermittently clear thinking and coherent or grossly confused, disoriented, and disorganized
    c. Reversed sleep-wake cycles and increased activity and confusion during the nighttime hours

3. Evaluation and management
    a. ABCs as required for all patients with a critical illness
    b. Pay careful attention to metabolic problems that may produce CNS disturbances
    c. Obtain laboratory evaluations for blood glucose, electrolytes, calcium, BUN, and LFTs, as well as ABGs or pulse-oximetry to rule out hypoxemia (a common cause of mental status changes in the ICU)
    d. Obtain an ECG to help rule out myocardial ischemia
    e. Give patients with unexplained mental status changes CT scanning or magnetic resonance imaging (MRI) of the brain followed by LP to rule out infectious or other causes
    f. Ensure careful review of the medications prescribed for the patient. Drugs commonly associated with delirium are depicted in the Box below.
    g. Whether or not the etiology is known, some simple interventions are often missed that may help to control the patient's confusion and behavior. For example, if the patient normally wears eyeglasses or a hearing aid, return these items. The old practice of placing delirious pa-

---

Drugs Commonly Associated with Delirium

Analgesics (e.g., morphine)
Antibiotics (e.g., aminoglycosides)
Antivirals (e.g., amantadine, acyclovir)
Anticholinergics (e.g., atropine)
Anticonvulsants (e.g., phenytoin)
Antiinflammatory agents (e.g., corticosteroids, nonsteroidal antiinflammatory drugs [NSAIDs])
Antineoplastic drugs
Cardiac drugs (e.g., beta-blockers, ACE inhibitors)
Drug withdrawal (e.g., ethanol, benzodiazepines)
Sympathomimetics (e.g., amphetamines, cocaine)
Miscellaneous (e.g., disulfiram, lithium)

tients together is not helpful and indeed, it may increase the aggressive behavior of both patients, thus making orientation almost impossible

h. Haloperidol is a highly potent antipsychotic agent that effectively calms agitation, sedates, and reduces hallucinations and paranoid thinking. For the patient with a mild level of delirium or agitation, a starting dose of 0.5-2 mg IV or IM is usually enough. However, for patients with severe agitation, a starting dose of 5-10 mg may be necessary. Allow an interval of 20-30 min between doses. After giving three doses of haloperidol with no improvement in symptomatology, give 1-2 mg lorazepam IV concurrently, or alternate with haloperidol q30min. Assuming the patient is calm, reduce the dose by 15% q24hr. *Note*: Haloperidol is not approved for IV use despite its common use for this indication. Large IV doses have been used in critically ill patients without evident harm or side effects. Doses as high as 100 mg IV bolus have been given to medically ill patients without evidence of respiratory depression

i. Delirium should prompt neuropsychiatric consultation for recommendations in evaluation and therapy

Selected readings

American Nimodipine Study Group: Clinical trial of nimodipine in acute ischemic stroke. *Stroke* 1992; 23:3-8.

Bleck TP, Smith MC, Pierre-Louis SJC et al: Neurologic complications of critical medical illness. *Crit Care Med* 1993; 21:98-103.

Cold GE, Holdgard HO: Treatment of intracranial-hypertension in acute head injury with special reference to the role of hyperventilation and sedation with barbiturates: a review. *Intensive Care World* 1992; 9:172-8.

Doyle DJ, Mark PWS: Analysis of intracranial pressure. *J Clin Monit* 1992; 8:81-90.

Dutka AJ, Hallenbeck JM: Pharmacologic therapy for ischemic cerebrovascular disease. *Neurol Clin* 1980; 8:161-76.

Hund EF, Borel CO, Cornblath DR et al: Intensive management and treatment of severe Guillain-Barré syndrome. *Crit Care Med* 1993; 21:433-46.

Jafar JJ, Johns LM, Mullan SF: The effect of mannitol on cerebral blood flow. *J Neurosurg* 1986; 64:754-9.

Kelly BJ, Luce JM: Current concepts in cerebral protection. *Chest* 1993; 103:1246-54.

Knekt P, Reunanen A, Aho K et al: Risk factors for a subarachnoid hemorrhage in a longitudinal population study. *J Clin Epidemiol* 1991; 44:933-9.

Leppik IE: Status epilepticus—the next decade. *Neurology* 1990; 40(suppl2):4-9.

Pascual J, Sedano NJ, Polo JM et al: Intravenous lidocaine for status epilepticus. *Epilepsia* 1988; 29:584-9.

Ropper AH: The Guillain-Barré syndrome. *N Engl J Med* 1992; 326:1130-6.

Rosner MJ, Coley IB: Cerebral perfusion pressure, intracranial pressure, and head elevation. *J Neurosurg* 1986; 65:636-41.

Saul TG, Ducker TB: Effect of intracranial pressure monitoring and aggressive treatment on mortality in severe head injury. *J Neurosurg* 1982; 56:498-503.

Teres D, Brown RB, Lemshaw S: Predicting mortality of intensive care unit patients: the importance of coma. *Crit Care Med* 1982; 10:86-95

12 Nutrition

Pamela R. Roberts

AIMS OF NUTRITIONAL SUPPORT

1. Preserve tissue mass and decrease usage of endogenous nutrient stores.
2. Decrease catabolism.
3. Maintain/improve organ function.
   a. Immune
   b. Renal
   c. Hepatic
   d. Muscle
4. Improve wound healing.
5. Decrease infection.
6. Maintain gut barrier (decrease translocation).
7. Decrease morbidity/mortality
   a. Decrease ICU/hospital stay
   b. Decrease hospital costs

TIMING OF INSTITUTION OF NUTRITIONAL SUPPORT

1. Optimal timing remains controversial.
   a. Some patients tolerate short periods of starvation by using endogenous stores to support body functions
   b. Well-nourished patients (nonstressed) have actually survived without food for 6 weeks (ingesting only water)
   c. Hypermetabolic and hypercatabolic critically ill patients can probably tolerate only a few weeks of starvation before death
   d. There appears to be no benefit of total starvation
2. Accumulating data suggest that outcome can be improved with early and optimal nutritional support.
   a. Early nutritional support blunts the hypercatabolic/hypermetabolic response to injury
   b. In a growing number of studies, patients randomized to receive early vs delayed feeding had decreased infection rates, fewer complications, and a shorter length of stay in the hospital
   c. Animal studies report improved wound healing and improved hepatic function in several injury models with early feeding

12.3 **ROUTE OF NUTRITIONAL SUPPORT**

1. Parenteral nutrition
   a. Nutrients: amino acids, dextrose, soy-based lipids, vitamins, minerals, and trace elements (see Table 12-1)
   b. Delivery via peripheral or central vein
   c. Major complications
      (1) Central line placement (pneumothorax, hemothorax, carotid artery perforation)
      (2) Metabolic derangements (hyperglycemia, electrolyte disturbances)
      (3) Immune suppression
      (4) Increased infection rates (catheter-related sepsis, pneumonia, abscesses)
      (5) Liver dysfunction (fatty infiltration, cholestasis, liver failure)
      (6) Gut atrophy (diarrhea, bacterial translocation)
      (7) Venous thrombosis
      (8) Overfeeding
   d. Other problems include the lack of some conditionally essential amino acids that are not stable in solution (e.g., glutamine, cysteine)
   e. Glucose to fat ratio
      (1) Usually 60:40 to 40:60 (ratio of calories from each source)
      (2) Large amounts of glucose (>60% of calories) can
         (a) Increase energy expenditure
         (b) Increase CO_2 production and increase pulmonary workload (may delay ventilator weaning)
         (c) Produce liver steatosis
         (d) Lead to immune compromise
2. Enteral nutrition
   a. Nutrients (see Table 12-1)
      (1) Nitrogen sources: amino acids, peptides, or intact proteins (e.g., casein, whey, soy, lactalbumin)

Table 12-1 Comparison of nutrients in enteral vs parenteral nutrition

Nutrient	Enteral	Parenteral
Nitrogen source	Intact proteins, peptides, or amino acids	Amino acids*
Carbohydrates	Simple sugars or complex carbohydrates (e.g., starch and fiber)	Simple sugar (dextrose)
Lipids	Long- and medium-chain triglycerides, or long-chain fatty acids (ω-3 or ω-6)	Soy-based lipids
Vitamins	Present	Can be added
Minerals and trace elements	Present	Can be added

*Lacks some conditionally essential amino acids (e.g., glutamine and cysteine).

      (2) Carbohydrates: simple sugars or complex carbohydrates (e.g., starch and fiber)

      (3) Lipids: long- or medium-chain triglycerides, ω-3 or ω-6 long-chain fatty acids

      (4) Vitamins

      (5) Minerals and trace elements

   b. Delivery

      (1) Oral

      (2) Gastric tube (i.e., nasogastric, gastric)

      (3) Small bowel feeding tube (i.e., nasoduodenal, gastroduodenal, jejunal)

   c. Major complications

      (1) Aspiration (pneumonia, chemical pneumonitis, acute respiratory distress syndrome [ARDS])

      (2) Metabolic derangements (e.g., electrolyte disturbances, hyperglycemia) are less common with enteral nutrition than with parenteral nutrition

      (3) Diarrhea

      (4) Misplaced feeding tubes (e.g., pneumothorax, empyema, bowel perforation)

      (5) Overfeeding

3. Enteral vs parenteral nutrition

   a. Enteral nutrition is required for optimal gut function (i.e., maintenance of gut barrier, gut-associated immune system, IgA secretion, mucin layer)

   b. Total parenteral nutrition (TPN) is associated with

      (1) Immunosuppression (thought to be related to IV lipids which are high in ω-6 long-chain fatty acids)

      (2) Increased infection rates (compared to enteral) in patients following trauma, burns, surgery, and cancer chemotherapy/radiotherapy

      (3) Higher mortality in patients receiving chemotherapy/radiotherapy and after burn injury

   c. TPN is not superior to enteral nutrition in patients with inflammatory bowel disease or pancreatitis

   d. TPN may be beneficial in patients with short-gut syndromes and some types of gastrointestinal (GI) fistulas

   e. Enteral nutrition is the preferred method of feeding in patients receiving chemotherapy/radiotherapy, and following surgery, burns, trauma, sepsis, renal failure, liver failure, and respiratory failure

   f. Parenteral nutrition is indicated when enteral nutrition is not possible (i.e., inadequate small bowel function)

12.4 GI FUNCTION DURING CRITICAL ILLNESS

1. Oral nutrition remains the best form of nutritional support; however, in many critically ill patients this is not possible.

2. Decreased motility of the stomach and colon is common and typically lasts 5-7 days in a critically ill patient (longer if the patient remains critically ill).

   a. Gastric paresis is best assessed and monitored by measuring gastric residuals

b. Gastric residuals of ≥150 ml are usually considered abnormal
c. Patients with gastric residuals ≥150 ml should be fed in the small bowel (postpyloric) to decrease the risk of aspiration
3. Motility and nutrient absorptive capability of the small bowel is usually preserved (even after severe trauma, burns, or major surgery).
4. Bowel sounds are a poor index of small bowel motility.

12.5 **NUTRIENT REQUIREMENTS (QUANTITY)**

1. Energy
   a. Caloric content of major nutrients
      (1) Lipids provide 9 kcal/g
      (2) Carbohydrates provide 4 kcal/g
      (3) Proteins provide 4 kcal/g
   b. Studies show that most critically ill patients expend 25-35 kcal/kg/day
   c. Resting metabolic expenditure (RME) can be estimated using the Harris-Benedict equation (see Table 12-2)
   d. RME can also be measured by indirect calorimetry (metabolic cart)
   e. Some authors recommend adjusting RME by multiplying it by a correction factor (see Table 12-3); however, correction factors frequently overestimate energy needs

Table 12-2 Harris-Benedict equation

Men	Women
RME (kcal/day) = 66 + (13.7 × W) + (5 × H) − (6.8 × A)	RME (kcal/day) = 665 + (9.6 × W) + (1.7 × H) − (4.7 × A)

Key: RME: resting metabolic expenditure
  W: weight in kg
  H: height in cm
  A: age in years

Table 12-3 Energy expenditure correction factors

Starvation	0.7
Confined to bed	1.2
Out of bed	1.3
Fever	1 + 0.13/degree C
Elective surgery	1-1.2
Multiple fractures	1.2-1.4
Sepsis	1.4-1.8
Burns	
<20% BSB*	1-1.5
20-40% BSB	1.5-1.9
40-100% BSB	1.9-2.1

*BSB: body surface area burned

    f. The authors prefer to initially administer 25 kcal/kg/day (see Table 12-4)

       (1) Approximately 20% protein (% refers to % of total daily calories)

       (2) Approximately 30% lipids

       (3) Approximately 50% carbohydrates

    g. Patients with organ failure/disease states may have increased or decreased needs and should be considered individually

    h. Overfeeding (with either enteral or parenteral nutrients) is associated with more adverse side effects than slightly underfeeding during most critical illnesses

2. Protein

    a. Most critically ill patients need 1.2-2 g/kg/day

    b. Protein requirements increase in patients with severe trauma, burns, and protein-losing enteropathies

3. Water

    a. Must be individualized as needs vary greatly among patients (differences in insensible losses, GI losses, and urine losses)

    b. Initially estimate 1 ml water/kcal of energy in adults

4. Vitamins

    a. Fat-soluble vitamins: A, D, E, and K

    b. Water-soluble vitamins: ascorbic acid (C), thiamine (B_1), riboflavin (B_2), niacin, folate, pyridoxine (B_6), cyanocobalamin (B_{12}), pantothenic acid, and biotin

    c. Published recommended daily allowances (RDAs) are based on oral intake in healthy individuals

    d. Vitamin needs for critically ill patients have not been determined

    e. See Table 12-5 for estimates of nutritional requirements

    f. Commercial enteral formulas generally supply the RDA of vitamins (if patients receive their caloric needs)

    g. An adult parenteral vitamin formulation was approved by the FDA in 1979 and is available for addition to TPN solutions; this should be added just before administration since degradation can occur

Table 12-4 Macronutrient nutritional requirements

Nutrient	% of total calories	Quantity of nutrients	Example for 70-kg patient
Total calories		25 kcal/kg/day	1750 kcal/day
Protein/amino acids	15-25	1.2-2 g/kg/day	95 g/day (380 kcal/day [based on 1.35 g/kg/day])
Carbohydrates	30-65	50% of calories (avg pt)	220 g/day (880 kcal/day)
Fats	15-30	30% of calories (avg pt)	55 g/day (495 kcal/day)

Table 12-5 Micronutrient nutritional requirements

Micronutrient	Enteral Nutrition	Parenteral Nutrition	Example for TPN for a 70-kg Patient
Minerals			
Sodium	60-140 mmol/day	60-120 mmol/day	80 mmol/day
Potassium	50-140 mmol/day	50-120 mmol/day	50 mmol/day
Magnesium	8-15 mmol/day	8-12 mmol/day	10 mmol/day
Phosphorus	25 mmol/day	14-16 mmol/day	15 mmol/day
Calcium	20 mmol/day	7-10 mmol/day	10 mmol/day
Trace elements			
Iron	10 mg/day	1-2 mg/day	None
Zinc	15 mg/day	2-5 mg/day	5 mg/day
Copper	2-3 mg/day	0.5-1.5 mg/day	1 mg/day
Chromium	50-200 mcg/day	10-20 mcg/day	10 mcg/day
Selenium	50-200 mcg/day	80-150 mcg/day	100 mcg/day
Iodine	150 mcg/day	120 mcg/day	120 mcg/day
Manganese	2.5-5 mg/day	0.2-0.8 mg/day	0.5 mg/day
Vitamins*			
Vitamin A	RDA: 4000-5000 IU/day	ND†	3300 IU/day
Vitamin D	RDA: 200-400 IU/day	ND†	200 IU/day
Vitamin E	RDA: 12-15 IU/day	ND†	10 IU/day
Vitamin K	RDA: 60-80 mcg/day	ND†	10 mg/week‡
Thiamine	RDA: 1.1-1.4 mg/day	ND†	3 mg/day
Riboflavin	RDA: 1.2-1.7 mg/day	ND†	5 mg/day
Niacin	RDA: 13-19 mg/day	ND†	40 mg/day
Pantothenic acid	4-7 mg/day§	ND†	15 mg/day
Pyridoxine	RDA: 1.6-2 mg/day	ND†	4 mg/day
Folic acid	RDA: 0.4 mg/day	ND†	0.4 mg/day
Vitamin B_{12}	RDA: 3 mcg/day	ND†	5 mcg/day
Vitamin C	RDA: 40 mg/day	ND†	100 mg/day
Biotin	RDA: 30-100 mcg/day	ND†	60 mcg/day

*Enteral requirements should always exceed parenteral requirements; most recommend supplying 1-3 × the RDA of each vitamin to patients with critical illness. (Requirements are probably increased by stress, infection, disease). However, the exact requirements are not known.
†ND: Not defined.
‡None if anticoagulation is used.
§RDA is not established.

5. Minerals (Na$^+$, K$^+$, Ca^{++}, Phosphorus, Mg^{++})
    a. See Table 12-5 for estimates of daily nutritional requirements
    b. Present in sufficient quantities in enteral products (special formulas limit electrolytes for renal failure)
    c. Must be supplemented in TPN
6. Trace elements (iron, copper, iodine, zinc, selenium, chromium, cobalt, manganese)
    a. Needs in critically ill patients have not been determined (see Table 12-5 for estimates of requirements)
    b. Sufficient quantities are thought to be present in enteral products
    c. Must be supplemented in TPN (all except iron can be added to solution)
        (1) Deficiency states reported in long-term TPN patients
        (2) Specifics are best managed by specially trained nutritional support teams

12.6   **ROLE OF SPECIFIC NUTRIENTS (QUALITY)**

1. Nitrogen sources
    a. Choices
        (1) Amino acids
        (2) Hydrolyzed protein (peptides)
        (3) Intact proteins
    b. Evidence suggests that peptides generated from the diet possess specific physiologic activities
    c. Nitrogen is best delivered as intact protein (if digestion and absorption are intact) or hydrolyzed protein (in case of impaired digestion)
    d. Protein is absorbed primarily as peptides (60%) and amino acids (33%)
    e. Essential amino acid formulas should *not* be used
    f. Some amino acids become essential during critical illness
        (1) These are called conditionally essential amino acids
        (2) Examples include glutamine, cysteine, arginine, and taurine
    g. Some amino acids appear to have specific roles
        (1) Glutamine is a fuel for the GI tract and immune system
        (2) Arginine is required for optimum wound healing and is important in immune function
        (3) Cysteine is needed for synthesis of glutathione
        (4) Branched-chain amino acids (BCAA) may improve mental status in patients with hepatic encephalopathy; these are primarily metabolized by peripheral muscle rather than the liver
        (5) Note that glutamine and cysteine are not stable (or present) in TPN solution
2. Lipids
    a. Linoleic acid
        (1) Essential fatty acid (need 7%-12% of total calories supplied as linoleic acid)
        (2) ω-6 polyunsaturated, long-chain fatty acid (immunosuppressive)
        (3) Precursor to membrane arachidonic acid
    b. ω-3 polyunsaturated fatty acids (PUFA)
        (1) Fish oils and linolenic acid

    (2) Decrease production of dienoic prostaglandins (i.e., PGE_2), tumor necrosis factor, interleukin-1, and other proinflammatory cytokines

  c. Medium chain triglycerides

    (1) Good energy source

    (2) Water-soluble

    (3) Enter circulation via the GI tract

  d. Short-chain fatty acids (SCFA)

    (1) Examples: butyric and propionic acid

    (2) Major fuel for the gut (especially the colon)

    (3) Derived from metabolizable fiber

  e. High-fat formulas

    (1) If the patient is not overfed, these have little effect on CO_2 production (despite being marketed for decreasing the respiratory quotient [RQ])

    (2) Poor GI tolerance

3. Carbohydrates

  a. Starches and sugars are good for energy

  b. Fiber

    (1) Metabolizable fiber (i.e., pectin, guar) is converted to SCFA in the colon by bacteria

    (2) Bulk increases stool mass, softens stool, adds body to stool, and provides some stimulation of gut mass

4. Dietary nucleic acids may be important for immune function

12.7 MONITORING RESPONSES TO NUTRITIONAL SUPPORT

1. Visceral proteins

  a. Prealbumin

    (1) Half-life approximately 2 days

    (2) Normal range: 10-40 mg/dL

  b. Transferrin

    (1) Half-life approximately 8-9 days

    (2) Normal range: 160-355 mg/dL

  c. Albumin

    (1) Half-life approximately 20 days

    (2) Normal range: 3.2-5 mg/dL

2. Visceral protein levels are affected by nutritional intake as well as by the disease state (especially in the presence of inflammation)

3. Increasing levels of visceral proteins suggest that nutritional support is adequate

4. Nitrogen balance

  a. Determined from 12-24 hr urine collections and measurements of total urinary nitrogen (more accurate than total urea nitrogen) compared to total nitrogen intake

  b. May be inaccurate

    (1) In patients with renal failure

    (2) If urine is not correctly collected by the staff

    (3) If the patient has increased losses of nitrogen in stool or from wounds (e.g., burns)

   c. Nitrogen balance: protein intake (g/day)/6.25 − (total urinary nitrogen [g/day] + 2)

   d. Negative nitrogen balance is not necessarily detrimental over the short term (i.e., 1-2 weeks)

   e. Improvement in nitrogen balance suggests that nutritional support is adequate

   f. Be aware that nitrogen balance may improve as catabolism decreases despite inadequate nutritional support

5. Indirect calorimetry (metabolic cart)

   a. Measures oxygen consumption and CO_2 production for 15-30 min, estimates energy expenditure, then extrapolates to 24 hr

   b. Keep RQ <1 (values >1 suggest lipogenesis from excessive caloric intake; values of approximately 0.7 are found in starvation and reflect fat oxidation)

6. Other nutritional parameters not generally useful in the critically ill

   a. Weight

   b. Skin-fold thickness

   c. Delayed cutaneous hypersensitivity (DCH)

   d. Lymphocyte counts

12.8   NUTRITION FOR SPECIFIC DISEASE PROCESSES

1. Acute renal failure (ARF)

   a. Use intact protein or peptide formula with moderate fat

   b. Do not restrict protein; it is required for healing and other organ functions

   c. May limit fluid intake with double-strength formula (2 cal/ml)

   d. Watch K^+, Mg^{++}, Phosphorus levels

2. Hepatic failure

   a. Use intact protein or peptide formula

   b. Usually 1-1.2 g/kg/day of protein are needed to support repair and immune function

   c. BCAA may be of value if encephalopathy persists following the use of intact protein or peptide diets

3. Inflammatory bowel disease/pancreatitis

   a. Postpyloric enteral feeding of a peptide-based diet is usually well tolerated

   b. Enteral nutrition should be attempted before initiating TPN

4. Multiorgan failure

   a. Nutritional support is usually of marginal value

   b. Nutritional support needs to be started before organ failure develops

12.9   NASODUODENAL FEEDING TUBE PLACEMENT

1. Use in patients who do not tolerate oral or gastric feeding

2. Patients with abdominal surgery should have a tube placed during surgery under direct visualization

   a. Anesthesiologist inserts the tube into the stomach

   b. Surgeon locates the tube and directs it into the duodenum or jejunum

   c. Eliminates the need for confirmatory x-rays

    d. Allows immediate feeding upon admission into the ICU

    e. Feeding tubes may also be placed into the small bowel using a gastrostomy or jejunostomy

3. Tubes placed into the stomach will rarely (5%-15%) migrate spontaneously into the small bowel in critically ill patients (due to gastroparesis)

4. Bedside method

    a. Place the patient in the right lateral decubitus position (if possible)

    b. Lubricate the nostril with generic lubricant or 2% viscous lidocaine

    c. Insert 8-10 French small-bore feeding tube (containing wire stylet) into the nostril and gently advance through the nasopharynx into the esophagus and then into the stomach

    d. If resistance is met or the patient coughs, becomes agitated, or decreases oxygen saturation

      (1) Pull the tube back into the nasopharynx

      (2) Repeat step 3 and reinsert the tube into the stomach

      (3) Alternatively the position of the neck may be changed (slightly flex or extend) before re-attempting insertion

    e. Confirm the position of the tube in the stomach

      (1) Auscultate over the abdomen

      (2) Aspirate gastric contents (pH approximately 2-5 unless on H_2 blocker)

    f. Remove wire stylet and place a 45° bend approximately 1″ from the distal end of the wire

    g. Gently re-insert the wire stylet (it should not meet resistance)

    h. Slowly advance the tube while rotating in a clock-wise direction

    i. Check the position q 10-15 cm

      (1) Auscultation will reveal higher pitched sounds when the tube is in the pylorus and proximal small bowel

      (2) Bile may be aspirated from the tube in the small bowel

      (3) Bile/small bowel secretions have a pH of approximately 6-7

      (4) Abdominal x-ray

        (a) Can confirm small bowel location

        (b) May not be cost-effective

        (c) Will avoid feeding into the lung in rare cases of a misplaced feeding tube

5. With this bedside method the authors successfully place >90% of attempted small bowel tubes into the duodenum or jejunum (see references for more details)

6. Aggressive surgical and bedside placement allows the authors to feed enterally >97% of critically ill patients within 24-48 hr of admission into the ICU

7. If bedside placement is not possible, place the feeding tube into the small intestine using

    a. Endoscopy

    b. Fluoroscopy

12.10 RECOMMENDATIONS FOR TPN USE

a. Use *only* when enteral nutrition is not possible (e.g., short-gut syndrome, chylothorax)

    (1) Failure of the stomach to empty is not an indication for TPN but rather for a small bowel feeding tube

    (2) Most patients with diarrhea can be managed with enteral nutrition

b. Initial TPN orders may be based on recommendations in Tables 12-4 and 12-5

c. Overall TPN management is best performed by specially trained nutritional support teams

d. For more specifics, the reader is referred to entire texts written about TPN

12.11   APPROACH TO ENTERAL FEEDING

1. Initiate enteral nutritional support within 12-48 hr of admission to the ICU

2. The oral route is preferred (but frequently not possible)

3. The gastric route is the second choice and should be tried in most patients before placing a small bowel tube

4. Patients at high risk for aspiration or who have known gastric paresis should be fed with a small bowel tube

5. Do *not* dilute feeding formulas

6. Keep the head of the bed elevated 30° to decrease the risk of aspiration

7. Start feeding at 25-30 ml/hr and increase by 25 ml/hr q 1-4 hr as tolerated by gastric residuals (<150 ml) until caloric goal (25-30 kcal/kg/day) is achieved

8. If the protein goal is not achieved, use a formula with a higher protein:calorie ratio or add protein to the formula

9. Monitor gastric residuals q4hr

10. If the gastric residual is >150 ml, hold feeds for 2 hr and then resume

11. Feeds may be increased at a slower rate (i.e., approximately 10 ml/hr q 6-12 hr) but often this is not necessary

12. The goal for the rate of infusion should be met by the third day of therapy (frequently earlier)

13. Monitor nutritional response by measuring visceral protein levels

    a. Measure prealbumin and transferrin levels on day 1 and q3days thereafter during initial therapy

    b. Increasing levels suggest that the patient is receiving adequate nutritional support

    c. Levels usually normalize in 1-2 weeks if the disease process is controlled and nutritional support is adequate

    d. If levels fail to increase

        (1) Consider underlying infection, inflammation, or other disease processes

        (2) Re-evaluate the adequacy of nutritional support

        (3) Nitrogen balance and energy balance (i.e., indirect calorimetry) may be informative

        (4) Consult nutritional support service

14. Several flow diagrams (for specific patient populations and using enteral products currently on the authors' formulary) are given as examples

    a. For isolated head injury see Fig. 12-1

    b. For multitrauma, burns, sepsis, and abdominal surgery see Fig. 12-2

    c. For severe malnutrition see Fig. 12-3

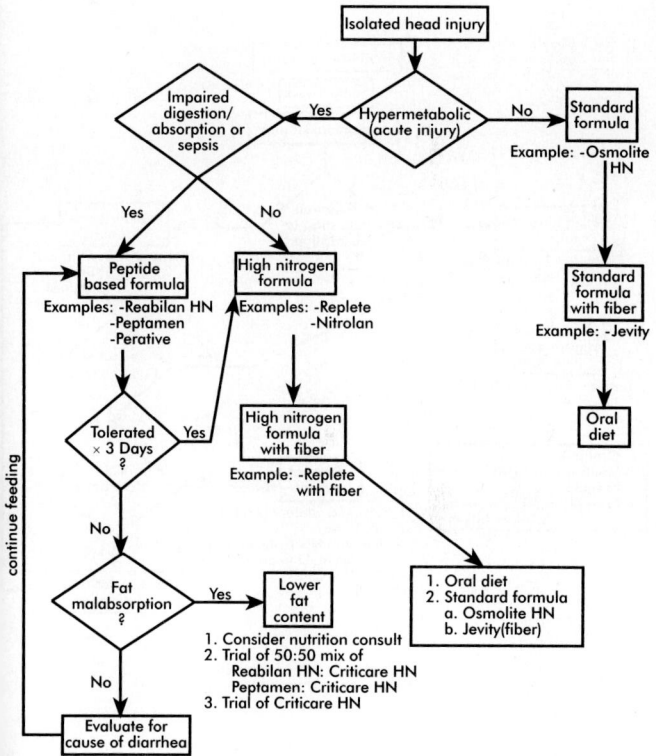

Figure 12-1
Flow diagram for nutritional support in patients with isolated head injury.

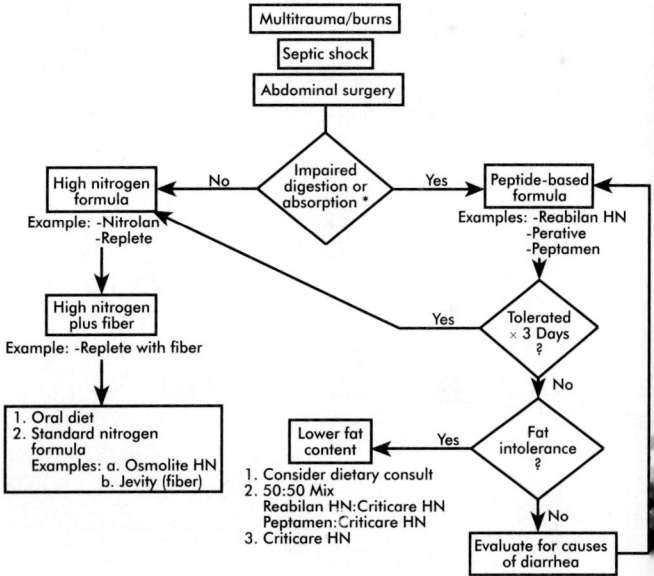

*Shock, resuscitation, major abdominal surgery, gut or
pancreatic injury, sepsis, acute hypoalbuminemia (<2g/dL)

Figure 12-2
Flow diagram for nutritional support in patients with multiple trauma, burn injury,
sepsis/septic shock, or abdominal surgery.

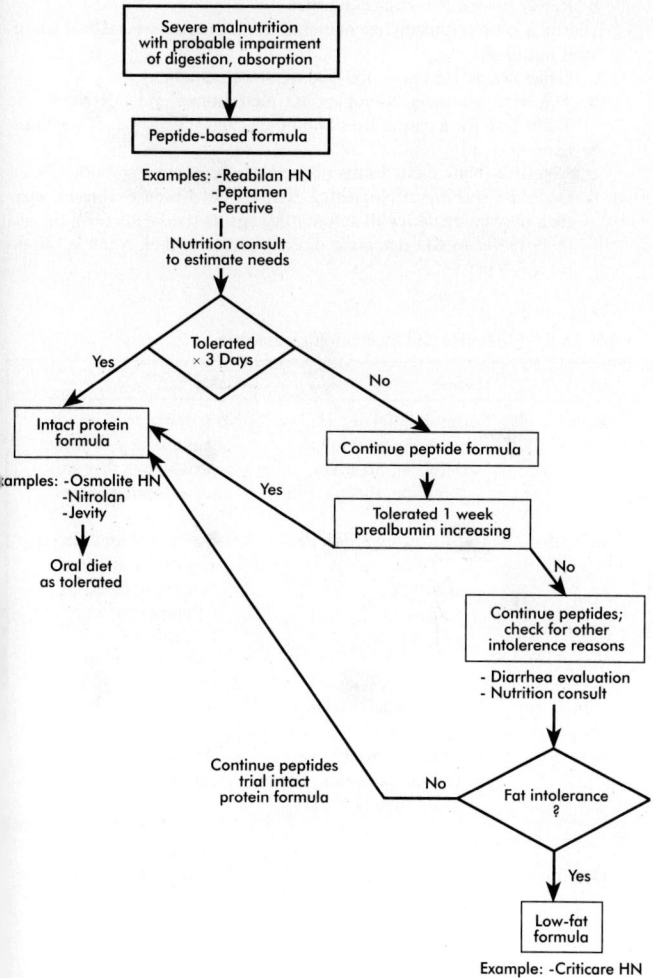

Figure 12-3
Flow diagram for nutritional support in patients with severe malnutrition.

15. If peptide-based diets are not available, use intact protein diets
16. Formula osmolality
    a. 300-600 mOsm/kg H_2O
    b. Rarely causes intolerance/diarrhea
17. Diarrhea is unfortunately encountered in patients on enteral and parenteral nutrition
    a. Generally defined as >300-500 ml stool output/day
    b. The most common etiologies are medications and infections (see Table 12-6 for a partial list of etiologies and suggestions for preliminary workup)
    c. Note that many elixir forms of medications contain sorbitol
    d. Once the specific etiologies of diarrhea have been evaluated, diarrhea may be treated with antimotility agents (i.e., narcotics); the authors prefer to add paregoric directly to the feeding formula (30-60 ml q 4-6 hr)

Table 12-6   Etiologies and evaluation of diarrhea

Causes	Examples	Workup
Drugs	Sorbitol, antacids, H_2 blockers, antibiotics, lactulose, laxatives, quinidine, theophylline	No specific workup; discontinue any of these medications that are not absolutely necessary
Infections	1. *Clostridium difficile*	1. Specific stool culture, *C. difficile* toxin assay, sigmoidoscopy/ colonoscopy for evidence of pseudomembranes
	2. Infectious diarrhea (e.g., typhoid fever, shigellosis)	2. Fecal leukocytes, culture
	3. Other: bacterial overgrowth, parasites, systemic infection, HIV	3. As relevant (e.g., look for ova and parasites although these rarely cause new diarrhea in the critically ill)
Osmotic		Measure stool osmotic gap* (SOG); SOG >100 suggests osmotic diarrhea
Impaction	May be secondary to narcotics	Rectal exam
Other causes	Inflammatory bowel disease, pancreatic insufficiency, short-gut syndrome	See other references for workup

*SOG: stool osmolality $- 2$ (stool $Na^+ + K^+$).

Selected readings

American College of Chest Physicians: Report of the consensus committee on nutrition in the ICU. *Chest* (in press).

American College of Physicians: Parenteral nutrition in patients receiving cancer chemotherapy. *Ann Intern Med* 1989; 110:734-6.

Bower RH: Nutrition during critical illness and sepsis. *New Horizons* 1993; 1:348-52.

Detsky AS, Barker JP, O'Rourke K, et al: Perioperative parenteral nutrition: a meta-analysis. *Ann Intern Med* 1987; 107:195-203.

Grant JP: *Handbook of total parenteral nutrition,* ed 2, Philadelphia, 1992, WB Saunders Company.

Kudsk KA, Croce MA, Fabian TC, et al: Enteral versus parenteral feeding: effects on septic morbidity after blunt and penetrating abdominal trauma. *Ann Surg* 1992; 215:503-11.

Moore F, Feliciano DV, Andrassy RJ, et al: Early enteral feeding, compared with parenteral, reduces postoperative septic complications: the results of a meta-analysis. *Ann Surg* 1992; 216:172-83.

Veterans Affairs Total Parenteral Nutrition Cooperative Study Group: Perioperative total parenteral nutrition in surgical patients. *N Engl J Med* 1991; 325:525-32.

Zaloga GP: Bedside method for placing small bowel feeding tubes in critically ill patients. *Chest* 1991; 100:1643-6.

Zaloga GP: *Nutrition and prevention of systemic infection.* In Taylor RW, Shoemaker WC, editors: *Critical care—state of the art,* Fullerton, CA, 1991, Society of Critical Care Medicine.

Zaloga GP, editor: *Nutrition in critical care,* St. Louis, 1994, Mosby–Year Book.

13

Oncologic
Critical Care

Luviza Santos, Cynthia Curioso, J. Gabriel Martinez, and

Arthur H. Combs

Enhanced critical care capabilities have contributed substantially to improved survival of cancer, the second leading cause of death in the United States. Critical care may be needed on a short-term basis for the complications of the underlying malignancy or for aggressive antineoplastic therapy. Postoperative critical care has greatly facilitated major extirpative cancer surgery as well as being an implicit part of other approaches such as bone marrow transplantation.

This chapter considers different types of cancer patients likely to need and benefit from treatment in the intensive care unit (ICU). Clinical judgement regarding the appropriate use of critical care services is required in all patient populations and the decision to admit and technologically support critically ill cancer patients should be individualized.

13.1 CENTRAL NERVOUS SYSTEM

Altered mental status

Alteration in mental status is the most common CNS presentation for cancer patients in the ICU. The common differential diagnoses are considered below. If these can be excluded, and the patient has not received excessive sedative or narcotic-analgesic agents, the patient should be treated presumptively for sepsis. Altered mental status is a reliable, though nonspecific, sign of sepsis, which carries a high mortality rate in cancer patients.

1. *Intracranial mass lesions:* A history of headache, nausea, vomiting, or seizure activity, with papilledema and other signs of raised intracranial pressure (ICP), suggests an intracranial mass lesion. A moderate increase in ICP alone is relatively well tolerated; however, when ICP becomes critical, brain substance shifts in the direction of least resistance with resultant herniation through the tentorium or foramen magnum

2. *Primary tumors of the CNS* present with focal neurologic signs depending on location

3. *Secondary (metastatic) tumors:* approximately 15%-30% present with

232

new-onset seizures. Common malignancies associated with cerebral metastases include breast, lung, kidney, and melanoma

4. *Cerebral hemorrhage* associated with acute promyelocytic leukemia, as a direct complication of brain metastases or related thrombocytopenia

5. *Subdural hematoma* presents with fluctuation in the level of consciousness and hemiparesis

6. *Brain abscess* accounts for 30% of CNS infections in cancer patients
   a. Clinically apparent raised ICP and neurologic deficits are late signs
   b. Usually presents with fever, headache, drowsiness, confusion, and seizures
   c. Typically seen in patients with leukemias or head and neck tumors

Other causes of altered mental status in critically ill cancer patients

1. Leptomeningeal metastases
   a. May present with signs of raised ICP and hydrocephalus
   b. Acute leukemias, lymphomas, and breast carcinomas are frequent causes

2. Cerebrovascular accident (CVA) commonly occurs in cancer patients. As in all patients, the CVA may be thrombotic, hemorrhagic, or embolic in nature
   a. Most patients present with focal neurologic signs and headaches
   b. Seizures are common, especially in hemorrhagic CVA
   c. Embolic CVA in cancer patients may be related to septic emboli, especially in patients with known fungal infection (e.g., aspergillosis)

3. Metabolic encephalopathies: Lethargy, weakness, somnolence, coma, agitation or psychosis, and focal or generalized seizures can all result from metabolic abnormalities. Lack of focal neurologic signs suggests a metabolic encephalopathy. Examples include
   a. Hypercalcemia (see below)
   b. Hyponatremia
   c. Hypomagnesemia
   d. Hypoglycemia
   e. Uremia

4. Seizures/postictal state: Primary and secondary tumors (especially hemispheric) commonly present with seizures
   a. Differential diagnosis includes CVA, CNS infection or narcotic withdrawal as causes
   b. In the immediate postictal period findings may include evidence of tongue biting, loss of bladder/bowel control, and extensor plantar responses
   c. The presence of lateralized focal signs suggests that seizures may have a focal origin
   d. Prolonged coma after a generalized seizure, or transient hemiparesis (Todd's paralysis) following a jacksonian, focal, or generalized seizure is more common in patients with seizures secondary to mass lesions than in those with seizures secondary to other conditions

5. Cerebral leukostasis: Patients with hyperleukocytosis (defined as a peripheral white blood cell count [WBC] count >100,000/mm^3) may

present with blurred vision, dizziness, ataxia, stupor, coma, or intracranial hemorrhage

  a. Hemorrhage results from leukostatic plugging of arterioles and capillaries with endothelial cell damage, capillary leak, and small-vessel disruption

  b. Retinal hemorrhages are suggestive of intracranial hemorrhage; thus, fundoscopic examination should be performed frequently

6. Hyperviscosity syndrome (HVS): Excessive elevations of serum paraproteins or marked leukocytosis can result in elevated serum viscosity, sludging, and decreased perfusion of the microcirculation with stasis. HVS can affect any organ system; however, characteristic clinical findings occur in the lungs and CNS

  a. Patients may present with visual disturbances or visual loss

  b. Characteristic retinopathy is present with venous engorgement ("sausage-link" or "boxcar" segmentation), microaneurysms, hemorrhages, exudates, and occasionally papilledema

  c. Similar vascular changes may be seen in the bulbar conjunctivae

  d. Other clinical findings may include headache, dizziness, jacksonian and generalized seizures, somnolence, lethargy, coma, and auditory disturbances (including hearing loss)

7. CNS infections: Patients with cancer are susceptible to a variety of CNS infections including meningitis, brain abscess (see above), and encephalitis

  a. Meningitis is most frequently encountered in patients with impaired cell-mediated immunity and is typically caused by *Cryptococcus neoformans* or *Listeria monocytogenes*

  b. Meningitis presents with fever, headache, and altered mental status

  c. All cancer patients with fever and altered mental status should have a lumbar puncture (LP) preceded by a head computed tomography (CT) scan (if a cerebral mass lesion is suspected)

  d. Encephalitis is most often caused by herpes viruses (simplex or zoster) or *Toxoplasma gondii*

  e. Patients with encephalitis commonly present with signs of meningeal irritation (fever, headache, nuchal rigidity) and evidence of altered mental status. Confusion may progress to stupor and coma; focal neurologic signs and seizures are common

Spinal cord compression. Significant cord compression results from epidural metastases and is most frequently seen in breast, lung, or prostate cancer with disseminated disease. Classically, the chief complaint is back pain (90% of patients) that may be associated with weakness, autonomic dysfunction, sensory disturbances, ataxia, and flexor spasms. The neurologic deficit is determined by the level of the involved spinal cord.

1. Compression from metastases typically arises from three locations

  a. Vertebral column (85%)

  b. Paravertebral spaces (10%-15%)

  c. Epidural space (rare)

2. The distribution throughout the spine is approximately

  a. Thoracic (70%)

  b. Lumbar (20%)

  c. Cervical (10%)

CNS diagnostic evaluation in the ICU

1. History, physical examination and careful neurologic evaluation emphasizing lateralizing signs, fundoscopy, and evidence of raised ICP
2. Laboratory should include
   a. Arterial blood gases (ABG)
   b. Serum electrolytes, glucose
   c. Calcium, magnesium, phosphorus
   d. Renal and hepatic function tests
   e. Determination of serum viscosity, especially in cases of multiple myeloma or other paraprotein-producing tumors
3. Head CT is the diagnostic test of choice for mass lesions, midline shift, intracranial hemorrhage, or hydrocephalus
4. Magnetic resonance imaging (MRI) is a sensitive test to detect intracerebral metastases and to differentiate between vascular and tumor-related masses. It is also the examination of choice for the evaluation of intramedullary, intradural, and extramedullary spine lesions
5. Myelography provides an indirect image of the spinal cord and nerve roots from the foramen magnum to the sacrum. It is the "gold standard" in the evaluation of spinal cord involvement by tumor
6. LP is most useful for the diagnosis of meningeal carcinomatosis, CNS leukemia, and CNS infections

CNS acute management in the ICU (see also Chapter 11)

1. Raised ICP with impending herniation
   a. Glucocorticoid therapy improves neurologic deficits in 70% of patients with symptomatic brain metastases by reduction of vasogenic brain edema. An initial dose of 10 mg dexamethasone may be given intravenously, followed by 16 mg/day in 3 or 4 divided doses by the most appropriate route. Patients who do not respond to the standard dosage may improve when the dosage is increased to 100 mg/day
   b. Initiate osmotherapy with agents such as urea or mannitol to produce rapid reduction of ICP in patients with known or suspected intracranial metastases showing signs of herniation.
      Mannitol 1.5-2 g/kg as a 20% solution can be administered by slow IV infusion. Total dosage should not exceed 120 g/day
   c. Hyperventilation may be instituted in patients who present with signs of brain herniation. These patients should be intubated expeditiously and ventilated to maintain an arterial P_{CO_2} of 25-30 torr
   d. Neurosurgical consultation is appropriate for in the majority of patients
2. Seizures
   a. Position patient laterally to prevent aspiration and protect the airway
   b. Correct any metabolic alteration or hypoxemia
   c. If the seizure is sustained, acute control is achieved with diazepam 5-10 mg IV, which may be repeated in 5-10 min up to 30 mg. Alternatively, lorazepam 1-10 mg IV or by continuous infusion can be used
   d. Long-term seizure control can usually be established with intravenous phenytoin. The loading dose is 15 mg/kg IV (50 mg/min)
   e. Treat intracerebral metastases with corticosteroids, chemotherapy, radiation, or surgery as indicated by the specific lesion

3. Spinal cord compression: palliation is generally accepted as a reasonable goal in the management of these patients
   a. Radiotherapy and surgical decompression are the cornerstones of management
   b. Chemotherapy with nitrogen mustard or cyclophosphamide has been effectively used, generally in combination with radiation, for the management of cord compression caused by lymphoma or Hodgkin's disease
4. Other modalities
   a. Leukophoresis is one of the therapeutic options for severe symptomatic leukocytosis with leukostasis
   b. Manage hydrocephalus by emergent relief and shunting
   c. Radiotherapy is currently the most commonly employed therapeutic modality for palliation of cerebral metastases
5. General supportive care
   a. Stress ulcer prophylaxis in the form of antacids, sucralfate, or H_2-receptor antagonists
   b. Deep venous thrombosis (DVT) prophylaxis should include (if no contraindication exists) the use of subcutaneous heparin and/or the use of sequential compressive devices (SCDs) on the lower extremities
   c. Provide nutrition for repletion of malnourished patients and for maintenance of good nutrition in patients at risk for malnutrition due to cancer or its therapy
   d. Appropriate antimicrobial therapy (see below)

13.2 PULMONARY

The lungs are commonly involved in cancer patients with 75-90% of pulmonary complications being secondary to infection. Noninfectious complications include those due to chemotherapy (e.g., bleomycin), thoracic irradiation, and pulmonary resections. Respiratory failure in cancer patients requiring mechanical ventilation is associated with a 75% mortality rate.

Pulmonary infiltrates:
In patients with systemic cancer, the differential diagnosis of pulmonary infiltrates seen on a routine chest film is extensive.
1. Localized infiltrates that are confined to a lobe or segment in a patient with a compatible history most frequently represent a bacterial process
2. Diffuse bilateral infiltrates are suggestive of opportunistic infection, treatment-induced lung injury, or lymphangitic spread of carcinoma
3. Bilateral perihilar infiltrates suggest a diagnosis of fluid overload in patients who have rapidly gained weight
4. Pulmonary infiltrates following bone marrow transplantation
   a. Life-threatening infections generally occur within the first 100 days post-transplant
   b. Within the initial 30 days the most common pathogens for pneumonia are bacterial or fungal
   c. Interstitial pneumonia (diffuse nonbacterial pneumonia) is the predominant problem following transplantation with the syndrome consisting of dyspnea, nonproductive cough, hypoxemia, diffuse bilateral infiltrates, and occurrence 30-100 days after transplant

e. Cytomegalovirus (CMV) pneumonia comprises the majority of interstitial pneumonitis. The incidence of CMV infection appears to be related to the loss of immunity during pretransplant conditioning and to the development of graft-versus-host disease

Diagnosis

1. Chest X-ray (CXR) is never diagnostic of any single entity
2. Routinely obtain cultures of sputum and special stains of tracheobronchial secretions (KOH, India ink). Colonization of the upper respiratory tract as well as the inadequacy of sputum production may make identification of the offending organism(s) difficult
3. Blood cultures for fungal and bacterial organisms
4. Viral titers (especially CMV)
5. Daily determination of serum lactate levels may be of some value for patients with respiratory failure. An increase in the serum lactate level may precede the deterioration of ABG and the development of diffuse infiltrates typical of adult or acute respiratory distress syndrome (ARDS)
6. Bronchoscopy with bronchoalveolar lavage has a diagnostic sensitivity of 80%-90% and is the procedure of choice in cancer patients with diffuse infiltrates
   a. Bronchoalveolar lavage is most helpful in diagnosing opportunistic infection (i.e., *Pneumocystis carinii,* viruses [CMV], fungus, and mycobacteria)
   b. This procedure is also useful for the diagnosis of intraparenchymatous pulmonary hemorrhage
   c. Bronchoalveolar lavage is safe in thrombocytopenic and mechanically ventilated patients who may not tolerate transbronchial biopsy
7. Open lung biopsy is reserved for selected patients due to its attendant morbidity, discomfort, and financial cost

Management

1. Early empiric use of broad-spectrum antibiotics (see Chapter 10)
2. Amphotericin B has been shown to reduce the mortality rate due to infection in patients who remain persistently febrile despite the use of antibiotics
3. Gancyclovir and hyperimmune globulin have recently been shown to improve survival in patients with interstitial pneumonia

Pulmonary leukostasis

Definition

Leukostasis, with obstructed flow in small pulmonary vessels, is the consequence of the intravascular accumulation of immature, rigid myeloblasts, observed predominantly in acute myelogenous leukemia (AML) and chronic myelogenous leukemia (CML) patients in blast phase. Vascular stasis and distention result in local hypoxia. The release of intracellular enzymes and procoagulants leads to vascular and pulmonary parenchymal damage.

1. Signs and symptoms: progressive dyspnea and/or altered mental status (see above discussion on CNS)
2. Diagnosis
   a. Complete blood cell count (CBC): WBC count is usually $>150,000$ cells/mm^3

b. ABGs: true hypoxemia develops as a result of impaired pulmonary gas exchange. Spurious low values for Pao_2 may be consistently obtained because the large number of blasts consume oxygen within the ABG specimen itself. The longer the interval between the collection and analysis, the lower the measured Pao_2. This may make assessment of gas exchange difficult

c. Pulse oximetry may be of benefit to follow the adequacy of arterial oxygenation

d. CXR may be normal or show diffuse nodular infiltrates

3. Management

a. Myeloblast counts $>50,000/mm^3$ warrant prompt treatment for reduction of the total WBC count to 20%-60% within hr of recognition of the syndrome

b. Leukophoresis

c. Chemotherapy (i.e., daunorubicin, cytosine arabinoside, hydroxyurea)

d. Adequate hydration

e. Initiate urate nephropathy prevention with allopurinol and urine alkalinization

f. Hemodynamic monitoring is suggested

g. When ARDS results from leukostasis, the following should be carried out expeditiously

(1) Fluid resuscitation to restore blood volume

(2) Optimize cardiac output and hemodynamics through volume enhancement and inotropic agents as needed

(3) Treat pulmonary vasoconstriction with a combination of volume expansion, inotropic agents, and supplemental O_2

(4) Monitor Do_2 and Vo_2 frequently and optimize to ≥ 600 ml $O_2/min/m^2$ and ≥ 150 ml/O_2/min/m^2 respectively

(5) Institute mechanical ventilation when needed to achieve normal pH, Pco_2, and Po_2 >60 on nontoxic FIo_2 (see Chapter 4)

Treatment-induced lung injury

Chemotherapy-induced lung injury

A large number of chemotherapeutic agents can produce pulmonary toxicity actively or delayed for years after therapy. Commonly used agents with known pulmonary toxicity include alkylating agents (i.e., cyclophosphamide, carmustine, chlorambucil, melphalan, busulfan), antimetabolites (i.e., methotrexate, azathioprine), antitumor antibiotics (i.e., bleomycin, mitomycin), and alkaloids (i.e., vincristine). Pulmonary toxicity may take the following forms:

1. Noncardiogenic pulmonary edema (ARDS)
2. Chronic pneumonitis and fibrosis
3. Hypersensitivity pneumonitis (i.e., procarbazine, methotrexate, bleomycin)

Radiation-induced lung toxicity
Definition
Radiation pneumonitis is a clinical syndrome of dyspnea, cough, and fever developing in association with indistinct, hazy pulmonary infiltrates that may

progress to dense alveolar consolidation following treatment with ionizing radiation.

1. The likelihood of developing radiation-induced lung injury is influenced by a number of variables including the total dosage, fractionation of doses, volume of lung irradiated, and history of prior irradiation and chemotherapy
2. Pathophysiology includes:
   a. Direct effect of ionizing particles on alveolar structure
   b. Generation of high-energy oxygen free radicals in excess of what normal enzymatic systems (e.g., peroxidase, superoxide dismutase) can remove
   c. Release of vasoactive substances such as histamine and bradykinin affect capillary permeability and pulmonary vascular resistance. The resultant pulmonary damage can exceed the area of radiation
3. 5%-15% of patients develop radiation pneumonitis
4. Symptoms may occur 1-6 months following completion of thoracic irradiation

13.3 CARDIOVASCULAR

Cardiac tamponade (see also Chapter 5)
Definition
Cardiac tamponade is a life-threatening condition caused by increased intrapericardial pressure resulting in limitation of ventricular diastolic filling and decreased stroke volume and cardiac output. Common etiologies in cancer patients include:

1. Metastatic tumors of the pericardium
   a. Much more commonly produce tamponade than primary tumors of the pericardium
   b. Cause tamponade by producing either effusions or constriction
   c. Cancer of the lungs and breast, lymphoma, leukemia, and melanoma, accounting for 80% of metastatic causes of cardiac tamponade
2. Primary tumors of the pericardium
3. Postirradiation pericarditis with fibrosis. The pericardium is the most frequent site injured by radiation. The latent period between radiotherapy and onset of clinical pericardial disease may be years
4. Encasement of the heart by the tumor

Clinical findings
1. Symptoms are often nonspecific but commonly include sensation of fullness in the chest, pericardial or interscapular pain, apprehension, dyspnea, and orthopnea
2. Clinical signs include altered mental status, hypotension, tachycardia, narrow arterial pulse pressure, distant heart tones with diminished apical impulse, tachypnea, oliguria, and diaphoresis. Other signs include
   a. Pulsus paradoxus
   b. Ewart's sign (area of dullness at angle of left scapula)
   c. Kussmaul's sign (neck veins bulge on inspiration)

Diagnosis
1. Clinical suspicion: the key to recognizing tamponade is considering the diagnosis

2. CXR
   a. Large globular heart shadow ("water bottle" configuration). If pericardial fluid is <250 ml, the cardiac silhouette may be normal
   b. Lung fields are usually clear
   c. Pleural effusions are common associated findings
3. Electrocardiogram (ECG)
   a. Sinus tachycardia
   b. Low voltage QRS (<5 mV)
   c. Electrical alternans results from the heart oscillating in the filled pericardial sac. Alternation of the QRS complexes is most specific for pericardial effusion
4. Echocardiography makes a quick and definitive diagnosis of tamponade. 2D echo is more sensitive than M-mode. Findings include
   a. Prolonged diastolic collapse or inversion of right atrial free wall
   b. Early diastolic collapse of the right ventricular free wall
   c. Effusions as small as 30 ml are detected early by echocardiography (seen as an echo-free space)
5. Pulmonary artery (PA) catheterization (Swan-Ganz)
   a. Elevated pulmonary capillary wedge and right atrial pressures with a prominent **x** descent with no significant **y** descent ("square root sign")
   b. Decreased cardiac output, stroke volume, systemic arterial pressure, and mixed venous oxygen saturation (SvO_2)
   c. Equalization of all pressures in diastole
6. MRI is also diagnostic, but is expensive and time-consuming compared with echocardiography
7. Diagnostic pericardiocentesis
   a. Cytology to detect presence of malignant cells.
   b. Gram's stain and acid-fast bacilli (AFB) smear, culture and sensitivity, cell count, and differential
   c. Protein, lactate dehydrogenase (LDH) content

Therapy
1. Perform therapeutic pericardiocentesis immediately in hemodynamically compromised patients
   a. 2D-echocardiography–guided pericardiocentesis is successful in 95% of cases with no major complications
   b. Reaccumulation of fluid is likely to occur in malignant effusions but can be prevented with chemical sclerosis (i.e., tetracycline), radiation therapy, or surgery (i.e., pleuropericardial window or pericardiectomy)

Myocardial tissue injury
Common etiologies in cancer patients
1. Anthracycline antibiotics (e.g., doxorubicin and daunorubicin)
2. Mitoxantrone: total dose of more than 100-140 mg/m^2 can cause congestive heart failure and exacerbate pre-existing anthracycline-induced cardiomyopathy
3. Cyclophosphamide: dosage of >100-120 mg/kg over 2 days can result in congestive heart failure and hemorrhagic myocarditis/pericarditis and necrosis
4. Busulfan: conventional oral daily dosage may cause endocardial fibrosis
5. Interferons: in conventional dosage may exacerbate underlying cardiac disease

6. Mitomycin C: standard dosage can cause myocardial damage
7. Radiation-induced cardiomyopathy causes a dose-dependent endocardial and myocardial fibrosis that can result in a restrictive cardiomyopathy

Diagnosis
1. Endomyocardial biopsy is valuable for establishing etiology of cardiac injury in patients who may have received chemotherapy and for detecting subclinical cardiac damage. The anthracyclines cause characteristic degenerative changes in the myocytes
2. ECG-gated blood pool scan for precise measurement of ejection fraction and detecting regional and global myocardial dysfunction

Therapy
Treatment is the same as for congestive cardiomyopathy of any cause. There is no specific therapy directed at radiation- or chemotherapy-induced myocardial damage.

Cardiac dysrhythmias

1. Etiology
   a. Anthracycline antibiotics cause dysrhythmias unrelated to the cumulative dosage that can be seen hours or days after administration. Commonly observed dysrhythmias include supraventricular tachycardia, complete heart block, and ventricular tachycardia. Doxorubicin may also prolong the QT interval
   b. Amacrine produces ventricular dysrhythmias
   c. Taxol causes bradycardia and, in combination with cisplatin, may produce ventricular tachycardia
2. Diagnosis and treatment are the same as for rhythm disturbances of other etiologies

Superior vena cava syndrome

1. Etiology: ablation of blood flow from the superior vena cava (SVC) to the right atrium caused by extravascular compression or intravascular obstruction
   a. 95% of cases are secondary to extrinsic compression of the SVC by mediastinal malignancy (3% from benign disease)
   b. The most common tumors are bronchogenic carcinoma of small-cell type (48%) and lymphoma (21%)
2. Clinical manifestations
   a. Dyspnea aggravated by lying supine or leaning forward
   b. Tachypnea and signs of airway obstruction
   c. Signs and symptoms of increased ICP (i.e, dizziness, headache, visual disturbance, seizure, altered mental status)
   d. Dysphagia, hoarseness
   e. Neck vein distention, facial plethora, and edema
   f. Numerous, dilated, vertically oriented, and tortuous cutaneous venules or veins above the rib cage margin
   g. Upper-body edema with cyanosis and ruddy complexion
   h. Immediate causes of death are airway obstruction and intracranial hemorrhage. Thrombosis at the SVC may occur in 30% of these patients
3. Diagnosis
   a. Clinical suspicion

    b. CT scan with IV contrast is the diagnostic procedure of choice

    c. Transesophageal echocardiography is a safe bedside procedure excellent for evaluating the SVC and surrounding structures

    d. Angiography and radionuclide venography help to localize the obstruction

4. Therapy

    a. Symptomatic relief is the rule

    b. Operative bypass relieves symptoms faster than radiation and is indicated in patients with life-threatening respiratory compromise or advanced cerebral edema

    c. Radiation therapy is the mainstay of treatment for most malignant SVC obstructions, although in small-cell carcinoma and lymphomas chemotherapy is particularly useful

    d. Temporizing measures may be used in patients without significant airway or neurologic compromise. These include corticosteroids to decrease cerebral and laryngeal edema, diuretics, and elevation of the head

    e. Anticoagulation has no definitive role

13.4   GASTROENTEROLOGY

Neutropenic enterocolitis (ileocecal syndrome)

1. Incidence: commonly occurs in patients with hematologic malignancies (leukemia is the most common, with an incidence of 10%-40%) receiving chemotherapy

2. Pathophysiology: results from mucosal ulceration and necrosis of the ileum, cecum, or ascending colon with overgrowth and mural invasion by bacteria and/or fungi. Thrombocytopenia may predispose to hemorrhage into the bowel wall. Typically presents on the seventh day of severe neutropenia

3. Clinical manifestations

    a. Abdominal distention

    b. Right-sided abdominal tenderness

    c. Watery diarrhea

    d. Fever

    e. Thrombocytopenia and neutropenia

4. Diagnosis

    a. Clinical suspicion

    b. Plain radiographs of the abdomen may show ileus with distended cecum and pneumatosis coli

    c. CT of the abdomen: thickened bowel wall containing air

    d. Sigmoidoscopy

5. Differential diagnosis

    a. Appendicitis

    b. Pseudomembranous colitis

    c. Diverticulitis

    d. Other acute abdominal disorders

6. Medical therapy

    a. Nutritional support

    b. Nasogastric suction

  c. Broad-spectrum antibiotics with anaerobic, gram-negative, and *C. difficile* coverage
7. Surgical exploration is indicated for
  a. Perforation
  b. Severe bleeding
  c. Abscess
  d. Uncontrolled sepsis
  e. Failure to improve after 2-3 days of intensive conservative management

Gastrointestinal (GI) tract hemorrhage and perforation

1. GI hemorrhage
  a. The most common cause is hemorrhagic gastritis (32%-48%) followed by peptic ulcer disease
  b. Only 12%-17% bleeding is from the tumor per se (most commonly seen in GI lymphomas)
  c. Less common causes include esophageal varices, Mallory-Weiss tears, *Candida* esophagitis, and enteritis
2. Perforation: lymphomas are the most common malignancies to perforate during chemotherapy
3. Diagnosis: standard diagnostic workup to identify the source of bleeding with emphasis on endoscopy
4. Therapy
  a. Surgical
  b. Temporizing modalities to control bleeding include
    (1) Angiography, with or without vasopressin or embolization
    (2) Endoscopic intervention
    (3) These modalities may also be useful in patients with carcinomatosis and previously unresectable disease

13.5 | RENAL/METABOLIC

Many cancer patients develop metabolic abnormalities caused by tumor-produced factors (hormones or locally acting substances) or from tumor destruction by antineoplastic therapy.

Hypercalcemia

1. Causes of hypercalcemia in cancer patients
  a. Secondary to malignancy: 4%
  b. Etiologies other than the malignancy: 77%
  c. With coexistent hyperparathyroidism: 2%
  d. Vitamin D intoxication: 16%
  e. Idiopathic
2. Hypercalcemia is the most common metabolic abnormality of cancer patients (10%)
3. May occur with or without bone metastases
4. Breast cancer is associated with hypercalcemia in 27%-35% of patients. Mechanisms include widespread osteolytic metastases, production of parathormone-like hormone, PGE_2 (following hormonal therapy with estrogens or anti-estrogens), humoral osteoclast activating factor, and co-existing primary hyperparathyroidism

5. Lung cancer is associated with hypercalcemia in 12.5%-35% of patients. Frequently seen in squamous cell carcinoma and rarely in small-cell carcinoma. May occur early or late, with or without bone metastases. Mechanisms include production of osteoclast activating factor, transforming growth factor alpha, interleukin-1, and tumor necrosis factor

6. Multiple myeloma produces hypercalcemia in 20%-40% of patients. Hypercalcemia develops secondary to extensive osteolytic bone destruction, osteoclast activating factor, and lymphotoxin. 50% develop renal insufficiency that can aggravate the hypercalcemia

7. Lymphoma causes hypercalcemia by humoral mediation and local bone destruction

8. Head and neck malignancies have a 6% incidence of hypercalcemia that is humorally mediated. Hypercalcemia is associated with malignancies of the oropharynx (37%), hypopharynx (24.3%), and tongue (21.5%)

9. Squamous cell, transitional cell, bladder, renal, and ovarian carcinomas may also produce humoral hypercalcemia

Clinical presentation

1. Severity of illness depends on the degree of hypercalcemia, concurrent illness or debility, age, and associated metabolic disturbances

2. Hypercalcemia of malignancy usually has a rapid onset

3. Neuromuscular manifestations often predominate and include lethargy, confusion, stupor, and coma (occurs when serum calcium level is >13 mg/dL). Hallucinations and psychosis, weakness, and decreased deep tendon reflexes (DTRs) are also common

4. Cardiovascular manifestations include increased cardiac contractility, increased sensitivity to digitalis, and dysrhythmias

5. Renal manifestations include polyuria and polydipsia (earliest symptoms), dehydration, decreased glomerular filtration, loss of urinary concentrating ability, and renal insufficiency

6. GI signs and symptoms include nausea and vomiting, anorexia, obstipation/constipation, ileus, and abdominal pain

7. Skeletal involvement is the hallmark of hypercalcemia from osteolytic metastases or humorally mediated bone resorption resulting in pain, pathologic fractures, deformities, or necrosis

Diagnosis

1. Laboratory studies
   a. Total and ionized serum calcium
   b. Electrolytes, blood urea nitrogen (BUN), creatinine
   c. Serum phosphorus and alkaline phosphatase
   d. Measures of urinary calcium and cAMP (excretion)
   e. High alkaline phosphatase level

2. Radiologic studies
   a. Radionuclide bone scan
   b. Skeletal surveys
   c. Baseline CXR

3. Perform ECG to look for characteristic changes including prolonged PR and QRS intervals and shortened QT

Treatment

Hypercalcemia is often fatal if left untreated, especially when symptomatic or if serum calcium is >13 mg/dL. Treatment goals include promoting urinary calcium excretion, inhibiting bone resorption, and reducing entry of calcium into the extracellular fluid compartment.

1. Hydration to restore intravascular volume and increase the urinary output
   a. Initially 5-8 L of normal saline IV over the first 24 hr; then, adequate IV fluids to maintain a urine output of 3-4 L/day
   b. Monitor electrolytes during normal saline infusion
   c. Monitor urine output and cardiac status to avoid fluid overload
2. Loop diuretics (e.g., furosemide) promote calciuresis by blocking calcium reabsorption in the ascending loop of Henle and augment the calciuretic effect of normal saline
   a. Furosemide in doses of 40-80 mg IV may be given after adequate hydration
   b. Monitor electrolytes and urine output to avoid overdiuresis
3. Promptly initiate inhibitors of bone resorption in symptomatic hypercalcemia
   a. Mithramycin is an antitumor antibiotic with a direct toxic effect on osteoclasts. Usual dose is 25 mcg/kg IV over 6 hr. It generally decreases serum calcium within 6-48 hr; may be repeated if there is no response within 2 days. Restrict use to emergency treatment of severe hypercalcemia. Complications include thrombocytopenia, myelosuppression, hypotension, and hepatic and renal toxicity
   b. Disodium etidronate (EHDP) is an analog of pyrophosphate that blocks osteoclastic bone resorption and formation of bone crystals. Dosage: 7.5 mg/kg/day in 250 ml saline infused over 2-6 hr for 3-7 days, followed by 20 mg/kg/day PO. Onset of action is slow with normocalcemia achieved in 4-7 days 75% of the time. Contraindicated in patients with renal failure
   c. Glucocorticoids (e.g., prednisone) are most effective in hematologic malignancies (especially multiple myeloma) and breast carcinoma; they are of little value in solid tumors. These agents lower serum calcium by inhibition of calcium absorption and the action of vitamin D. Prednisone in a dosage of 1-2 mg/kg/day has an onset of action in 3-5 days. Adverse effects include GI bleeding, hyperglycemia, and osteopenia
   d. Calcitonin inhibits osteoclastic bone resorption and enhances calcium excretion. Dosage: 4-8 IU/kg q6hr IM or SQ. It may lower calcium by 2-3 mg/dl over 2-3 hours. Adverse reactions include nausea and vomiting, flushing, and hypersensitivity reactions (initial skin testing is recommended before administration)
4. Hemodialysis is useful in patients who present with renal failure or who are unable to be treated with normal saline diuresis
5. Initiate specific antineoplastic therapy in patients for whom treatment exists. It is the most effective means of achieving long-term correction of cancer-related hypercalcemia

Tumor lysis syndrome

Seen when cytotoxic chemotherapy induces rapid tumor cell lysis in patients with a large malignant cell burden of an exquisitely chemosensitive tumor.

Intracellular metabolites are released in quantities that exceed the excretory capacity of the kidneys.

1. Classically occurs in patients with Burkitt's and non-Hodgkin's lymphomas, acute lymphoblastic and nonlymphoblastic leukemias, and chronic myelogenous leukemia
2. May occur spontaneously in patients with lymphomas and leukemias or following treatment with chemotherapy, radiation, glucocorticoids, tamoxifen, and/or interferon

Manifestations

1. Related to metabolic abnormalities
   a. Hyperkalemia: generalized weakness, irritability, decreased DTRs, paresthesias, paralysis, cardiac dysrhythmias, and cardiac arrest. The classic ECG changes include peaked T waves, diminished R waves progressing to widened QRS, prolonged PR, loss of P wave, sine wave pattern as terminal event
   b. Hypocalcemia (related to hyperphosphatemia): muscle spasms, carpopedal spasms, facial grimacing, laryngeal spasm, irritability, depression, psychosis; intestinal cramps, chronic malabsorption; and seizures and respiratory arrest. Chvostek's and Trousseau's signs are present in some patients. ECG reveals prolonged QT interval
   c. Hyperuricemia: gouty arthritis, nephrolithiasis, and urate nephropathy
2. Precipitation of calcium salts in tissues
3. Acute renal failure

Prevention and treatment (see Box on p.247.)

1. To prevent acute renal failure, patients who are to undergo treatment for malignancies should receive
   a. Vigorous IV hydration, often with diuretics or renal dose dopamine to ensure adequate urine output
   b. Alkalinization of the urine during the first 1-2 days of cytotoxic therapy to increase the solubility of uric acid
   c. Allopurinol to decrease the formation of uric acid

Other common metabolic abnormalities in cancer patients

1. Syndrome of inappropriate antidiuretic hormone secretion (SIADH). See Chapter 6.
   a. Occurs in 1%-2 % of cancer patients
   b. Common in small-cell carcinoma of the lungs as well as prostatic, pancreatic, ureteric, and bladder carcinomas
   c. Occasionally seen in lymphomas and leukemias
2. Hypoglycemia
   a. Insulinomas: insulin-secreting, benign, islet cell tumors
   b. Non–islet cell tumors (i.e., mesothelioma, fibrosarcoma, hemangiopericytoma, hepatoma, adrenocortical carcinoma, leukemia and lymphoma, pseudomyxoma, pheochromocytoma, anaplastic carcinoma)

13.6   **HEMATOLOGY**

Cancer itself, antineoplastic therapy, and the acute conditions that occur in cancer patients all result in hematologic abnormalities. Red blood cells, white blood cells, platelets, and coagulation factors may all be adversely affected

Management of Patients at Risk for Tumor Lysis Syndrome

When No Metabolic Aberration Exists

1. Allopurinol 500 mg/m^2 BSA/day; reduce to 200 mg/m^2 BSA/day 3 days into chemotherapy
2. Hydration 3000 ml/m^2 BSA/day
3. Chemotherapy initiated within 24-48 hr of admission
4. Monitor electrolytes, BUN, creatinine, uric acid, calcium, phosphorus q12-14hr

When Metabolic Aberration Exists

1. Allopurinol initiated as above, reduce dose if hyperuricemia is controlled, reduce dosage for renal insufficiency
2. Hydration as above, add nonthiazide diuretics as needed
3. Urinary alkalinization (urine pH >7)
   - Sodium bicarbonate 100 mEq/L IV solution initially; adjust as needed
   - Discontinue when uric acid is normal
4. Chemotherapy postponed until uric acid is controlled or dialysis begun
5. Monitor same studies, q 6-12 hr until stable (at least 3-5 days)
6. Replace calcium as Ca^{++} gluconate by slow IV infusion for symptomatic hypocalcemia or severe ECG changes
7. Treat hyperkalemia with exchange resins, bicarbonate

Criteria for Hemodialysis in Patients Unresponsive to the Above Measures

1. Serum potassium ≥6 mEq/L
2. Serum uric acid ≥20 mg/dL
3. Serum phosphorus rapidly rising or ≥10 mg/dL
4. Fluid overload
5. Symptomatic hypocalcemia

quantitatively, qualitatively, or both. Bleeding and infection are the primary life-threatening events in critically ill cancer patients, and they are both the cause and result of hematologic abnormalities. An extensive discussion of these entities can be found in Chapter 9.

13.7 CHEMOTHERAPY-INDUCED HYPERSENSITIVITY REACTIONS

Etiology and presentation

1. Asparaginase has the highest incidence of hypersensitivity reactions (6%-43%). The incidence is higher when the drug is given intravenously and as a single agent. Common manifestations include
   a. Hypotension or hypertension
   b. Laryngospasm, respiratory distress
   c. Agitation

    d. Facial edema

    e. Reactions can be life-threatening and are more likely to occur after 2 or more weeks of treatment

2. Cisplatin is the second most common antineoplastic agent that causes hypersensitivity reactions (1%-20%). Potentially fatal reactions occur in 5% of patients

3. Alkylating agents are a much less common cause of hypersensitivity reactions

    a. Melphalan causes anaphylactic reactions in approximately 2%-3% of patients

    b. Bleomycin causes febrile illness in 20%-25% of patients, and in some cases progresses to a life-threatening syndrome (confusion, chills, respiratory distress, hypotension). It is seen especially when administered IV to lymphoma patients

    c. Doxorubicin may also cause anaphylaxis

Therapy

1. Severe reactions

    a. Stop the antineoplastic drug infusion immediately

    b. Epinephrine: 0.5-0.75 ml (1:1000 in 10 ml normal saline) IV push q 5-15 min

    c. Aminophylline for acute bronchospasm

    d. Diphenhydramine (or other antihistaminic agent) 25-50 mg IV

    e. Hydrocortisone: 500 mg IV initially and repeated q6hr for prolonged reactions

13.8   IMMUNE COMPROMISE

The patient with cancer (especially while undergoing chemotherapy) must be considered an immunocompromised host. A number of immune defects are recognized in these patients:

1. Defects in cellular and humoral immunity

    a. T-lymphocyte mononuclear phagocyte defect: Hodgkin's disease, lymphoma, cytotoxic chemotherapy

    b. Decreased or absent B-cell function in patients with multiple myeloma, chronic lymphocytic leukemia

2. Neutropenia

    a. Most common immunologic defect in patients with neoplastic diseases

    b. Risk for bacteremia and fungal infection with absolute neutrophil counts (ANC) <1000/mm^3

    c. Most common cause is myelotoxic chemotherapy; also seen with leukemia, aplastic anemia, drug reactions, and when the bone marrow is destroyed by tumor or radiation

3. Disruption of the integument or mucosal surfaces

    a. Diagnostic procedures entailing skin puncture and biopsies

    b. Invasive procedures such as the placement of indwelling central venous and pulmonary artery catheters, urinary catheters, and endotracheal tubes

    c. Loss of the physical, chemical, and immunologic barrier functions of the gut lining

4. Hyposplenism or postsplenectomy states
    a. Decreased host responses to infections from encapsulated organisms such as *S. pneumoniae*, *H. influenzae* and *N. meningitidis*

Clinical evaluation

1. Pay careful attention to the patient's history of antineoplastic therapies
2. Investigate recurring infections, exposure to contagious diseases, and recent travel
3. Thoroughly investigate the presence of fever without an obvious source by evaluating
    a. Blood, urine, and sputum
    b. Indwelling catheters
    c. Surgical or other skin wounds
    d. Cerebrospinal fluid (CSF)
    e. Stool
    f. Possibility of undrained collections and abscesses
4. Skin lesions should be inspected carefully. *Ecthyma gangrenosum* is a characteristic skin lesion associated with bacterial and fungal sepsis
5. The oral cavity is another potential source in immunocompromised hosts. Sinusitis and periodontitis may be sources, especially in orotracheally or nasotracheally intubated patients and in those with nasogastric tubes
6. Fundoscopic examination is essential for detection of fungal infection, especially in patients with central venous and urinary catheters
7. Perianal lesions may cause severe infection
8. Panculture is indicated in all febrile patients. Remove and replace all indwelling vascular appliances

The diagnosis and treatment of specific infections in the immunocompromised host is covered in Chapter 10.

Selected readings

Attie M: Treatment of hypercalcemia. *Endocrinol Metab Clin North Am* 1989; 18:807.

Ayala K, Chandrasekaran K, Karalis DG et al: Diagnosis of superior vena caval obstruction by transesophageal echocardiography. *Chest* 1992; 101:874-6.

Bajorunas D: Clinical manifestations of cancer-related hypercalcemia. *Semin Oncol* 1990; 17(suppl):16-25.

Callahan JA, Seward JB, Nishimura RA et al: Two-dimensional echocardiographically guided pericardiocentesis: experience in 117 consecutive patients. *Am J Cardiol* 1985; 55:476-9.

Cohen LF, Balow JE, Magrath IT et al: Acute tumor lysis syndrome: a review of 37 patients with Burkitt's lymphoma. *Am J Med* 1980; 68:486.

Hildebrand FL, Rosenow EC, Habermann TM et al: Pulmonary complications of leukemia. *Chest* 1990; 5:1233-9.

Howland W, Carlon GC: *Acute respiratory failure in cancer patients.* In Howland W, Carlon GC, editors: *Critical care of the cancer patient.* Chicago, 1985, Year Book Medical Publishers.

Kiehm T: Bacteremia and fungemia in the immunocompromised patient. *Eur J Clin Microbial Infect Dis* 1989; 8:832-7.

Lazarus HM, Creger RJ, Gerson SL: Infectious emergencies in cancer patients. *Semin Oncol* 1989; 16:543-60.

Pruitt A: Central nervous system infections in cancer patients. *Neurol Clin* 1991; 9:867-88.

Ritch P: Treatment of calcium-related hypercalcemia. *Semin Oncol* 1990; 2:26-33.

Rosen A, Reichert N, Lieberman Y: Superior vena cava syndrome: the myth—the facts. *Am Rev Respir Dis* 1990; 141:114-8.

Rosenberg A, Brown A: Infection in cancer patients. *Dis Mon* 1993; 39:510-69.

Schneider SM, Distelhorst CW: Chemotherapy-induced emergencies. *Semin Oncol* 1989; 16:572-8.

Silverman P, Distelhorst CW: Metabolic emergencies in clinical oncology. *Semin Oncol* 1989; 16:504-15.

Spain RC, Whittlesey D: Respiratory emergencies in patients with cancer. *Semin Oncol* 1989; 16:471-89.

Stellato TA, Shenk RR: Gastrointestinal emergencies in the oncology patient. *Semin Oncol* 1989; 16:521-31.

Whimbey E, Kiehn TE, Brannon P, et al: Bacteremia and fungemia in patients with neoplastic disease. *Am J Med* 1987; 82:723-30.

Pregnancy

14

Robert J. Carpenter, Jr.

Many patients presenting to an intensive care facility are pregnant, have diseases peculiar to pregnancy, and need critical care support. Others, however, have underlying medical diseases (see the Box below), some of which require consideration of the passenger (fetus) who has created many changes in maternal physiology. The hormonal milieu created by the placenta—progesterone and, to a lesser extent, estrogen—is responsible for the multifaceted changes in system function.

One change seen early in pregnancy is in pulmonary function. Fig. 14-1 shows the changes in graphic form while Table 14-1 depicts the modifications. The kidney is another organ system with significant change. Table 14-2 reflects the serial changes in function. The Box on p. 254 demonstrates the differential risk of both acquired and congenital heart disease during pregnancy.

Since many books on obstetrical critical care have been published and a full review of the many changes and diseases is beyond the scope of this chapter, a disease process that reflects the complexity of the severely ill gravida within the intensive care unit (ICU) has been chosen.

Preexistent Medical Diseases*

Asthma
Cardiac disease, New York Heart Association class III/IV
   Prosthetic valve replacements
   Critical mitral stenosis
   Aortic stenosis
   Eisenmenger's syndrome
Cystic fibrosis
Diabetes mellitus (insulin-dependent)
Chronic renal failure
Hypertension
Renal, hepatic, cardiac transplants
Systemic lupus erythematosus
Thyrotoxicosis / thyroid storm

---

*Treatment of these conditions during pregnancy should remain unchanged.

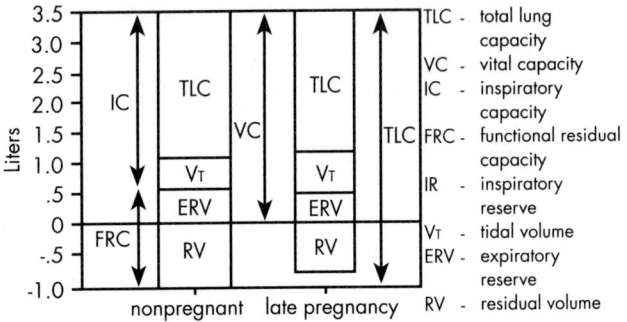

Figure 14-1
Lung volumes in nonpregnant women and in pregnant women.

Table 14-1 Lung volumes and capacities in pregnancy

	Definition	Change in Pregnancy
Respiratory rate (RR)	Number of breaths per min (bpm)	Unchanged
Vital capacity (VC)	Maximum amount of air that can be forcibly expired after maximum inspiration (IC + ERV)	Unchanged
Inspiratory capacity (IC)	Maximum amount of air that can be inspired from resting expiratory level (TV + IRV)	Increased 5%
Tidal volume (VT)	Amount of air inspired and expired with normal breath	Increased 30%-40%
Inspiratory reserve volume (IRV)	Maximum amount of air that can be inspired at end of normal inspiration	Unchanged
Functional residual capacity (FRC)	Amount of air in lungs at resting expiratory level (ERV + RV)	Decreased 20%
Expiratory reserve volume (ERV)	Maximum amount of air that can be expired from resting expiratory level	Decreased 20%
Residual volume (RV)	Amount of air in lungs after maximum expiration	Decreased 20%
Total lung capacity (TLC)	Total amount of air in lungs at maximal inspiration (VC + RV)	Decreased 5%

From Cruikshank DP, Hays PM: *Maternal physiology in pregnancy.* In Gabbe SG, Niebyl JR, Simpson JL, editors: *Obstetrics: normal and problem pregnancies,* ed 2, New York, 1991, Churchill Livingstone.

Table 14-2 Serial changes in renal hemodynamics

	Seated Position ($N = 25$)				Left Lateral Recumbent Position ($N = 17$)	
	Nonpregnant	16 wk	26 wk	36 wk	29 wk	37 wk
Effective renal plasma flow (ml/min)	480 ±72	840 ±145	891 279	771 ±175	748 ±85	677 ±82
Glomerular filtration rate (ml/min)	99 ±18	149 ±17	152 ±18	150 ±32	145 ±19	138 ±22
Filtration fraction	0.21	0.18	0.18	0.20	0.19	0.21

From Cruikshank DP, Hays PM; *Maternal physiology in pregnancy.* In Gabbe SG, Niebyl JR, Simpson JL, editors: *Obstetrics: normal and problem pregnancies,* ed 2, New York, 1991, Churchill Livingstone.

Table 14-3 Hemodynamic changes of pregnancy

Parameter	Change
Cardiac output	Increases 30%-40%
Heart rate	Increase 10-15 BPM
Stroke volume	Increases
Blood volume	Increases 30%-40%
Systemic blood pressure	Decreases
Pulse pressure	Increases
Systemic resistance	Decreases
Pulmonary artery pressure	No change
Pulmonary resistance	Decreases
Myocardial function	Improves

Table 14-4 Hemodynamic effects of labor and delivery

Parameter	Effect
Cardiac output	Increases with contractions
Blood volume	Increases
Heart rate	Variable
Peripheral resistance	No change
Systemic artery pressure	Increases

Pregnancy Risk with Cardiac Disease

Category 1: Low Risk During Pregnancy

Small left-to-right shunts
Pulmonary stenosis <50 mm Hg gradient
Mild mitral/aortic insufficiency
Mild aortic stenosis
Mitral valve prolapse
Rheumatic fever or endocarditis history
Postoperative patients, normal hemodynamics

Category 2: Moderate Risk During Pregnancy

Large left-to-right shunts, low pulmonary pressure
Moderate pulmonary stenosis
Aortic stenosis (30-60 mm Hg gradient)
Mild hypertrophic cardiomyopathy
Cardiac valve prosthesis
Mild mitral stenosis
Palliated cyanotic heart disease
Moderate aortic/mitral regurgitation

Category 3: High Risk During Pregnancy

Large left-to-right shunts, mild pulmonary hypertension
Severe aortic/pulmonary stenosis
Mild mitral stenosis with atrial fibrillation
Moderate mitral stenosis
Cardiomyopathy in early stages
Moderate to severe idiopathic hypertrophic subaortic stenosis (IHSS)
Cyanotic congenital heart disease, unoperated
Mild Epstein's disease
Postcardiac surgery, mild residual problems

Category 4: Pregnancy Contraindicated

Congestive heart failure
Pulmonary hypertension
Eisenmenger's syndrome
Severe cyanosis
Advanced coronary artery disease
Marfan syndrome

Hemodynamic changes during pregnancy and maternal physiologic changes occurring during labor should be kept in mind (see Tables 14-3 and 14-4).

14-1   PREGNANCY-INDUCED HYPERTENSION (PIH)

Definition

The presence of elevated blood pressure (BP) with evidence of end-organ dysfunction, most commonly seen as edema and proteinuria. The Box on p.255 presents many of the synonyms for this process. The classification of preeclampsia (PIH) is depicted in Table 14-5.

Etiology

No causative agent has been isolated for the development of preeclampsia (PIH). It is most commonly believed to be an end product of antigen-antibody interaction with abnormal ratios of vasoactive agents such as prostacyclins and thromboxanes. The relationship of other agents such as lipid peroxides is under active investigation. Regardless of the exact etiology, the process reflects a diffuse systemic endothelial dysfunction intimately associated with platelet dysfunction. This is seen in the classic HELLP (hemolysis, elevated liver enzymes, low platelets) syndrome in which many organ systems have reflected the disease and, without assiduous management, severe maternal morbidity or mortality may occur. The top Box on p. 257 reflects the panorama of disease manifestations. The center Box on p. 257 depicts those subsets of pregnant women at greatest risk for the disease process. The bottom Box on p. 257 presents the frequency of preeclampsia in the highest risk populations.

Patients with prior PIH who have underlying chronic hypertension have a 50%-75% probability of developing PIH in pregnancy. No method exists to predict the severity or to time the onset of the PIH process.

Approach to the preeclamptic patient

1. Obtain patient history
   a. Current gestational age (LMP [last menstrual period])
   b. Past medical history: renal or chronic hypertensive diseases, systemic lupus erythematosus (SLE)
   c. Family history of preeclampsia/eclampsia
   d. Symptoms of disease
      (1) Headache, blurred vision, and scotomas
      (2) Blindness and diplopia
      (3) Weight gain >2 lbs/week
      (4) RUQ pain, epigastric pain, and diffuse abdominal pain (ruptured liver)
      (5) Tetanic contractions *(abruptio placentae)*
      (6) Nausea and emesis
      (7) Unconsciousness or seizure activity
      (8) Vaginal bleeding
      (9) Fetal movement

Table 14-5   Classification of preeclampsia

	Mild	Severe*
Blood pressure	130/80 to 140/95	>160/110 mm Hg
Absolute	Systolic ≥140 mm Hg Diastolic ≥90 mm Hg	
Relative	Systolic increased >30 mm Hg Diastolic increased >15 mm Hg	
Clinical findings	1+ edema	3-4+ edema
	Normal reflexes	3-4+ reflexes
	No visual symptoms	Scotomas/papilledema, diplopia
		May have seizures, altered consciousness
		Severe headaches
		Severe right upper quadrant abdominal pain or tenderness
		HELLP*
		Congestive heart failure
		Pulmonary edema
		Oliguria <400 cc/24hrs
Weight		>5 pounds/week
Lab		
Proteinuria	≥300 mg/24 hr	≥5 g/day; 3+/4+ semi-quantitative
Platelets	Normal	May be <150,000
Liver function	Normal	Elevated asparate aminotransferase (AST)/ alanine aminotransferase (ALT)
Clotting studies	Normal	May be prolonged
Bilirubin	Normal	May be elevated
Anticonvulsants	Intrapartum: yes	Antepartum: yes Intrapartum: yes
Abdominal pain	Absent	May be present in epigastrium or right upper quadrant

*HELLP syndrome reflected by hemolysis, elevated liver enzymes, and low platelet count comprises the greatest risk group for mortality and morbidity.

Synonyms for Pregnancy-Induced Hypertension

Toxemia of pregnancy
PIH
Preeclampsia
Eclampsia
Peripartum hypertension
Edema, proteinuria, hypertension (EPH) gestosis

Pregnancy-Induced Hypertension: Associated Complications

Hypertensive crisis
Pulmonary edema: acute respiratory distress syndrome (ARDS)
Eclampsia
Intracranial hemorrhage
Amaurosis
Cerebral edema
Acute renal failure
Cortical necrosis
Ruptured liver
Microangiopathic hemolytic anemia
Thrombocytopenia
Disseminated intravascular coagulation (DIC)
HELLP syndrome

Factors Associated with PIH

Nulligravida
Prior preeclampsia/eclampsia
Family history preeclampsia/eclampsia
Multifetal pregnancies
Molar pregnancies
Hydrops fetalis (any etiology)
Chronic hypertension/renal disease
Diabetes mellitus (insulin-dependent)

Frequency of Preeclampsia

7% of all pregnancies
  70% nulligravidas
  30% multigravidas

Twins	30%
Molar pregnancies	up to 70%
Hydrops fetalis	up to 50%
Diabetes mellitus	up to 50%
Chronic hypertension	20%
Prior severe PIH	up to 50%

2. Physical examination
   a. Maternal BP,* pulse, and respiratory rate
   b. Fetal heart rate (FHR) by continuous electronic monitoring
   c. Extensive cardiopulmonary examination
   d. Eyes: scleral icterus, ecchymoses, and petechiae
   e. Fundoscopic examination, retinal artery spasm, papilledema, and hemorrhages (acute vasospasm is often seen; arteries may be only 50% diameter of veins)
   f. Abdominal examination
      (1) Upper quadrant tenderness
      (2) Uterus size, tone, soft, noncontracting, or rigid contracting
      (3) Distention: is there suggestion of ascites?
   g. Extremities/face: evidence of pathologic edema
   h. Pelvic examination: cervical softness, dilatation, position effacement, and fetal presentation
   i. Patellar reflexes: persistent clonus reflects central nervous system (CNS) hyperactivity and significant potential for seizure activity
3. Laboratory evaluation
   a. Type/Rhesus blood factor (Rh), indirect Coombs', rapid plasma reagin (RPR), hepatitis B surface antigen (HB_sAg), and rubella (if not previously obtained)
   b. Complete blood cell count (CBC), platelets, microscopic examination
   c. Blood urea nitrogen (BUN), creatinine, AST, ALT, glucose, electrolytes, uric acid

---

*Note that BP may be taken in both supine and lateral positions. Arm elevation when the patient is turned to the lateral decubitus results in a fall in BP commensurate with the distance in centimeters above the atrial level roughly 13.6 mm Hg/10 cm of hydrostatic pressure. This change in pressure is frequently suggested to be the "real" blood pressure. A patient may then be considered normal when in fact hypertension exists. Table 14-6 reflects these changes in the best study done in normal pregnant patients. (Mean arterial pressure [MAP] is unchanged.)

Remember that because of the vasodilation of pregnancy and decreased systemic vascular resistance (SVR), patients, especially teenagers, with BPs of <140/90 may be significantly hypertensive.

Table 14-6 Hemodynamic alterations in response to position change late in third trimester of pregnancy

Hemodynamic Parameter	Left Lateral	Supine	Sitting	Standing
MAP (mm Hg)	90 ± 6	90 + 8	90 ± 8	91 ± 14
Cardiac output (L/min)	6.6 ± 1.4	6.0 ± 1.4*	6.2 ± 2.05	4 ± 2.0*
Pulse (bpm)	82 ± 10	84 ± 10	91 ± 11	107 ± 17*
Systemic vascular resistance (dyne/cm/sec^{-5})	1210 ± 266	1437 ± 338	1217 ± 254	1319 ± 394
Pulmonary vascular resistance (dyne/cm/sec^{-5})	76 ± 16	101 ± 45	102 ± 35	117 ± 35*
Pulmonary capillary wedge pressure (mm Hg)	8 ± 2	6 ± 3	4 ± 4	4 ± 2
Central venous pressure (mm Hg)	4 ± 3	3 ± 2	1 ± 1	1 ± 2
Left ventricular stroke word index (g/m/m²/beat)	43 ± 9	40 ± 9	44 ± 5	34 ± 7*

*Pulse < 0.05, compared with left lateral position.
Modified from Clark SL, Cotton DB, Pivarnik JM, et al: Position change and central hemodynamic profile during normal third-trimester pregnancy and postpartum, *Am J Obstet Gynecol* 1991; 164:883-7.

    d. Coagulation studies: prothrombin time (PT), partial thromboplastin time (PTT), fibrinogen, Fibrin split products (FSPs)
    e. Plasma oncotic pressure (COP) decreases in pregnancy secondary to hemodilution (see Table 14-7)
    f. Urinalysis with rapid screen for proteinuria in ICU
    g. Chest x-ray (CXR) only if pulmonary symptoms or physical examination suggests the need
    h. Obstetrical ultrasound (in ICU) for fetal age and number, estimated fetal weight, position of fetus(s), and placental position
    i. Continuous FHR monitoring
    j. 24-hr urine collection for creatinine clearance and protein excretion

Table 14-7   Colloid osmotic pressure

Nonpregnant	28 mm Hg
Pregnant: term	23 mm Hg
Postpartum	17 mm Hg
Preeclampsia (PIH)	13.7 mm Hg

Table 14-8   Magnesium toxicity

Manifestations	Level (mEq/L)
Loss of patellar reflex	(8-12 mEq/L)
Feeling of warmth, flushing	(9-12 mEq/L)
Somnolence	(10-12 mEq/L)
Slurred speech	(10-12 mEq/L
Muscular paralysis	(15-17 mEq/L)
Respiratory difficulty	(15-17 mEq/L)
Cardiac arrest	(30-35 mEq/L)

Modified from Sibai, BM: Preeclampsia-eclampsia: valid treatment approached, *Contemporary OB/GYN* 1990; 35:84-100.

Medical therapy

1. The presentation of a patient with PIH may range from a mild to a life-threatening disease process. The process can be ended only by delivery. The decision to continue or to deliver the pregnancy is made by consultation between medical and obstetrical personnel

2. A true rule is that the disease may rapidly progress. Follow-up of all maternal and fetal biophysical parameters on a routine basis is required. The frequency will be determined by the severity of disease

3. Most preeclamptic patients have vasoconstriction and hemoconcentration. After initial therapy, volume expansion and hemodilution occur

4. Magnesium sulfate ($MgSO_4$) is considered the standard therapy as a prophylaxis for seizure activity. The loading dose is 4-6 g $MgSO_4 \cdot 7H_2O$ in 100 cc D5 0.25 normal saline over 15-20 min. A constant infusion of 1-2 g $MgSO_4$/hr is maintained depending on urine output and reflex activity, which are checked on a q1hr basis. Table 14-8 lists the potential effects of the magnesium ion and the average serum level at which they may occur. When $MgSO_4$ is infused, normally both a Buretrol and an infusion pump are used to enhance patient safety, thus preventing a massive infusion of $MgSO_4$ that could cause maternal death or severe morbidity

5. Detailed intake and output (I&O) records must be maintained. Since renal function is frequently impaired, an increase in total body water can result in pulmonary edema. In rare cases, if hyponatremia is allowed to occur, cerebral edema may be observed

6. Post-delivery I&O must be assiduously maintained to prevent hypovolemia and renal hypoperfusion

---

Acquired Obstetrical Disease That May Require Invasive Hemodynamic Monitoring

Amniotic fluid embolism
Hemorrhagic shock
   Abruptio placentae
   Placenta previa
   Abdominal pregnancy
Pneumonias
   Viral
   Bacterial
Septic shock
Chorioamnionitis
Pyelonephritis
Septic abortion

---

7. Even in mild disease, diplopia may indicate the development of cerebral edema. Standard therapy with mannitol plus or minus furosemide (Lasix®) may be used (see Chapter 11). Nimodipine, a specific cerebral Ca^{++} channel blocker, may be given 30-60 mg PO q6hr with substantial improvement in cerebral autoregulation

8. Severe pulmonary edema and ARDS may occur in preeclamptic patients as in any other acutely ill patient. Indications for ventilator support are unchanged in this population (see also Chapter 15)

9. Disseminated intravascular coagulation, especially associated with the HELLP syndrome, may require extensive blood product transfusion. In preeclampsia, because of vasoconstriction and the increased risk of pulmonary edema, cryoprecipitate is often preferred to fresh frozen plasma (FFP). This reduces the volume of infused blood products. **Note:** There is a higher risk of hepatitis with increasing number of donor exposures

10. When platelets and FFP are required, it is always advisable to use *jumbo* packs of each to decrease multiple donor exposure

11. Swan-Ganz catheter: invasive pulmonary artery catheter monitoring is sometimes required with preeclampsia, especially when complicated by abruptio placentae, hemorrhage, and ARDS/pulmonary edema. Knowledge of the hemodynamic changes in pregnancy is required in the selection of therapy (see Tables 14-3 and 14-4)

12. A Swan-Ganz catheter may also be required in other obstetrical disorders

13. Development of seizures (eclampsia) may occur pre or post treatment with $MgSO_4$. If pre-therapy, 4 g of $MgSO_4$ (8 cc of $MgSO_4 \cdot 7H_2O$ - 50% solution) may be rapidly infused. If post-treatment, a second dose of $MgSO_4$ may be given; or some physicians choose to give diazepam, 2.5-5 mg as an IV push as the agent of choice. If the patient does not awaken and become responsive within 60 min, then the possibility of an intracranial hemorrhage must be considered and worked up (see Chapter 11)

14. Pulse oximeters and recording dynamaps may be used in many patients. If any concern for an atypical or severe manifestation of PIH is present, an arterial pressure catheter should be placed. Repetitive lab studies can be drawn and continuous BP recording can be achieved
15. Interactive dialogue among all members of the health care team will achieve optimum outcome for both mother and child

Major complications of preeclampsia/eclampsia

1. Hypertensive crises
   a. BP > 200 systolic or 120 diastolic
   b. May be associated with pulmonary edema, intracranial hemorrhage, or cerebral edema
   c. Rapid critical treatment (see Table 14-9): an acute reduction of elevated BP should initially be limited to a 20% reduction in MAP. A more substantial reduction may create severe uteroplacental hypoperfusion and precipitate acute fetal death or asphyxia. This is especially true if the diastolic BP is acutely dropped to 90 mm Hg or less
   d. These patients frequently warrant placement of invasive monitoring systems such as pulmonary artery catheters and peripheral arterial cannulas
2. CEREBRAL EDEMA
   a. Initiate fluid restriction
   b. Instigate monitoring
   c. IV mannitol 1-2 g/kg of a 20% solution (100 qms) of mannitol in 500cc of D_5W given over 10-20 min followed by a maintenance dosage of 50-300 mg/kg IV q6hr is effective; the serum osmolality should *not* be allowed to exceed 330-340 mOsm
   d. Complications of the use of osmotic agents include
      (1) Osmotic diuresis with dehydration and hypernatremia
      (2) Rebound increase in intracranial pressure
      (3) Acute volume expansion
   e. Nimodipine, a new calcium channel blocker, has been found to be very effective in cases of subarachnoid hemorrhage associated with cerebral edema to decrease death and permanent neurologic damage. A dosage of 60 mg PO q 4-6 hr may be given. It can be given via a nasogastric tube if required
   f. If the patient is intubated, hyperventilation may be used (see Chapter 11)
3. HEPATIC RUPTURE
   a. Massive intraabdominal hemorrhage results with the need for
      (1) Massive blood volume support
      (2) Correction of DIC
      (3) Invasive cardiovascular monitoring
   b. Instigate exploration and surgical repair when "stable" patient present Repeat procedures are frequently necessary (see Fig. 14-2). Because of liver dysfunction/damage, packing of rupture site is often accomplished
   c. Potential for automatic cell saver at operation can reduce total transfusion requirements

Table 11-5 Antihypertensive drugs in pregnancy

Drug	Onset of Action	Duration	Dosage	Mechanism	Side Effects
Methyldopa	3-6 hr	7-16 hr	IV 250-500 mg q6hr PO 250-500 mg q6-8 hr	Vasodilation	Sedation, dry mouth, nasal congestion, occasional depression, postural Coombs' + hemolytic anemia reflex
Hydralazine	15-20 min	3-6 hr	5-10 mg q30min	Direct smooth muscle relaxation	Reflex tachycardia Headache
Nicardipine*	1-5 min	3-6 hr	IV drip 2 mg/hr, increase by 2 mg/hr each hr; maximum dosage 10 mg/hr	Vasodilation Ca$^+$ channel blocker	Headache, nausea, vomiting, hypotension
Nifedipine†	1-5 min	3-5 hr	10 mg capsule sublingual 10-20 mg PO, q6hr	Vasodilation Ca^{++} channel blocker	Headache, palpitations, fluid retention Potential for respiratory failure when used with MgSO$_4$ Potential for neuromuscular blockage or potential other drug effects
Labetalol	5-10 min	3-6 hr	20 mg by slow IV injection over 2 min. May repeat dose q10-15 min to achieve desired pressure. Maximum dosage 300 mg	Beta-blocker 7:1 vasodilator Ratio of beta-blocker to alpha blocker (7:1) with IV administration	Hypotension, dizziness, fatigue, nausea, bronchoconstriction in some patients with asthma Fetal side effects may include bradycardia, poor temperature control, hypoglycemia, and decreased short-term variability

Continued.

Table 14-9 cont'd   Antihypertensive drugs in pregnancy

Drug	Onset of Action	Duration	Dosage	Mechanism	Side Effects
Sodium Nitroprusside	Immediate	<3 min	50 mg/500 ml D5W Rate of 0.2-0.8 mcg/kg/min Titrate to desired BP (light sensitive). Average of 3 mcg/kg/min will usually decrease pressure to desired value	Vasodilation	Nausea, severe hypotension if not closely watched, thiocyanate toxicity (even when required antepartum, cyanide poisoning does not usually occur)
Trimethaphan	Immediate	10-15 min	500 mg/500 ml D5W Titrate to desired BP	Ganglionic blocker	Tachycardia, severe hypotension if not carefully titrated Cycloplegia Tachyphylaxis Potential for neuromuscular blockage when >6 mg/min infusion rate May prolong effect time of other neuromuscular blocking drugs

*Newer agent, effective, but not much data in pregnancy.

†Perforate or crush capsule; patient may chew capsule to release contents.

WARNING: Ca++ channel blockers, when used with MgSO₄, may create profound cardiac dysfunction and hypotension!

‡A reduction of 20% in MAP should be maximal initial target. Following maternal and fetal response to therapy, further decrease in MAP may be desired.

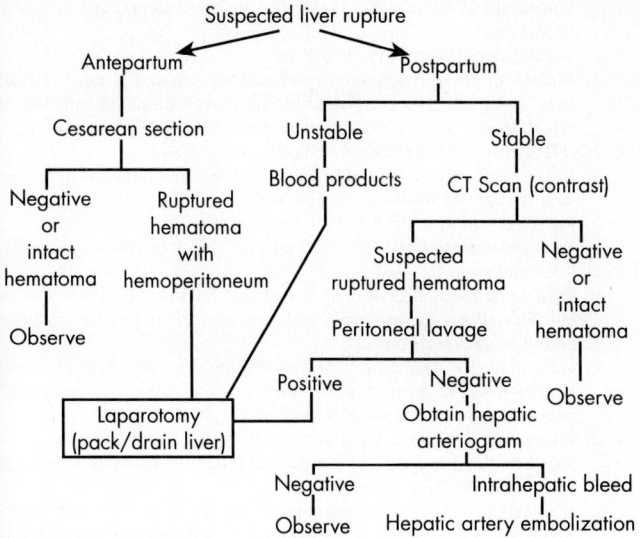

Figure 14-2
Algorithm for management of hepatic capsular rupture and hemorrhage during pregnancy.

4. ABRUPTIO PLACENTAE
   a. Frequently associated with fetal distress
   b. Often accompanied by coagulopathy with prolonged PT, PTT, low fibrinogen, and low platelet count
   c. Vigorous/massive transfusion support may be required
   d. Four major complications of hypovolemia and shock in these patients are
      (1) Acute tubular necrosis
      (2) Cortical renal necrosis
      (3) Sheehan's syndrome with acute pituitary insufficiency
      (4) **ARDS!** This has been a major cause of death in the authors' OB ICU

14-2   THERAPEUTIC MODALITIES

1. Magnesium sulfate
   a. Distribution of extracellular space, bones, and intracellular space
   b. Unbound to protein
   c. Excretion by kidney, filtered load excretes T_{max} for reabsorption in most patients treated
   d. Excretion half-life is approximately 4 hr
   e. When used in normal patients for treatment of preterm labor, the earliest manifestation of excessive Ca^{++} antagonism is the ocular symp-

    tom of visual disturbance (blurring of vision, diplopia, and difficulty in focusing)

  f. $MgSO_4$ does not usually change BP

  g. Measurements of magnesium levels can be achieved in most clinical labs. There is a poor correlation between levels observed and clinical effect; therefore, no precise level can be stated to be therapeutic

2. ANTIHYPERTENSIVE THERAPY: (see Table 14-9)

  a. In most circumstances, drug therapy in pregnancy-induced hypertension is reserved for those patients with

    (1) Persistent systolic BP >180 mm Hg or

    (2) Persistent diastolic BP >110 mm Hg (105 mm Hg in some institutions)

  b. Prior to delivery, it is desired to maintain the diastolic BP >90 mm Hg. This allows for continued perfusion pressure to provide adequate uteroplacental perfusion

  c. If diastolic BP decreases <90 mm Hg, the decreased uteroplacental perfusion will frequently precipitate acute fetal distress that may progess to an in utero death or to perinatal asphyxia

  d. Postdelivery, an acute, rapid decrease in BP usually means substantial blood loss and *not* cure of the disease process. Likewise, a nadir of 90 mm Hg diastolic BP is desired

  e. Medical control of hypertension is often required only for a short period (usually days). No study has ever demonstrated a beneficial long-term outcome with prolonged antihypertensive therapy

  f. The use of calcium channel blockers in a setting of $MgSO_4$ therapy should be considered a significant therapeutic step that may create an adverse impact on cardiovascular function; therefore, an intensive care setting with knowledgeable personnel (internal medicine, OB/GYN maternal fetal medicine, or OB anesthesia) capable of responding to these problems should be present

| 14.3 | AMNIOTIC FLUID EMBOLISM

Definition

Vascular transfer of amniotic fluid containing lanugo hairs, vernix, meconium, and thromboplastic substances to pulmonary circulation. This is a rare (1 in 8000 pregnancies) event that is catastrophic and often associated with death.

1. Unpreventable; most frequent in second stage of labor
2. Mortality rate (80%), 25% of deaths occur in the first 60 min post-event
3. Old animal models of disease are not applicable to human pathology

Clinical presentation

Sudden onset of maternal distress

1. Severe dyspnea, bronchospasm, and tachypnea
2. Tachycardia, hypotension, and arrhythmias
3. Cyanosis; severe hypoxia
4. Acute cardiovascular collapse; often cardiac arrest

5. Disseminated intravascular coagulation
6. Seizures and coma

Risk factors

1. Multiple pregnancy
2. Large fetuses
3. Short, tumultuous labors
4. Oxytocin (Pitocin) administration
5. Late rupture of membranes with unengaged presenting part

Symptoms

1. Restlessness
2. Sweating
3. Anxiety
4. Coughing
5. Air hunger

Pathophysiology

1. Pulmonary hypertension; decreased cardiac output
2. Cor pulmonale with pulmonary edema
3. Severe hypoxemia and tissue hypoxia
4. If acute respiratory distress allows survival, thromboplastins yield DIC
5. Swan-Ganz data reveal predominant left heart failure/dysfunction: $2°$ to hypoxic injury

Differential diagnosis

1. Acute pulmonary embolism
2. Air embolism
3. Myocardial infarction
4. Acute aspiration of gastric contents
5. Massive pneumothorax (uni/bilateral)
6. Reaction to local anesthetic

Acute treatment

1. Place endotracheal tube
2. Mechanical ventilation/positive end expiratory pressure (PEEP)
3. Volume support with or without blood products
4. Peripheral and pulmonary arterial catheterization
5. Monitor central venous pressure
6. No specific drug therapy; vasopressors and/or bronchodilators of choice

Hemodynamic observations in humans

1. Mild to moderate increase in pulmonary artery pressure
2. Variable increase in central venous pressure
3. Elevated pulmonary capillary wedge pressure

Selected readings

Barton JR, Hiett AK, Conover WB: The use of nifedipine during the postpartum period in patients with severe preeclampsia. *Am J Obstet Gynecol* 1990; 162:788-92.
Barton JR, Rogers RC, Wilson DA, et al: Nifedipine pharmacokinetics and pharmaco-

dynamics during the postpartum period in patients with preeclampsia. *Am J Obstet Gynecol* 1991; 165-:951-4.

Barton JR, Sibai BM: Acute life-threatening emergencies in preeclampsia-eclampsia. *Clin Obstet Gynecol* 1992; 35:402-13.

Belfort MA, Carpenter RJ, Moise KJ et al: The use of nimodipine in a patient with eclampsia: color Doppler demonstration of retinal artery relaxation. *Am J Obstet Gynecol* 1993; 169:204-6.

Berkowitz RL, editor: *Critical care of the obstetric patient,* New York, 1983, Churchill Livingstone.

Carbonne B, Jannet D, Touboul C et al: Nicardipine treatment of hypertension during pregnancy. *Obstet Gynecol* 1993; 81:908-14.

Clark SL, Cotton DB, Hankins GDV et al, editors: *Critical care obstetrics,* ed 2, Boston, 1992, Blackwell Scientific Publications.

Clark SL, Cotton DB, Lee W, et al: Central hemodynamic assessment of normal term pregnancy. *Am J Obstet Gynecol* 1989 161:1439-1442.

Clark SL, Cotton DB, Pivarnik JM et al: Position change and central hemodynamic profile during normal third-trimester pregnancy and postpartum. *Am J Obstet Gynecol* 1991; 164:883-7.

Cunningham FG: *Hypertension disorder in pregnancy.* In *Williams obstetrics,* ed 19, Norwalk, Connecticut, 1993, Appleton & Lange.

Cunningham FG, Lindheimer MD: Hypertension in pregnancy. *N Eng J Med* 1992; 326:927-32.

Diaz JH: *Perinatal anesthesia and critical care,* Philadelphia, 1991, WB Saunders.

Donaldson JO: *Eclampsia.* In Sir John Walton, editor: *Neurology of Pregnancy,* ed 2, London, 1991, WB Saunders.

Dunn R, Lee W, Cotton DB: Evaluation by computerized axial tomography of eclamptic women with seizures refractory of magnesium sulfate therapy. *Am J Obstet Gynecol,* 1986, 155:267-8.

James FM III, Wheeler AS, Dewar DM: *Obstetric anesthesia: the complicated patient,* ed 2, Philadelphia, 1988, FA Davis.

Mabie WC, Gonzalez AR, Sibai BM et al: A comparative trial of labetalol and hydralazine in the acute management of severe hypertension complicating pregnancy. *Obstet Gynecol* 1987; 70:328-33.

Management of Preeclampsia, *American College of Obstetrics and Gynecology Technical Bulletin #91* 1986.

Richards AM, Moodley J, Graham DI et al: Active management of the unconscious eclamptic patient. *Br J Obstet Gynaecol* 1986, 93:554-62.

Roberts JM, Redman CWG: Pre-eclampsia: more than pregnancy-induced hypertension. *Lancet,* 1993; 341:1447-54.

Ryan G, MB, Lange IR, Naugler MA: Clinical experience with phenytoin prophylaxis in severe preeclampsia. *Am J Obstet Gynecol* 1989; 161:1297-1304.

Hypertension in Pregnancy, In Sibai Baha M, editor: *Clinics in perinatology, Vol 18, 4 December 1991* Philadelphia, WB Saunders.

In Sibai Baha M, editor: Hypertension in pregnancy, *Clin Obst Gynecol* Vol 35(2):315-436 1992.

Sibai BM: The HELLP syndrome (hemolysis, elevated liver enzymes, and low platelets): much ado about nothing? *Am J Obstet Gynecol* 1990; 162:311-16.

Sibai BM: Magnesium sulfate is the ideal anticonvulsant in preeclampsia-eclampsia. *Am J Obstet Gynecol* 1990; 162:1141-5.

Sibai BM: Preeclampsia - eclampsia. *Current Problems in Obstetrics, Gynecology, and Infertility* 1990; 13:3-45, 1990.

Sibai BM, Akl S, Fairlie F et al: A protocol for managing severe preeclampsia in the second trimester. *Am J Obstet Gynecol* 1990; 163:733-8.

Smith LG, Moise KJ, Dildy GA III et al: Spontaneous rupture of liver during pregnancy: current therapeutic modalities. *Obstet Gynecol* 1991; 77:171-5.

Pulmonary
Disorders

15

Mauricio A. Reinoso

15.1 **CHRONIC OBSTRUCTIVE PULMONARY DISEASE (COPD)**

1. Definition

A disorder characterized by expiratory flow limitation that does not change markedly over a period of several months of observation. The term *COPD* includes:

a. Chronic bronchitis: clinical diagnosis made when chronic cough with sputum production is present on most days for at least 3 months of the year for at least 2 consecutive years. Major pathologic findings include airway inflammation and enlargement of the submucosal mucous glands

b. Emphysema: defined pathologically as an abnormal permanent enlargement of the air spaces distal to the terminal bronchiole, accompanied by destruction of the wall without obvious fibrosis. This clinically correlates with a reduction in the diffusing capacity of lung for carbon monoxide (DL_{CO})

c. Various degrees of both chronic bronchitis and emphysema coexist in most patients with COPD. The term *COPD* should not be used for other forms of obstructive lung disease such as bronchiectasis, cystic fibrosis, or major airway obstruction

2. **Etiology and risk factors**

The pathogenesis of most cases of COPD remains unclear. The main risk factor associated with COPD is cigarette smoking but most smokers do not develop COPD. Less than 1% of patients with emphysema have alpha$_1$-antitrypsin deficiency (serum A_1AT <5 μmol - normal values 20-48 μmol).

3. **Diagnostic evaluation**

a. Clinical presentation

(1) Cough, sputum production, and dyspnea that have been present usually for several years. Symptoms consistent with severe COPD in a young and/or nonsmoking adult should prompt the consideration of other conditions such as alpha$_1$-antitrypsin deficiency, uncontrolled asthma, or other less common causes of obstructive lung disease (i.e., cystic fibrosis, immotile-cilia syndrome,

Young's syndrome [obstructive azoospermia with chronic bronchitis/bronchiectasis], congenital or acquired Ig deficiency)

(2) During an acute decompensation of COPD there is an increase in dyspnea, cough, and changes in sputum volume, color, and consistency. Physical examination may reveal
   (a) Pursed-lip breathing
   (b) Rapid, shallow breathing
   (c) Use of respiratory accessory muscles (i.e., sternocleidomastoid, pectoralis, or abdominal muscles)
   (d) Thoracoabdominal paradoxical breathing pattern
   (e) Wheezes, coarse crackles, and almost undetectable breath sounds in severe cases
   (f) Increased jugular venous distention, hepatomegaly, peripheral edema, right-side third heart sound (S_3), and increased pulmonic second sound (P_2) are characteristic of patients with cor pulmonale due to severe COPD
   (g) Various degrees of changes in mental status may be present and related to hypoxemia, hypercapnia, infection, and/or drugs.

(3) Other conditions that are commonly associated with or precipitate a worsening of COPD are depicted in the Box below.

b. Laboratory findings
   (1) Pulmonary function testing (PFT)
      (a) Spirometry reveals an obstructive pattern (reduction in the ratio of forced expiratory volume in the first second [FEV_1] to forced vital capacity [FVC]: normal for a 50-year-old person is 70%). The severity of the expiratory airflow limitation can be assessed by the FEV_1 (as % of normal predicted according to sex, race, and height). Commonly used values to assign severity of functional impairment are shown in Table 15-1.
      (b) The interrupter technique can be used in intubated, mechanically ventilated patients to diagnose airflow limitation and to

---

Common Conditions Associated with COPD Decompensation

- Respiratory infections: viral upper and lower respiratory tract (i.e., pharyngitis, tracheobronchitis, pneumonitis), aspiration, and bacterial pneumonia
- Narcotics and sedatives
- Inappropriately high fraction of inspired oxygen (FIo_2) (mainly in "CO_2 retainers")
- Heart failure
- Excessive diuresis with metabolic alkalosis and compensatory CO_2 retention
- Pneumothorax (i.e., rupture of a bleb)
- Hypophosphatemia, hypomagnesemia
- Hypermetabolic states (i.e, sepsis, fever)

assess the improvement of expiratory flow in response to bronchodilators

(2) Radiologic studies

  (a) Chest x-ray (CXR) may demonstrate evidence of emphysema

    (i) Flattening of the diaphragm

    (ii) Increased retrosternal air space

    (iii) Irregular areas of vascular attenuation and radiolucency (bullae: lucent areas in the lung parenchyma >1-2 cm in diameter)

    (iv) Typical smoker's emphysema is mainly of apical distribution. Predominant lower lung zone changes are consistent with emphysema due to alpha$_1$-antitrypsin deficiency

  (b) Chest computed tomography (CT) is the most sensitive way to detect emphysema although it is not routinely recommended as a diagnostic test

  (c) The roentgenographic features of chronic bronchitis are *nonspecific* and may include increased lung markings ("dirty lungs") and thickening of bronchial walls

  (d) CXR during an acute COPD exacerbation can be helpful in the detection of associated processes such as pneumonia, atelectasis, or pneumothorax

(3) Arterial blood gases (ABGs)

  (a) Various degrees of hypoxemia with increased $P(A\text{-}a)o_2$ gradient are typical of COPD patients

  (b) Chronic hypercapnia with compensatory metabolic alkalosis is seen in severe cases (CO_2 retainers)

  (c) Finding chronic CO_2 retention in moderate COPD with FEV$_1$ >1-1.3 L is unusual and should raise the question of concomitant neuromuscular or sleep apnea disorders

  (d) Common acid-base disturbances seen during an acute exacerbation of COPD include

    (i) Acute respiratory acidosis

    (ii) Partially compensated respiratory acidosis (acute-on-chronic)

    (iii) Chronic respiratory acidosis (mild exacerbation in CO_2 retainers)

    (iv) Metabolic alkalosis induced by diuretics or continuous nasogastric aspiration may be a cause of persistent or worsening hypercapnia in COPD

Table 15-1 Degree of impairment in COPD based on FEV$_1$

Severity	FEV$_1$ (% Predicted)
Mild	<LLN* (i.e., <70%) ≥60%
Moderate	<60% − 40%
Severe	<40%

*LLN: lower limit of normal.

4. Management of acute COPD exacerbation
   a. Assure adequate oxygenation and ventilation
      (1) For most patients the goal is to maintain a Pao_2 of 55-60 mm Hg (arterial oxyhemoglobin saturation of 88%-90%). In patients with concomitant coronary artery disease an arterial saturation $>90\%$ is desirable
         (a) Spontaneously breathing patients with acute COPD exacerbation can usually achieve those levels using a Venturi mask set to deliver 24%-35% oxygen (preferred in mouth breathers) or nasal cannula with oxygen flow of 1-2 L/min (see Chapter 4)
         (b) Hypercapnia will develop or worsen in some COPD patients during O_2 therapy. A reduction of the hypoxic respiratory drive and a worsening of ventilation/perfusion (V/Q) mismatch are the underlying mechanisms thought to mediate that response
      (2) Patients with significant acidemia, inadequate Pao_2, hypercapnia with changes in mental status, or hemodynamic instability should be assisted with mechanical ventilation (MV)
         (a) Noninvasive positive pressure ventilation (NIPPV) as the initial form of ventilatory assistance has been reported to be effective in selected patients with acute respiratory failure. Candidates for NIPPV should
            (i) Tolerate a facial or nasal mask
            (ii) Cooperate with this form of therapy
            (iii) Have an intact upper airway function without excessive secretions, regurgitation, or vomiting
            (iv) Be hemodynamically stable
         (b) In addition, NIPPV may be offered to patients who require endotracheal intubation and decline invasive procedures
         (c) NIPPV can be administered using a volume-cycled or pressure-controlled ventilator (i.e., BiPAP in S/T mode IPAP 10 cm H_2O, EPAP 5 cm H_2O, rate 10 bpm). Close observation with frequent ABGs and continuous Sao_2 monitoring is recommended to determine NIPPV efficacy and to avoid delays in endotracheal intubation
         (d) When volume-cycled MV is instituted in intubated COPD patients, a major goal is to minimize dynamic hyperinflation (autoPEEP) and its hemodynamic consequences. In general, set the ventilator to lower the mean expiratory flow (V_T/T_e) through increases in inspiratory flow (i.e., 90 L/min) and expiratory time (reductions in machine rate, I:E ratio, or even sedation that leads to failure to trigger) and reductions in tidal volume (i.e., 8 ml/kg)
   b. Bronchodilators
      (1) Inhaled $beta_2$-agonists, when delivered by metered dose inhalers (MDI) and used with a spacer device, are as effective as nebulizers in intubated or spontaneously breathing patients. Albuterol 2-4 puffs may be administered initially q20 min $\times$ 3, followed by q 1-2 hr until improvement occurs, and then q 4-6 hr. The dose for

albuterol nebulization is 2.5 mg (0.5 cc of 0.5% solution in 2-3 cc of normal saline)

(2) Anticholinergics: ipratropium bromide has been shown to be at least as effective as beta$_2$ agonists with potentially fewer side effects. Ipratropium bromide 2-6 puffs q6hr should be added to inhaled albuterol during COPD exacerbations. Recently, ipratropium bromide solution has been approved for use in the United States. The recommended dose is 500 mg q6hrs (via nebulizer)

(3) Methylxanthines: the role of theophylline is still controversial. There is no conclusive evidence for its routine use during COPD exacerbations. Potential drug interactions (i.e., erythromycin, ciprofloxacin, cimetidine, isoniazid, Ca^{++} channel blockers); increased toxicity in the elderly, acutely ill COPD patient; and the need for frequent blood-level measurements should be considered when prescribing the drug during an acute exacerbation. In patients already taking theophylline, a loading dose of 1 mg/kg (ideal body wt) of aminophylline for each 2 mcg/ml of desired increase in serum theophylline to achieve a target concentration of 12-15 mcg/ml followed by a continuous infusion (0.5-0.6 mg/kg/hr assuming normal half-life) is recommended. For elderly patients and patients with heart or liver disease the maintenance dosage should be reduced to 0.1-0.3 mg/kg/hr. When switching to the oral route, 80% of the total 24-hr aminophylline infusion that gives a therapeutic level is given as theophylline in divided doses

c. Corticosteroids
Unconfirmed trials have shown benefits from administration of steroids in acute COPD exacerbations. Methylprednisolone 0.5 mg/kg IV q6hr or prednisone 40-60 mg/day PO for 3 days and then tapered over a 2-week period is recommended

d. Antibiotics
A recognized upper or lower respiratory infection should be treated adequately. Empiric antibiotic therapy (i.e., trimethroprim-sulfamethoxazole, doxycycline, or amoxicillin for 7-10 days) in acute COPD exacerbation has been associated with an earlier resolution and fewer relapses

e. Correct precipitating or associated problems (see Box on p. 270)

| 15.2 | ASTHMA |

1. Definition
   a. Asthma is a clinical syndrome characterized by increased responsiveness of the tracheobronchial tree to a variety of stimuli with slowing of forced expiration that changes in severity either spontaneously or as a result of therapy
   b. Status asthmaticus is a severe episode of asthma that does not respond to usually effective treatment and requires more aggressive therapy for reversal

2. Pathophysiology
   The key feature of asthma is airway inflammation with hyperresponsiveness leading to airway obstruction and, in severe cases, to hyperinfla-

tion, increased ratio of dead-space volume to tidal volume (V_D/V_T), and V/Q mismatch with subsequent hypoxemia and respiratory insufficiency.

3. Diagnostic evaluation
   a. Clinical presentation
      Dyspnea, wheezing, and coughing are the most common symptoms during an asthma attack. Other diagnostic considerations, especially when a prior history of asthma is absent, should include
      (i) Heart failure and ischemia with diastolic dysfunction
      (ii) Aspiration of foreign bodies
      (iii) Epiglottitis and croup
      (iv) Pulmonary embolism (rare)

The Box below shows several adverse prognostic indicators obtained by history, physical examination, and routine tests in acute life-threatening asthma
   b. Laboratory evaluation
      (1) Spirometry: bedside spirometry shows an obstructive pattern (see above section on COPD). Serial FEV_1 determinations are indicated to objectively evaluate the response to treatment. If spirometry is not available, monitoring peak expiratory flow using a peak flowmeter is recommended
      (2) ABGs: hypoxemia may be seen in cases complicated by respiratory failure, pneumonia, or pneumothorax. The most common acid-base abnormality is acute respiratory alkalosis. Normocapnia or acute respiratory acidosis indicates impending or established respiratory failure
      (3) CXR: may show evidence of hyperinflation, increased bronchial markings, or associated conditions such as pneumonia or pneumothorax
      (4) Other tests: in addition to the usual admission tests, theophylline level, as well as blood and sputum cultures, should be done if clinically indicated

4. Management of asthma attacks
   a. Assure adequate oxygenation
      (1) During an acute attack most asthma patients will maintain Sao_2

Factors Associated with Severe Acute Asthma Attacks

- Previous episode(s) of severe asthma (especially if associated with respiratory failure)
- Changes in mental status
- Use of accessory muscles of respiration
- Very diminished or absent breath sounds
- Pulsus paradoxus >10 mm Hg
- Tachycardia >130 bpm
- Cyanosis
- Hypoxemia
- Hypercapnia or normocapnia in the setting of tachypnea
- FEV_1 <20% predicted pretreatment

>90%-92% with low concentration of supplemental oxygen (Venturi mask or nasal cannula 2 L/min). Monitor the patient with a pulse oximeter and supplement O_2 as necessary

(2) Mechanical ventilation: Most patients with severe asthma respond to aggressive medical management and do not require ventilatory support. The ventilatory strategy in patients with severe airway obstruction is to provide adequate oxygenation and at the same time to minimize the risk of barotrauma through the use of small V_T (i.e., 5-8 ml/kg) and minute ventilation (even if $Paco_2$ is allowed to climb: "controlled hypoventilation"). As in the case of COPD with expiratory flow limitation, reducing the ventilator's mean expiratory flow (V_T/Te) improves air trapping with its deleterious consequences (see Section 15.1 on COPD and Section 15.5 on respiratory failure, p. 283)

b. Beta-adrenergic agonists

These are the first line of therapy for acute asthma episodes. Selective beta$_2$-agonists such as albuterol and terbutaline administered by MDI with a holding chamber or by nebulization titrated to maximun effect are preferred (see above section on COPD for dosage). When drug delivery by aerosol is inadequate, subcutaneous (SQ) epinephrine (0.3 ml 1:1000 q20min × 3 maximum) or terbutaline (0.25 mg q20min × 2 maximum) can be used

c. Corticosteroids

Methylprednisolone 40 mg q6hr IV or prednisone 60 mg PO q8hr are recommended for the first 36-48 hr. Significant clinical benefits are usually present 6 hr later. When stable, a prednisone tapering program may consist of 60 mg/day for 4 days, then reducing the dose to 40 mg/day, and then by 10 mg/day q4 days. At the same time the patient should be started on inhaled corticosteroids (i.e., triamcinolone acetonide 6-8 puffs bid)

d. Methylxanthines

The controversy continues. A recent study showed that aminophylline (theophylline), when added to the above therapy, may benefit hospitalized acute asthma patients. (For dosages and monitoring, see Section 15.1, p. 273)

e. Complicating factors

Treat any obvious associated precipitant or complicating conditions such as pneumonia or pneumothorax.

f. Other forms of therapy

Other interventions that have been used in status asthmaticus but are not considered standard therapy include magnesium sulfate, general anesthetics, and bronchial lavage of thick secretions

15.3 PULMONARY EMBOLISM (PE)

1. Clinical presentation and risk factors

a. The clinical findings of PE are nonspecific. It most commonly presents as the acute onset of dyspnea with or without pleuritic chest pain, minor hemoptysis, and tachypnea. CXR may be normal or abnormal. Other forms of presentation include

(1) Acute *cor pulmonale* (>40% of circulation compromised)

      (2) Insidious onset of dyspnea (recurrent, unrecognized PEs)
      (3) Syncope, wheezing, fever, dysrhythmias, cardiopulmonary arrest
      (4) Asymptomatic

b. PE originates from deep venous thrombosis (DVT) of the lower extremities in most cases. Important risk factors for venous thromboembolism include

      (1) Prolonged immobility or paralysis
      (2) Surgery (mainly orthopedic—hip, knee, and lengthy procedures)
      (3) Trauma
      (4) Malignancy
      (5) Congestive heart failure (CHF), recent myocardial infarction (MI)
      (6) Advanced age
      (7) Obesity
      (8) Pregnancy and estrogen therapy
      (9) Prior history of DVT/PE
          Less often, DVT/PE is caused by antithrombin III, protein S and protein C deficiencies, or lupus anticoagulant syndrome

c. CXR abnormalities may be subtle or even absent

      (1) Pulmonary infiltrates
         (a) Only a minority represent pulmonary infarction and these usually resolve over few days
         (b) A pleural-based triangular infiltrate (Hampton's hump) may be seen with infarction. It usually persist for weeks
      (2) Pleural effusion(s)
      (3) Elevated hemidiaphragm
      (4) Plate-like atelectasis
      (5) Oligemia (Westermark's sign)

d. ABGs

         (a) Hypoxemia in most cases (but 15% of PEs have Pao_2 >80 mm Hg)
         (b) $P(A-a)o_2$ gradient widened
         (c) Hypocapnia

e. ECG

      (1) Nonspecific QRS and ST-T changes
      (2) Sinus tachycardia
      (3) Atrial dysrhytmias (multifocal atrial tachycardia [MAT], atrial flutter)
      (4) S_1-Q_3-T_3 pattern (only 10% of cases)
      (5) Pulseless electrical activity (PEA or EMD) in massive PE

2. Diagnostic tests

a. Ventilation/perfusion (V/Q) scan

A normal V/Q scan practically rules out pulmonary embolism. On the other hand, an abnormal V/Q scan is nonspecific and should be considered in the context of the clinical probability (see Fig. 15-1). The V/Q scan and simultaneous CXR findings are categorized as normal/ near normal, low, intermediate, or high probability as depicted in the Box on p. 278.

b. Lower extremity venous studies (LEs)

      (1) Duplex ultrasound (DU) is doppler ultrasound combined with real-time, two-dimensional ultrasound to study the venous system.

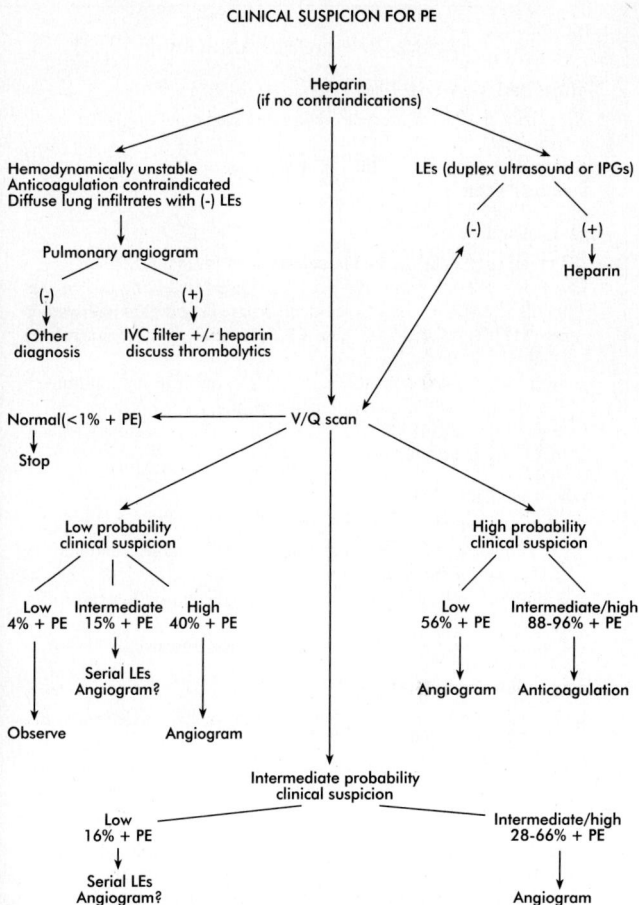

CLINICAL SUSPICION FOR PE

Heparin
(if no contraindications)

Hemodynamically unstable
Anticoagulation contraindicated
Diffuse lung infiltrates with (-) LEs

Pulmonary angiogram

(-) → Other diagnosis

(+) → IVC filter +/- heparin discuss thrombolytics

LEs (duplex ultrasound or IPGs)

(-)

(+) → Heparin

Normal(<1% + PE) → Stop

V/Q scan

Low probability clinical suspicion

Low 4% + PE → Observe

Intermediate 15% + PE → Serial LEs Angiogram?

High 40% + PE → Angiogram

High probability clinical suspicion

Low 56% + PE → Angiogram

Intermediate/high 88-96% + PE → Anticoagulation

Intermediate probability clinical suspicion

Low 16% + PE → Serial LEs Angiogram?

Intermediate/high 28-66% + PE → Angiogram

Figure 15-1
Diagnostic and therapeutic algorithm for PE.
%+PE = incidence of PE by angiography (based on the PIOPED study).

When available, it is the method of choice for diagnosing proximal DVT (positive predicted value of 94%). Diagnostic criteria of DVT include the inability to collapse the vein and to visualize the clot. DU can also assess flow augmentation, valvular incompetence, and other causes of pain and swelling (e.g., popliteal cysts and hematomas)

V/Q Scan Interpretation Categories

Normal and Very Low Probability

- No perfusion defects present (ventilation study and/or CXR may be abnormal)
- ≤3 small segmental (<25% of a segment) perfusion defects with normal CXR

Low Probability

- >3 small segmental perfusion defects with normal CXR
- Large or moderate segmental perfusion defect involving no >4 segments in one lung, no >3 segments in one lung region with *matching* ventilation defects, and CXR normal with abnormalities smaller than the perfusion defects
- Nonsegmental perfusion defect (small pleural effusion, cardiomegaly, enlarged aorta, mediastinum, and hila)
- One moderate segmental (>25%, <75%) perfusion defect with normal CXR mismatch)

High Probability

- ≥2 large segmental (>75%) perfusion defects without corresponding ventilation or CXR abnormality; or with smaller ventilation or CXR abnormalities (mismatch)
- ≥2 moderate segmental and one large segmental perfusion/ventilation mismatches
- ≥4 moderate segmental perfusion/ventilation mismatches

Intermediate Probability

- Includes all V/Q scans not listed in the above categories (borderline or difficult to categorize)

Modified from the PIOPED Study: Value of ventilation/perfusion scan in acute pulmonary embolism. *JAMA* 1990;263:2753-9.

(2) Impedance plethysmography (IPG) determines the changes in electrical impedance of the calf in response to blood volume changes produced by inflating a pneumatic thigh cuff. It is very sensitive for occlusive proximal DVT but insensitive for calf vein thrombosis. False positive results may be found in mechanically ventilated patients, CHF, and severe arterial insufficiency

(3) Venography is considered the "gold standard" for the diagnosis of leg DVT. Disadvantages include its invasiveness, cost, and potential allergic reactions of patients to contrast media. Definitive diagnostic findings include filling defects in a well-opacified vein and/or partially occluding defects surrounded by contrast media

(4) Other methods

    (a) Radiolabeled fibrinogen scan is very sensitive for below-the-knee DVT but definitive results take 6-72 hr

(b) Isotope venography is good for above-the-knee DVT (including the inferior vena cava [IVC]). It can give a perfusion lung scan at the same time

c. Pulmonary arteriography

In general it is a safe procedure (mortality <0.2%, morbidity 4%) even in patients with significant pulmonary hypertension. Definitive angiographic signs include the presence of intraluminal filling defects or cutoffs of pulmonary arteries. It is indicated in patients with suspected PE and the following:

(a) Contraindications for anticoagulation (considering IVC filter)

(b) Hemodynamically unstable (considering thrombolytic therapy or embolectomy)

(c) High clinical suspicion for PE with other than a high-probability V/Q scan and negative leg venous studies

(d) Extensive pulmonary parenchymal disease or CHF

3. Treatment of acute thromboembolism

a. Anticoagulation

Start anticoagulation as soon as the clinical suspicion for PE is high enough to initiate a diagnostic evaluation

(1) Heparin: initial bolus of 10,000 U IV followed by a continuous infusion of 1300 U/hr (20,000 U in 500 ml D_5W at 33 ml/hr). Check first activated partial thromboplastin time (aPTT) in 6 hr and maintain it between 1.5-2.5 × control. Modify heparin infusion according to the following

(a) If aPTT >2.5 control, stop the infusion for 1 hr, reduce the dosage by 100-200 U/hr, and recheck in 4-6 hr

(b) If aPTT is 1.25-1.5 control, increase the dosage by 100 U/hr and recheck in 4-6 hr

(c) If aPTT <1.25 control, rebolus with 5000 U IV, increase the dosage by 200 U/hr, and recheck in 4-6 hr

(d) For most patients, continue heparin for at least 5 days (provided that sodium warfarin [Coumadin] was started on day 1 or 2). Seven to 10 days of heparin infusion are recommended for patients with massive PE or extensive iliofemoral thrombosis

(2) Coumadin: oral anticoagulation started on day 1 or 2 at a dosage of 10 mg/day is recommended. The goal is to prolong the PT to an International Normalized Ratio (INR) of 2-3. Continue coumadin for at least 3 months in most patients. For those with a continuing risk factor or recurrent thromboembolism, anticoagulation should be given indefinitely. In cases where coumadin may be contraindicated (e.g., pregnancy during the first and third trimester), adjusted-dose SQ heparin can be effectively used

b. Thrombolytic therapy

Thrombolytic drugs dissolve thrombi by activating plasminogen to plasmin that in turn degrades fibrin (see Chapter 9). In contrast to thrombolytic therapy for MI, complete emboli resolution in the pulmonary vessels is not frequently accomplished. Although a reduction in PE mortality has not been shown with this form of therapy, it should be considered in patients with acute massive PE and hemodynamic instability without significant risk factors for bleeding. The role of thrombolytic therapy in DVT and submassive PE is less well established. Agents used for PE/DVT include

(1) Streptokinase (SK) 250,000 IU loading dose followed by 100,000 IU/hr for 24 hr in PE and 48-72 hr in DVT
(2) Urokinase (UK) 4400 IU/kg loading dose followed by 4400 IU/kg/hr for 12 hr in PE and 24-48 hr in DVT
(3) Tissue plasminogen activator (tPA) 100 mg over 2 hr
   The efficacy and bleeding complications of SK, UK, and tPA are equivalent. When using SK or UK, checking a thrombin time or an aPTT 2-4 hr into the infusion is recommended to verify a fibrinolytic state. Restart heparin when the aPTT <2 control

c. Inferior vena cava (IVC) filter
   Indications for placement of an IVC filter (Kimray-Greenfield, Mobin-Uddin, Bird's nest) include
   (1) Contraindications to anticoagulation
   (2) Acute massive PE
   (3) Recurrent PE on adequate anticoagulation therapy
   (4) Chronic thromboembolism with pulmonary hypertension
   (5) Following pulmonary embolectomy or thromboendarterectomy

d. Embolectomy
   May be considered for documented massive PE with hemodynamic instability despite heparin, fluids, and vasopressors, as well as for those patients with contraindications for thrombolytic therapy. This procedure is advised only if an experienced surgical team is immediately available

15.4   ACUTE RESPIRATORY DISTRESS SYNDROME (ARDS)

1. Definition
   ARDS is a form of acute lung injury characterized by a high permeability (noncardiogenic) pulmonary edema. In clinical practice it is defined by the presence of:
   a. Acute respiratory distress in a patient with predisposing conditions
   b. Diffuse bilateral infiltrates on CXR (pulmonary edema pattern)
   c. Hypoxemia (Pao_2 <55 mm Hg with FIo_2 >0.5) Pao_2/FIo_2 ≤200 mm Hg
   d. Reduced respiratory system static compliance ([Crs] <40-50 ml/cm H_2O)
   e. Low or normal pulmonary artery occlusion pressure (pulmonary capillary wedge pressure [PCWP] ≤18 cm H_2O)

2. Etiology
   ARDS is most commonly associated with:
   a. Sepsis
   b. Bronchial aspiration of gastric content
   c. Trauma
   d. Nosocomial pneumonia
      Major risk factors for the development of ARDS are listed in the Box on p. 281.

Conditions Associated with ARDS

- Air embolism
- Aspiration of gastric contents
- Burns
- Cardiopulmonary bypass
- Disseminated intravascular coagulation
- Drugs (cocaine, heroin, methadone, aspirin)
- Multiple fractures (fat embolism)
- Multiple transfusions
- Near-drowning
- Pancreatitis
- Pneumonia (bacterial, viral, fungal)
- Prolonged hypotension
- Sepsis
- Toxin inhalation
- Trauma

3. Pathophysiology
   The basic abnormality in ARDS is the disruption of the alveolar-capillary barrier. The endothelial injury in ARDS is frequently part of a more generalized permeability defect. An initial exudative phase is followed by proliferation of type II pneumocytes and fibrosis seen as early as the end of the first week.

4. Clinical presentation
   a. ARDS may develop insidiously over hours or even days after the initiating insult (e.g., pneumonia evolving into ARDS). Occasionally, it coincides with the precipitating event (e.g., gastric contents aspiration)
   b. The signs and symptoms of ARDS are non-specific and usually include
      (1) Dyspnea
      (2) Tachypnea (rapid, shallow breathing)
      (3) Coarse lung crackles
      (4) Cyanosis
      (5) Agitation
   c. Systemic manifestations of other organ dysfunctions may be related to the precipitating cause (e.g., burns, trauma) or may represent the generalization of the inflammatory response
      (1) Disseminated intravascular coagulation
      (2) Encephalopathy
      (3) Acute renal failure
      (4) Acute liver failure
      (5) Sepsis (gut bacterial translocation)
   d. ABGs show marked hypoxemia and hypocapnia with either acute respiratory alkalosis or acute metabolic acidosis
   e. Despite the CXR appearance of diffuse bilateral infiltrates, chest CT reveals a patchy, nonhomogeneous distribution of affected lung mixed

with normal parenchyma. Small pleural effusions can be seen in ARDS. Usually the cardiovascular silhouette on CXR is within normal limits

f. The pulmonary artery occlusion pressure or wedge pressure measured by a balloon-tipped, flow-directed catheter (Swan-Ganz) helps to detect a hydrostatic component of the pulmonary edema (cardiogenic). In pure ARDS the wedge pressure should be <16-20 cm H_2O

5. Management
   a. Treatment of the precipitating condition(s)
      Institute specific treatment for the underlying disorder as soon as possible (e.g., antimicrobials for infections and sepsis, drainage of abscesses, transfusion for hypovolemic shock)
   b. Supportive care
      (1) Ventilatory support (see Section 15.5 on acute respiratory failure)
      (2) Hemodynamic monitoring and support
          (a) A pulmonary artery catheter (Swan-Ganz) should be placed in patients with suspected or established ARDS. The information derived from hemodynamic monitoring is used in
              (i) Differentiation of cardiogenic vs noncardiogenic pulmonary edema
              (ii) Management of intravascular volume (avoiding volume overload)
              (iii) Assessment of cardiovascular effects of PEEP titration (cardiac index, stroke volume)
          (b) In severe cases of ARDS where high levels of extrinsic PEEP or dynamic hyperinflation (autoPEEP) are necessary to maintain adequate oxygenation, correct a reduced cardiac index with the use of inotropes (i.e., dobutamine or dopamine) to maintain an adequate oxygen delivery
      (3) Nutritional support (see Chapter 12)
      (4) Diagnosis and treatment of complications
          (a) Barotrauma (i.e., tube thoracostomy for pneumothorax)
          (b) Acute renal failure (i.e., hemodialysis)
          (c) Disseminated intravascular coagulation (DIC) (i.e., transfusions)
          (d) Infections: line sepsis, urinary tract infection (UTI), cellulitis (i.e., give antibiotics, change central lines)
   c. Other therapeutic modalities
      (1) Pharmacologic and immunologic agents targeted to arrest a specific step in the inflammatory cascade or the pathophysiologic process characteristic of ARDS and sepsis are currently being evaluated (e.g., monoclonal antibodies against bacterial lipopolysaccharide and tumor necrosis factor [TNF], soluble interleukin-1 and TNF receptors, prostaglandin E_1, pentoxifylline, nonsteroidal antiinflammatory drugs [NSAIDs; i.e., ibuprofen]), synthetic surfactant mixtures, inhaled nitric oxide)
      (2) Extracorporeal oxygenation and CO_2 removal (IVOX, ECCO$_2$R ECMO) as currently implemented have not demonstrated superiority to conventional supportive care

6. Prognosis
   a. The mortality rate of ARDS has remained 60%-80% in spite of advances in supportive therapy
   b. Early mortality is usually related to the underlying condition(s); later, mortality is mainly related to multiorgan failure rather than pulmonary dysfunction. (In a study by Montgomery et al <20% of deaths were attributed to irreversible respiratory failure)
   c. Most ARDS survivors have surprisingly minimal long-term impairment of lung function (mild restrictive and diffusion capacity [DL_{CO}] defects). Occasionally, reversible airway obstruction may develop

15.5   ACUTE RESPIRATORY FAILURE

1. Definition
   Acute respiratory failure is the inability to maintain adequate blood oxygenation and/or alveolar ventilation in the absence of an intracardiac shunt. Provided the baseline ABGs are close to predicted normal values, this usually means an acute increase in $Paco_2$ >50 mm Hg with arterial acidemia and/or a Pao_2 <55 mm Hg while breathing room air.
2. Classification and etiology
   Two distinct clinical and pathophysiologic types of acute respiratory failure can be described:
   a. Hypoxemic respiratory failure: the hallmark of this type of respiratory failure is the inability to adequately oxygenate the blood. The main pathophysiologic mechanisms involved are V/Q mismatch (response to 100% O_2) and intrapulmonary shunting (no significant improvement with 100% O_2). Patients exhibit a rapid, shallow breathing pattern and a low or normal $Paco_2$. This form of respiratory failure is commonly the result of a diffuse acute lung injury with high permeability pulmonary edema (ARDS), severe pneumonic infiltrates, or cardiogenic pulmonary edema
   b. Hypercapnic respiratory failure (pump failure): the hallmark of ventilatory pump failure is hypercapnia with acute respiratory acidosis. The $P(A-a)o_2$ gradient is useful in determining if the hypoxemia present in this form of respiratory failure is only due to hypoventilation (normal gradient) or if there is additional parenchymal lung disease (elevated gradient). The hypercapnia is the result of abnormalities in one or more of the determinants of the $Paco_2$ (Note: $\dot{V}E$ = minute ventilation)

$$Paco_2 = k\, \dot{V}co_2 / \dot{V}E\, (1 - V_D/V_T)$$

   (1) Increased CO_2 production ($\dot{V}co_2$) in patients with fever, sepsis, agitation, or excessive carbohydrate load, associated with a limited ventilatory capacity (high V_D/V_T, low VE)
   (2) Increased dead space (V_D/V_T) in severe COPD, cystic fibrosis, and severe asthma
   (3) Decreased total minute ventilation due to ventilatory pump dysfunction
       (a) Decreased central respiratory drive
           Cerebrovascular accident (CVA), drugs (narcotics, sedatives, anesthetics), central hypoventilation, and hypothyroidism

    (b) Abnormal respiratory efferents

        Spinal cord: trauma, poliomyelitis, amyotrophic lateral sclerosis, tetanus, and rabies. Neuromuscular: myasthenia gravis, multiple sclerosis, botulism, Guillain-Barré syndrome, hypophosphatemia, hypomagnesemia, drugs (i.e., streptomycin, amikacin, neuromuscular blockers), polyneuropathy of critical illness, and bilateral phrenic nerve injury

    (c) Abnormal chest wall and/or muscles

        Severe kyphoscoliosis, ankylosing spondylitis, massive obesity, muscular dystrophy, polymyositis, respiratory muscle fatigue, and acid maltase deficiency

    (d) Airways

        Upper airway obstruction: epiglottitis, fixed and variable upper-airway obstruction due to tumors, post-extubation, tracheomalacia, and bilateral vocal cord paralysis

3. Management

  The management of acute respiratory failure is initially supportive. It is aimed at the correction of hypoxemia or hypercapnia until specific actions are implemented to correct, if possible, the factors that led to the respiratory failure (i.e., antibiotics for pneumonia; diuretics, morphine, nitroglycerin, and afterload reducing agents for cardiogenic pulmonary edema; naloxone for narcotics overdose).

  a. Hypoxemic respiratory failure

    (1) Patients with V/Q mismatch abnormalities without significant intrapulmonary shunt usually respond to noninvasive O_2 supplementation (i.e., nasal cannula, Venturi mask).

    (2) In patients with cardiogenic pulmonary edema the use of continuous positive airway pressure (CPAP) 5-10 cm H_2O via face mask, in addition to oxygen supplementation, can be beneficial. This works by reducing the transmural pressure of the left ventricle (and therefore, afterload) and by decreasing the preload

    (3) Ventilatory management of patients with diffuse acute lung injury (i.e., ARDS) requires mechanical ventilation and should be viewed as a balance between adequate oxygenation on one hand, and risk for barotrauma and cardiovascular compromise on the other. The following pertains to specific aspects of the ventilatory management of ARDS

      (a) Adequate oxygenation

        For most patients with ARDS this means a Pao_2 of 55-60 mm Hg or oxygen saturation of 88%-90% with a cardiac index >2.5 L/min/m^2 and Hb ≥10 g/dl

        Arterial oxygen saturation can be increased in ARDS by

          (i) Raising the FIo_2: To avoid potential oxygen toxic effects, it is recommended not to use 100% O_2 for more than a few hr and to maintain an FIo_2 ≤0.6. Make a particular effort to decrease FIo_2 to the minimum acceptable in patients exposed to drugs that may increase oxygen toxicity (e.g., bleomycin, amiodarone)

          (ii) Increasing the end-expiratory lung volume to recruit collapsed or flooded alveoli can be achieved by adding extrinsic PEEP and/or setting the ventilator to create dynamic hyperinflation (autoPEEP). It is unclear if one strategy is more effective than the other in treating ARDS. The goal is to maximize oxygenation while at the same time avoiding hypotension, reduced cardiac pump function, and a plateau pressure >35 cm H_2O. With these considerations

- Extrinsic PEEP is usually started at a level of 5 cm H_2O and titrated in increments of 2 cm H_2O to a level of 15-20 cm H_2O along with the use of other strategies to minimize barotrauma (see below)
- Extended-ratio ventilation (prolonged I:E ratio, known as inverse ratio ventilation when I:E>1:1) is a technique used to increase mean alveolar pressure and transpulmonary pressure. It can be implemented with either volume-controlled or pressure-controlled ventilators. Increasing the inspiratory time (see Box below), increases the mean airway pressure (MAP) and allows the recruitment of lung units with long-time constants; therefore, it improves oxygenation. Extended-ratio ventilation is more easily implemented with volume-controlled ventilators than with pressure-controlled ventilators. Both require heavy sedation with or without paralysis (i.e., morphine sulfate; midazolam; lorazepam, or propofol by continuous infusion with or without vecuronium; or atracurium). Monitoring of plateau pressure to keep it <35 cm H_2O; autoPEEP (end-expiration occlusion method); and hemodynamics by a pulmonary balloon-tipped, flow-directed catheter (Swan-Ganz) are required

(b) Avoiding barotrauma

Barotrauma in the form of extraalveolar air or worsening of acute lung injury is the result of alveolar overdistention (increased transmural pressure or alveolar pressure [P_{ALV}] −

Prolonging Inspiratory Time (Ti) and I:E Ratio in Volume-Controlled Ventilators*

- Reduce inspiratory flow (i.e., to 40 L/min)
- Use decelerating inspiratory flow wave form
- Add an inspiratory pause (i.e., 0.2-0.5 second)
- Increase % inspiratory time†

---

*Applying these changes in a stepwise manner allows progressive extension of Ti and I:E ratio to the degree that is tolerated or needed. Adjustment in tidal volume (V_T) as recommended on p. 286 and monitoring of $P_{PLATEAU}$, autoPEEP, and its hemodynamic effects is required to avoid complications.

†Direct way of setting the I:E ratio (i.e., Siemens Servo ventilator).

pleural pressure [P_{PL}]); thus, it seems reasonable to avoid lung volumes above total lung capacity (TLC) to prevent lung damage

   (i) Because P_{ALV}, P_{PL}, and lung volumes are difficult to determine at the bedside, it is recommended to monitor the plateau pressure (end-inflation hold pressure) as the best approximation of the peak alveolar pressure

  (ii) Avoid a plateau pressure of ≥ 35 cm H_2O in the absence of significantly decreased chest wall compliance

 (iii) Peak airway pressure (P_{PEAK}) reflects not only the elastic but also the flow-resistive pressures of the respiratory system. It should be used only as a gross estimate for the risk of barotrauma (i.e., high P_{PEAK} may be due to a small endotracheal tube, bronchospasm, secretions, high inspiratory peak flow, or worsening of lung or chest wall compliance) that may or may not mean alveolar overinflation

 (iv) Determining V_T

   ARDS is a nonhomogeneous process with collapsed and flooded areas mixed with relatively normal aerated lung, resulting in a reduction in the TLC; thus, it makes sense to ventilate ARDS patients with smaller than conventional V_T. The V_T chosen should be one that prevents lung overinflation (i.e., plateau pressure <35 cm H_2O) and alveolar derecruitment at the end of expiration (inadequate oxygenation). This usually means an initial V_T of 7-8 ml/kg that may need to be reduced to 5 ml/kg

  (v) Setting the respiratory rate

   The machine rate is determined by considering the patient's metabolic demands, intrinsic rate, and desired I:E ratio. It is usually set to 25-40 bpm. Even with this rate (plus the low V_T used), minute ventilation may not be high enough for ARDS patients. Allowing CO_2 retention (i.e., 60 mm Hg) and respiratory acidemia (i.e., pH 7.2-7.25) in an effort to limit barotrauma is referred to as *permissive hypercapnia*

(c) Controlling the hemodynamic effects of mechanical ventilation

   The increase in end-expiratory lung volume and mean alveolar pressure produced by the ventilatory strategies described above can have deleterious hemodynamic consequences. It is important to document that a ventilator change aimed at increasing O_2 saturation does not reduce the total amount of oxygen delivered to the tissues via reduction in cardiac index. In severe cases, maintain the cardiac index >2.5 L/min/m^2 with the use of inotropic agents (dobutamine or dopamine if hypotension is present)

b. Hypercapnic respiratory failure

 The main goal in treating this form of failure is to improve alveolar ventilation through the use of mechanical ventilation. This is most commonly done through an endotracheal tube using a volume-controlled ventilator (usual initial settings are V_T 10 ml/kg, A/C mode, rate 8-10 bpm, and FIo_2 1). Check ABGs 10-20 min later to detect inadvertent and potentially life-threatening acute alkalosis secondary to overcorrection of the hypercapnia and to adjust the FIo_2. Noninvasive mechanical ventilation has been effective in patients with neuromuscular conditions. The management of hypercapnic respiratory failure in COPD and asthma is discussed in Sections 15.1 and 15.2, respectively.

15.6   BAROTRAUMA

1. Definition
   Lung injury related to high alveolar pressures and volumes. In the ICU setting it specifically refers to positive pressure ventilator-induced lung damage. Occasionally, a patient may be admitted to the ICU after a diving accident (sudden decompression) or foreign-body aspiration (ball-valve mechanism).
2. Clinical manifestations
   a. Classic mechanical ventilator–induced barotrauma is manifested by extraalveolar air in the form of
      (1) Pulmonary interstitial emphysema (PIE)
      (2) Subpleural air cysts
      (3) Pneumomediastinum
      (4) Pneumothorax (PTX)
      (5) Subcutaneous emphysema
      (6) Pneumopericardium
      (7) Pneumoretroperitoneum
      (8) Pneumoperitoneum
      (9) Gas emboli (main clinical manifestation in diving accidents)
   b. Tension PTX occurs in 30%-97% of all PTXs in mechanically ventilated patients and is characterized by worsening hypoxemia, hypotension, or even cardiovascular collapse with pulseless electrical activity (PEA). CXR shows lung collapse with hemithorax expansion and contralateral mediastinal shift
   c. Physical examination reveals
      (1) Absent breath sounds, hyperresonance to percussion, and decreased chest excursion on the affected side in cases of PTX
      (2) Crepitation on palpation or auscultation is found in cases of subcutaneous emphysema
      (3) Mediastinal "crunch" in pneumomediastinum
      (4) Changes in mental status or neurologic deficits are usually found in patients with gas embolism
   d. Development or worsening of diffuse lung injury (in the form of noncardiogenic pulmonary edema) also has been associated with positive pressure ventilation
3. Pathophysiology
   a. Alveolar rupture occurs at the site where alveoli attach to the bronchovascular sheath. From there, extraalveolar air may dissect the peribronchovascular tissues into different planes to produce the clinical

manifestations listed above. Alternatively, direct rupture of a subpleural cyst into the pleural cavity may also cause PTX

  b. Positive pressure mechanical ventilation has also been shown to produce

    (1) Increased lung microvascular permeability and filtration pressure

    (2) Alveolar epithelial injury

    (3) Alteration of surfactant function and turnover

4. Diagnosis

  a. A high index of suspicion should be maintained for those patients at risk for barotrauma (i.e. use of high V_T, high plateau pressure, peak pressure, PEEP, dynamic hyperinflation, extensive lung damage, and prolonged mechanical ventilation)

  b. CXR will usually confirm a diagnosis of extraalveolar air. PIE (seen as linear radiolucent streaks) is the first radiologic sign and should alert the physician for the risk of progression to PTX

  c. The classic radiologic sign of PTX (pleural line separated from the apicolateral chest wall) may not be present in ICU patients when a portable CXR is taken in the supine or semirecumbent position. For those patients, pay attention to the mediastinal and subpulmonic recesses where air accumulates

5. Management

  a. Extraalveolar air without PTX is managed conservatively. Obervation and avoidance of risk factors, if possible, are indicated (see Section 15.5, p. 285)

  b. In general, treat all PTXs in a mechanically ventilated patient with tube thoracotomy (see Chapter 17)

  c. The use of "prophylactic" tube thoracotomy for high-risk, mechanically ventilated patients is controversial and not recommended. Instead, it is advised to follow these patients closely and be prepared for immediate placement of a chest tube should PTX develop

  d. Persistent bronchopleural fistula(s), despite chest tube suction, should be managed with the lowest V_T, P_{PEAK}, and $P_{PLATEAU}$ that permit adequate ventilation. Consider high-frequency jet ventilation (HFJV), independent lung ventilation, or surgery if the air leak is massive and does not respond to the usual management

  e. Recompression in a hyperbaric chamber is indicated for diving accidents that result in air embolism (see Chapter 7)

| 15.7 | MASSIVE HEMOPTYSIS |

1. Definition

Hemoptysis is the expectoration of blood that originates from below the larynx. It is considered massive when the rate of bleeding is at least 400 ml in 6 hr or 600 ml in a 24-hr period.

2. Etiology

The most common causes of massive hemoptysis are

  a. Tuberculosis (rupture of Rasmussen's aneurysm)

  b. Bronchiectasis (erosion of bronchial vasculature)

  c. Bronchogenic carcinoma (invasion of pulmonary vessels)

d. Lung abscess (destruction of fairly normal vessels due to inflammation).

Other etiologies include: bronchial carcinoids, cystic fibrosis, broncholithiasis, aspergilloma, trauma, bronchovascular and AV fistulas, mitral stenosis, and pulmonary-renal syndromes

3. Evaluation
   a. Differentiate hemoptysis from hematemesis
      Hemoptysis is usually bright red blood, frothy, and with an alkaline pH. In contrast, hematemesis is usually darker with an acidic pH. At times this differentiation cannot be made easily because hematemesis may produce blood aspiration into the tracheobronchial tree that in turn causes "hemoptysis"; on the other hand, patients with hemoptysis may swallow blood and vomit it after coughing
   b. Localize the bleeding site
      Localization of the bleeding site is important to adequately plan any interventional procedure. Bleeding coming from the upper airways can be excluded by performing an ear, nose, and throat examination
      (1) CXR may suggest the bleeding site
         (a) Lung masses, apical cavitary lesions, or infiltrates in the CXR point to these places as sources of bleeding
         (b) A normal CXR is consistent with bleeding arising from the airways
         (c) Roentgenograms showing bilateral or diffuse disease are not helpful in pointing out the origin of bleeding
      (2) Perform a bronchoscopy to further identify the site and cause of bleeding, and to achieve temporary control. The type and timing of the procedure depend on the rate of bleeding
         (a) During flexible fiberoptic bronchoscopy (FFB) the patient must be intubated with a large endotracheal tube that may be used to tamponade the affected lung if necessary
         (b) Rigid bronchoscopy is the preferred temporizing method to evaluate and control massive bleeding. This procedure requires general anesthesia and must be performed by trained physicians
      (3) Angiography of the bronchial and pulmonary circulation is recommended when bronchoscopy cannot determine the bleeding site in more peripheral lesions
   c. Laboratory determinations
      Obtain ABGs, complete blood cell count, PT, PTT, bleeding time, creatinine, BUN, and request blood type and crossmatching.

4. Management
   a. Assure adequate ventilation and oxygenation
      This should be the main priority considering that the mode of death in massive hemoptysis is asphyxiation (as little as 150 cc of blood is needed to fill the airways)
      (1) Depending on the rate of bleeding, it may only be necessary to administer supplemental oxygen through nasal cannula or face mask. In the other extreme, perform endotracheal intubation (single or double lumen [Carlen's tube]) to aspirate the blood and ventilate the patient while definitive therapy is being prepared

(2) Position the patient on a lateral decubitus with the bleeding site down

b. Assure stable hemodynamic conditions
   (1) Obtain adequate venous access
   (2) Administer fluids as needed (normal saline or blood)

c. Suppress cough
   (1) Codeine 60 mg PO q6hr
   (2) Sedatives may be added (i.e., midazolam 2 mg or lorazepam 1 mg, IV q2hr prn)

d. Control the bleeding site
   (1) Bronchoscopic procedures include
       (a) Bronchial packing through a rigid bronchoscope
       (b) Tamponade of airway with a balloon-tipped catheter through a rigid bronchoscope or alongside a flexible bronchoscope
       (c) Bronchial lavage with cold saline through a rigid broncho-scope
       (d) Coagulation of visible lesions with a neodymnium-YAG laser (not helpful in very active, brisk bleeding)
   (2) Bronchial artery embolization is the method of choice for patients with massive or submassive hemoptysis and contraindications for surgery. Given its high success rate (90%), embolization has become a first-line treatment for all patients with massive or recurrent hemoptysis
   (3) Surgical resection is recommended for localized lesions that can be removed. It should not be offered to patients with
       (a) Widely metastatic lung cancer
       (b) Severe pulmonary or cardiovascular status
   (4) Correct coagulopathy if present (i.e., administer fresh frozen plasma [FFP] and vitamin K if PT is prolonged; transfuse platelets in severe thrombocytopenia).

5. Prognosis
   a. Although the underlying medical condition(s) affects the prognosis in massive hemoptysis, the best estimator of mortality is the rate of bleeding. A study by Crocco shows that hemoptysis of 600 cm^3 occurring over
      (1) 4 hr has 71% mortality
      (2) 4-16 hr has 45% mortality
      (3) 16-48 hr has 5% mortality
   b. Median operative mortality in massive hemoptysis is 17%. Actively bleeding patients at the time of the surgery have a higher mortality when compared with nonactively bleeding patients

Suggested readings

Anthonisen NR, Manfreda J, Warren CP et al: Antibiotic therapy in exacerbation of chronic obstructive pulmonary disease. *Ann Intern Med* 1987; 106:196-204.

Ashbaugh DG, Bigelow DB, Petty TL et al: Acute respiratory distress in adults. *Lancet* 1967; 2:319-23.

Crocco JA, Rooney JJ, Fankushen DS et al: Massive hemoptysis. *Arch Intern Med* 1968; 121:495-8.

Darioli R, Perret C: Mechanical controlled hypoventilation in status asthmaticus. *Am Rev Respir Dis* 1984; 129:385-7.

Ferguson GT, Cherniack RM: Management of chronic obstructive pulmonary disease. *N Engl J Med* 1993; 328:1017-22.

Gattinoni L, Pelosi P, Vitale G, et al: Body position changes redistribute lung computed-tomographic density in patients with acute respiratory failure. *Anesthesiology* 1991; 74:15-23.

Heijboer H, Buller HR, Lensing AW, et al: A comparison of real-time compression ultrasonography with impedance plethysmography for the diagnosis of deep-vein thrombosis in symptomatic outpatients. *N Engl J Med* 1993; 329:1365-9.

Huang D, O'Brien RG, Harman E, et al: Does aminophylline benefit adults admitted to the hospital for an acute exacerbation of asthma? *Ann Intern Med* 1993; 119:1155-60.

Hubmayr RD, Gay PC, Tayyab M: Respiratory system mechanics in ventilated patients: techniques and indications. *Mayo Clin Proc* 1987; 62:358-68.

Hyers TM, Hull RD, Weg JG: Antithrombotic therapy for venous thromboembolic disease. *Chest* 1992; 102(Suppl):408-25.

Macklin MT, Macklin CC: Malignant interstitial emphysema of the lungs and mediastinum as an important occult complication in many respiratory diseases and other conditions: an interpretation of the clinical literature in the light of laboratory experiment. *Medicine* 1944; 23:281-358.

Manning H: Peak airway pressure: why the fuss? *Chest* 1994; 105:242-7.

Maunder RJ, Pierson DJ, Hudson LD: Subcutaneous and mediastinal emphysema: pathophysiology, diagnosis and management. *Arch Intern Med* 1984; 144:1447-53.

McFadden ER, Jr: Dosage of corticosteroids in asthma. *Am Rev Respir Dis* 1993; 147:1306-10.

Montgomery AB, Stager MA, Carrico CJ, et al: Causes of mortality in patients with the adult respiratory distress syndrome. *Am Rev Respir Dis* 1985; 132:485-9.

Moser KM: Venous thromboembolism. *Am Rev Respir Dis* 1990; 141:235-49.

Murray JF, Matthay MA, Luce JM, et al: An expanded definition of the adult respiratory distress syndrome. *Am Rev Respir Dis* 1988; 138:720-3.

Reinoso MA, Gracey DR, Hubmayr RD: Interrupter mechanics of patients admitted to a chronic ventilator dependency unit. *Am Rev Respir Dis* 1993; 148:127-31.

Slutsky AS: ACCP consensus conference: mechanical ventilation. *Chest* 1993; 104:1833-59.

St John RC, Dorinsky PM: Immunologic therapy for ARDS, septic shock, and multiple organ failure. *Chest* 1993; 103:932-43.

Stein PD, Athanasoulis C, Alavi A, et al: Complications and validity of pulmonary angiography in acute pulmonary embolism. *Circulation* 1992; 85:462-8.

Stoll JF, Bettmann MA: Bronchial artery embolization to control hemoptysis: a review. *Cardiovasc Intervent Radiol* 1988; 112:63-9.

The Official Statement of the American Thoracic Society: Standards for the diagnosis and care of patients with chronic obstructive pulmonary disease (COPD) and asthma. *Am Rev Respir Dis* 1986; 136:225-44.

The PIOPED Investigators: Value of the ventilation/perfusion scan in acute pulmonary embolism. *JAMA* 1990; 263:2753-9.

Thompson AB, Teschler H, Rennard SI: Pathogenesis evaluation and therapy for massive hemoptysis. *Clin Chest Med* 1992; 13:69-82.

Renal and Fluid—
Electrolyte
Disorders

ACID-BASE DISTURBANCES

Definition

Acidosis is any process that tends (in the absence of buffering or compensation) to cause the accumulation of hydrogen ions (H^+). If the pH of the blood is lower than normal (<7.35), *acidemia* is present. Similarly, any process that tends to cause the accumulation of bicarbonate (HCO_3^-) is an alkalosis. An elevated blood pH (>7.45) is referred to as *alkalemia*. When the acid-base disturbance arises as a result of changes in the carbon dioxide tension (Pco_2) of the blood, a respiratory process is present. Conversely, when the acid-base disturbance occurs as a result of accumulation of nonvolatile acids or loss of HCO_3^- (or substances metabolized to HCO_3^-), a metabolic process is present. Acidosis and alkalosis can be either primary or compensatory for different acid-base problems.

1. APPROACH TO ACID-BASE DISTURBANCES
   a. The initial evaluation of acid-base disorders requires the simultaneous examination of arterial blood gases (ABGs) and serum electrolytes
   b. The typical patterns of blood pH, Pco_2, and HCO_3^- in various acid-base problems are listed in Table 16-1
   c. The adequacy of compensation for a primary acid-base abnormality can also be assessed
      (1) For patients with metabolic acidosis, the expected Pco_2 can be calculated as

$$Pco_2 = (HCO_3^- \times 1.5) + 8 \, (\pm 2)$$

      (a) If the actual Pco_2 is greater than expected, a simultaneous respiratory acidosis is present
      (b) If the measured Pco_2 is less than expected, a simultaneous respiratory alkalosis is present
      (2) For patients with metabolic alkalosis, the expected Pco_2 can be calculated as

$$Pco_2 = \{(HCO_3^- - 25) \times 0.7\} + 40 \, (\pm 2)$$

      (a) Respiratory compensation for a primary metabolic alkalosis is limited to a Pco_2 of approximately 55 mm Hg. Even this

Table 16-1 Systematic evaluation of acid-base disorders

Compensated Process

	pH	Pco$_2$	HCO$_3^-$
Metabolic acidosis	pH ↓	Pco$_2$ ↓	HCO$_3^-$ ↓
Respiratory acidosis	pH ↓	Pco$_2$ ↑	HCO$_3^-$ ↑
Metabolic alkalosis	pH ↑	Pco$_2$ ↑	HCO$_3^-$ ↑
Respiratory alkalosis	pH ↑	Pco$_2$ ↓	HCO$_3^-$ ↓

Uncompensated Process

	pH	Pco$_2$	HCO$_3^-$
Metabolic acidosis	pH ↓	Pco$_2$ —	HCO$_3^-$ ↓
Respiratory acidosis	pH ↓	Pco$_2$ ↑	HCO$_3^-$ —
Metabolic alkalosis	pH ↑	Pco$_2$ —	HCO$_3^-$ ↑
Respiratory alkalosis	pH ↑	Pco$_2$ ↓	HCO$_3^-$ —

Mixed Process

	pH	Pco$_2$	HCO$_3^-$
Metabolic/respiratory acidosis	pH ↓	Pco$_2$ ↑	HCO$_3^-$ ↓
Metabolic/respiratory alkalosis	pH ↑	Pco$_2$ ↓	HCO$_3^-$ ↑

limit may not be attained in patients with chronic pulmonary or hepatic disease, or congestive heart failure (CHF)

(3) Metabolic compensation for respiratory acid-base disturbances depends in part on the duration of the problem

  (a) For patients with chronic respiratory acidosis, the expected HCO$_3^-$ can be calculated as

$$HCO_3^- = (Pco_2 - 40) \times 0.35 + 25 \, (\pm 2)$$

  • The upper limit for this process is HCO$_3^-$ = 55 mEq/L
  • If the degree of compensation is inadequate, the possibility of a mixed acid-base disturbance or a superimposed acute process should be considered

  (b) The expected degree of compensation for acute respiratory acidosis is calculated as

$$HCO_3^- = (Pco_2 - 40) \times 0.10 + 25 \, (\pm 2)$$

The upper limit of compensation for acute respiratory acidosis is HCO$_3^-$ = 30 mEq/L

  (c) The expected metabolic response to chronic respiratory alkalosis can be estimated by

$$HCO_3^- = 25 - ([40 - Pco_2] \times 0.5) \, (\pm 2)$$

Inadequate compensation for chronic respiratory alkalosis should raise the possibility of a superimposed acute respiratory alkalosis or a mixed acid-base problem

  (d) The expected metabolic response to acute respiratory alkalosis can be calculated as

$$HCO_3^- = 25 - ([40 - Pco_2] \times 0.25) \, (\pm 2)$$

2. METABOLIC ACIDOSIS

The clinical consequences of metabolic acidosis are due to abnormalities of intracellular pH, transcellular ionic shifts, or both.

  a. Signs and symptoms include tachypnea, depressed cardiac function, fatigue, weakness, and altered mental status

b. Laboratory findings: hyperkalemia, calciuresis, and changes in carbohydrate and lipid metabolism

c. Other specific findings may occur due to the etiology of the underlying cause

d. Metabolic acidoses are classified based on whether the plasma anion gap (AG) is normal or elevated. Its value is calculated as

$$AG = Na^+ - (Cl^- + HCO_3^-) \ (nl = 10\text{-}15 \ mEq/L)$$

(Note: Na^+ = sodium; Cl^- = chloride; nl = normal)

e. The differential diagnosis of primary metabolic acidosis is listed in Table 16-2.

(1) In general, high AG metabolic acidoses are caused by the accumulation of an acid in the plasma in which the anion is something other than Cl^-. These acids can be endogenous (i.e., lactic acid, ketoacids, uremic acids), exogenous (i.e., salicylates), or the endogenous metabolic products of exogenous toxins (i.e., paraldehyde, methanol, ethylene glycol)

(2) The accumulation of these unmeasured acid anions should be stochiometrically equal to the observed decrease in HCO_3^-

(3) This equality will be preserved when the normal difference is maintained; thus, if a normal AG = 12 mEq/L and a normal HCO_3^- = 25 mEq/L, in a pure high AG metabolic acidosis

$$Na^+ - (Cl^- + 25) = 12; \ or$$
$$Na^+ - Cl^- = 37 \pm 3$$

If $(Na^+ - Cl^-)$ is significantly >37, then a coexistent metabolic alkalosis should be suspected. If the difference is significantly <37, then a coexistent normal AG acidosis is probably present

(4) The causes of metabolic acidosis with a normal AG are listed in Table 16-2. These so-called hyperchloremic acidoses occur due to either the administration of exogenous acids in which the anion is chloride (e.g., hydrochloric acid [HCl], ammonium chloride [NH_4Cl], calcium chloride [$CaCl_2$]) or the loss of a body fluid that is relatively low in chloride but high in bicarbonate or its metabolic equivalent

Table 16-2   Causes of metabolic acidosis

Elevated Anion Gap	Normal Anion Gap
Methanol	Urinary-enteric fistula
Uremia	Saline volume expansion
Ketoacidosis	Endocrinopathies
Paraldehyde	Diarrhea
Lactic acidosis	Carbonic anhydrase inhibition
Ethylene glycol	Acid-chloride administration
Salicylates	Renal tubular acidosis
	Mineralocorticoid antagonists

(a) In cases of normal AG metabolic acidosis, measurement of the urinary AG can be diagnostically useful. It is calculated as

$$AG_U = U_{Na} + U_K - U_{Cl}$$

The AG_U is inversely related to urinary ammonium (NH_4) excretion. Its value should be <0 in acidotic patients with gastrointestinal (GI) bicarbonate losses since renal ammoniagenesis ought to be well preserved. In patients with acidosis due to urinary bicarbonate losses, especially if caused by renal tubular acidosis (RTA), the AG_U should be >0

f. The primary therapy of metabolic acidosis is to treat the underlying disease

g. The use of exogenous $NaHCO_3$ in the therapy of metabolic acidosis (especially lactic acidosis) is somewhat controversial since evidence exists that such treatment can actually accelerate lactate production. However, it is generally accepted that severe acidemia (pH <7.20) of metabolic origin should be corrected with $NaHCO_3$. The amount of bicarbonate required can be calculated by

$$HCO_3^- \text{ deficit} = \text{body wt(kg)} \times 0.5 \times$$
$$(\text{target} - \text{actual } HCO_3^-)$$

(1). Administration of $NaHCO_3$ as an isotonic solution (i.e., 3 ampules of $NaHCO_3$/L of sterile water or D_5W) reduces the risk of hypernatremia in patients at particular risk

h. Dialysis is sometimes indicated not only for the correction of acidosis but also for the rapid elimination of certain toxins that cause acidosis, such as methanol and ethylene glycol, even if the blood urea nitrogen (BUN) and creatinine are normal

i. Treatment of chronic metabolic acidosis, especially if caused by RTA, includes oral alkali replacement as well as therapy for any associated electrolyte abnormalities

3. RESPIRATORY ACIDOSIS

a. The clinical effects of respiratory acidosis include findings compatible with intracellular acidosis in addition to syndromes caused by abnormal pulmonary gas exchange. Of these, the most important is hypoxemic encephalopathy. Signs of chronic pulmonary disease, including *cor pulmonale,* may be present

b. Some common causes of respiratory acidosis are listed in the Box on p. 296.

c. Chronic respiratory acidosis is seldom associated with severe acidemia (pH <7.20) even if marked hypercapnia ($P_{CO_2} >100$ mm Hg) is present. A superimposed acute metabolic or respiratory acidosis should be suspected if arterial pH is outside of this expected range

d. The most important aspect of treatment of acute respiratory acidosis is the immediate restoration of effective alveolar gas exchange

(1) This usually requires mechanical ventilation (see Chapter 4)

(2) If intubation is not immediately available, cautiously administer supplemental oxygen and $NaHCO_3$

e. Treatment of chronic respiratory acidosis depends mainly on the prevention and prompt recognition and therapy of intercurrent complications such as infections and CHF

Causes of Respiratory Acidosis

Central Nervous System (CNS) Disorders

Drugs (narcotics, anesthetics, tranquilizers)
Brain stem injury
Primary hypoventilation

Peripheral Nervous System Disorders

Infectious diseases (botulism, tetanus, polio)
Amyotrophic lateral sclerosis
Guillain-Barré syndrome
Spinal cord/phrenic nerve injury
Organophosphates poisoning

Primary Muscular Disease

Muscular dystrophy
Myasthenia gravis
Severe hypokalemia

Pulmonary Disease

Chronic obstructive lung disease
Pneumonia
Pulmonary edema
Smoke inhalation
Pulmonary embolism

Thoracic/Upper-Airway Disorders

Chest wall (flail chest, pneumothorax, kyphoscoliosis)
Airway obstruction (laryngospasm, foreign body)

Failure of Mechanical Ventilator

4. METABOLIC ALKALOSIS
   a. The clinical features of metabolic alkalosis are nonspecific
      (1) Evidence of neuromuscular irritability or latent tetany may be present
      (2) Cardiac dysrhythmias can occur
   b. Hypokalemia and hypochloremia are usually present
   c. The plasma AG is frequently elevated due partly to a slight increase in lactate levels but mainly due to release of H^+ ions from plasma proteins (especially albumin) as part of the buffering process
   d. Urine pH measurements are *not* helpful
   e. The most useful biochemical determination is the level of urinary chloride (U_{Cl}), which forms the basis for classification of metabolic alkaloses
      (1) Metabolic alkaloses associated with a U_{Cl} <10 mEq/L are termed *chloride-responsive,* whereas those with a U_{Cl} >20 mEq/L are termed *chloride-resistant*

Causes of Metabolic Alkalosis

Chloride-Responsive

Gastrointestinal disorders
   Gastric: vomiting, nasogastric suction
   Colonic: villous adenoma, chloride diarrhea
Renal disorders
   Diuretic therapy
   Posthypercapnic alkalosis
Cystic fibrosis

Chloride-Resistant

Hypermineralocorticoid states
Severe potassium depletion
Bartter's syndrome

Miscellaneous

Alkali administration (antacids, transfusions)
Hypercalcemia
Poorly absorbable anion administration (antibiotics)

    (2) In some cases, U_{Cl} falls between these levels and no definite classification is possible
  f. Causes of metabolic alkalosis are listed in the Box above.
  g. Since the kidney can ordinarily excrete a vast amount of HCO_3^-, acid loss (or base accumulation) alone does not usually result in a sustained alkalosis
    (1) If coexistent volume depletion is present, alkalosis can be persistent. This is by far the most common pathogenesis for metabolic alkalosis. This combination occurs when body fluids rich in NaCl and poor in $NaHCO_3$ are lost, usually from the intestinal tract or kidneys. Rarely, other sites of NaCl loss (e.g., skin losses in cystic fibrosis) may be present
    (2) Extracellular fluid volume contraction causes avid NaCl and $NaHCO_3$ reabsorption in all nephron sites with attendant decreases in U_{Cl} and perpetuation of the alkalosis
    (3) Hypokalemia occurs due to intracellular potassium (K^+) shifts and mineralocorticoid-induced urinary K^+ losses
    (4) Much less commonly, metabolic alkalosis occurs in the absence of significant volume depletion. This situation is most often associated with hypermineralocorticoidism as a primary feature. The excessive mineralocorticoid activity can be either endogenous (e.g., Conn's syndrome, Cushing's syndrome) or exogenous (e.g., licorice, chewing tobacco). In these cases, excessive renal reabsorption of $NaHCO_3$ and NaCl occurs in the absence of significant chloride deficits. Therefore, U_{Cl} levels remain relatively high
    (5) Severe total body K^+ deficits exceeding 1000 mEq may result in the inability to correct metabolic alkalosis but probably does not

cause the disorder in humans. Metabolic alkalosis with high U_{Cl} occurs in Bartter's syndrome, which is characterized by renal wasting of K^+ and Cl^-, normal blood pressure (BP), and partial response to prostaglandin inhibition

h. Some patients present with intermediate levels of chloride excretion (U_{Cl} 10-20 mEq/L). Many of these patients are found to have excessive alkali administration, especially in the form of antacids or citrate anticoagulation of blood products

i. The treatment of metabolic alkalosis depends on its cause

    (1) Identify and correct the underlying source of acid loss or base accumulation if possible

    (2) Administration of NaCl (and usually KCl as well) is mandatory for patients with chloride-responsive alkalosis

    (3) In some situations, urinary HCO_3^- excretion can be hastened with the use of the carbonic anhydrase inhibitor, acetazolamide. This may be of particular benefit in patients with diuretic-dependent CHF and associated alkalosis

    (4) In rare cases, infusion of HCl or NH_4Cl may be necessary

        (a) This therapy requires an ICU setting and use of a central venous catheter

        (b) It should only be considered in cases where the arterial pH >7.60

        (c) The target pH for treatment with IV acid is 7.55

        (d) The amount of acid required can be calculated by

$$\text{mEq HCl} = \text{body wt(kg)} \times 0.5 \times (\text{actual} - \text{target } HCO_3^-)$$

        (e) Infuse this solution over a period of 12-24 hr with frequent monitoring of blood chemistries and ABGs during therapy

    (5) In patients with severe alkalemia, complicating acute renal failure, or chronic renal failure, hemodialysis with an acid bath solution can be employed

5. RESPIRATORY ALKALOSIS

a. Symptoms and signs of respiratory alkalosis include

    (1) Neuromuscular irritability

    (2) Cardiac dysrhythmias and electrocardiographic changes of ischemia

b. Laboratory findings include

    (1) Mild hyponatremia, hypokalemia, and hyperchloremia

c. Some causes of respiratory alkalosis are listed in the Box on p. 299

d. Treatment of respiratory alkalosis depends on the cause

    (1) Supplemental O_2 is beneficial in hypoxemic patients

    (2) Rebreathing techniques are effective in patients with hyperventilation due to anxiety

    (3) Patients with respiratory alkalosis due to underlying CNS disease may require a period of intubation with paralysis and mechanical ventilation if the primary process is not directly treatable

    (4) Drug-induced hyperventilation can sometimes be treated with dialysis and other measures designed to accelerate drug elimination

Causes of Respiratory Alkalosis

Iatrogenic (Hemodialysis, Mechanical Ventilation)
Central Stimulation of Respiration

Anxiety/pain
Trauma
Infections (meningitis, encephalitis)
Intracranial tumors
Cerebrovascular accidents
Drugs (salicylates, exogenous catecholamines)
Miscellaneous (fever, cirrhosis)

Hypoxemic Stimulation of Respiration

Pneumonia
Volume overload/pulmonary edema
Pulmonary emboli
Decreased lung compliance
High altitude
Carbon monoxide intoxication

16.2 ACUTE RENAL FAILURE

Definition

Acute renal failure (ARF) is defined as a relatively sudden (over hours to days) decrease in renal function leading to serious derangements of body fluid homeostasis. It is usually classified as being due to prerenal, postrenal, or intrinsic renal disorders. Prerenal ARF is caused by renal perfusion defects. Postrenal ARF is caused by obstruction of the urinary tract. Intrinsic ARF is due to parenchymal disease of the kidneys.

1. PRERENAL ARF
   a. The causes of prerenal ARF are listed in the Box on p. 300
      (1) Prerenal ARF also occurs in situations characterized with renal hypoperfusion despite adequate or even expanded extracellular fluid (ECF) volume. This is due to global or local abnormalities in circulation leading to renal insufficiency. Frequent examples include CHF and decreased peripheral vascular resistance that may accompany the sepsis syndrome
      (2) Renal blood flow may be selectively impaired by certain drugs (especially nonsteroidal antiinflammatory drugs [NSAIDs] and angiotensin inhibitors) or in the hepatorenal syndrome
      (3) In any case where renal blood flow is severely curtailed, ischemic acute renal failure is a possibility
   b. The diagnosis of prerenal ARF can often be made on clinical grounds
      (1) History and physical examination are crucial
      (2) Assessment of serial weights and intake/output (I/O) records are valuable if available
      (3) Oliguria is a customary finding
      (4) Urinalysis (U/A) reveals urinary concentration (specific gravity >1.020) but is otherwise typically benign

---

Causes of Prerenal ARF

Absolute ECF Volume Depletion

Extrarenal volume losses
  GI losses
  Third-space losses
  Inadequate fluid intake
  Hemorrhage
Renal volume losses (diuretics)

Relative ECF Volume Depletion

CHF
Decreased peripheral vascular resistance

Changes in Renal Vascular Tone

Nonsteroidal antiinflammatory drugs
Angiotensin converting enzyme inhibitors
Hepatorenal syndrome

---

(5) A ratio of BUN:creatinine >20:1 is suggestive but *not* diagnostic of prerenal ARF
(6) The most helpful feature is evidence of avid sodium reabsorption in an oliguric patient
  (a) Sodium avidity can be assessed by determining the fractional excretion of sodium (FE_{Na}), calculated as
$$FE_{Na} = (U_{Na} \times P_{creat})/(P_{Na} \times U_{creat}) \times 100$$
  (b) Values <1% suggest prerenal azotemia in the appropriate clinical setting
(7) In occasional cases where doubt remains, measurement of central venous pressure or pulmonary capillary wedge pressure may be useful in guiding therapy
c. Treatment of prerenal ARF depends on correction of the underlying cause and replacement of any volume deficits
  (1) Identify and treat the cause of fluid losses if possible
  (2) Maximize left ventricular function if CHF is playing a role
  (3) Discontinue offending drugs
  (4) Hepatic transplantation may restore renal function to normal in the patients with hepatorenal syndrome
  (5) In addition to treatment of the underlying disease, volume expansion with appropriate IV fluids (usually normal saline or blood products) is required for patients who are unable to ingest sufficient sodium and water
2. POSTRENAL ARF
a. Some causes of postrenal ARF are listed in the Box on p. 301
b. The diagnosis of postrenal ARF can be suspected on the basis of history and physical examination
  (1) Alternating polyuria and oligoanuria is suggestive of subtotal uri-

Causes of Postrenal ARF

Urethral Obstruction
Urethral valves
Prostatic hypertrophy

Bladder Obstruction
Neurogenic bladder
Bladder tumors
Cystitis

Ureteric Obstruction
Intrinsic
 Ureteric stones
 Papillary necrosis

Extrinsic
 Tumors
 Retroperitoneal fibrosis
 Aortic aneurysm
 Pregnancy

   nary obstruction, as is a very large postvoiding residual urine volume
  c. Laboratory tests are usually nonspecific
    (1) The U/A may be normal or disclose evidence of hematuria, pyuria,
        or crystalluria
    (2) The best screening test for obstruction is renal ultrasound, with a
        specificity of over 90%
    (3) If obstruction is still suspected despite a negative ultrasound, ret-
        rograde pyelography can be performed
  d. Therapy of postrenal ARF largely depends on the site of obstruction
    (1) The coexistence of obstruction and urinary tract infection is a uro-
        logic emergency mandating broad-spectrum antibiotic coverage
        and immediate decompression of the urinary tract
      (a) Upper-tract disease can be effectively approached with in-
          dwelling stents or percutaneous nephrostomy
      (b) Lower urinary obstruction can be relieved with urethral or su-
          prapubic catheterization
    (2) After the patient's medical condition has stabilized, it is often pos-
        sible to undertake definitive repair of the obstructing lesion. Re-
        lief of even long-standing obstruction is generally indicated since
        some functional recovery may occur, even weeks or months later
3. INTRINSIC ARF
  a. Some causes of intrinsic ARF are listed in the Box on p. 302
  b. Acute tubular necrosis (ATN) is by far the most common cause of
     intrinsic ARF among hospitalized patients

Causes of Intrinsic ARF

Glomerular Diseases

Acute glomerulonephritis
Rapidly progressive glomerulonephritis

Tubulointerstitial Diseases

Acute tubular necrosis
  Drug-induced
  Ischemic
Acute interstitial nephritis
  Allergic/drug-induced
  Idiopathic

Vascular Diseases

Renal artery
  Thrombosis/embolus
  Dissection
  Trauma
Renal microcirculation
  Vasculitis
  Malignant hypertension
  Disseminated intravascular coagulation (DIC)/thrombotic
  thrombocytopenic purpura (TTP)
  Cholesterol atheroemboli
Renal vein thrombosis

---

(1) There are multiple drugs and toxins that can cause ATN, including aminoglycoside antibiotics, certain chemotherapeutic agents (i.e., cisplatin, mithramycin), and radiographic contrast materials

(2) Ischemia is another major factor causing ATN

(3) ATN is especially common in patients with major trauma, recent major surgery (particularly vascular operations), sepsis, or crush injury

c. Acute interstitial nephritis (AIN) is usually caused by exposure to a drug or allergen. Rare idiopathic cases are encountered

(1) NSAIDs are probably the most common drugs that cause AIN

(2) Other frequent agents include antibiotics (particularly penicillins, cephalosporins, and sulfa-derivatives), loop and thiazide diuretics, and cimetidine

(3) Recognition of this entity is especially important since effective therapy depends on withdrawal of the offending drug

d. Diagnosis of intrinsic ARF depends heavily on the history and physical examination with subsequent directed laboratory and radiographic evaluations

(1) Carefully review medications

(2) Examine the urine sediment. It is valuable to note that intrinsic ARF is almost invariably accompanied by abnormalities on U/A. The absence of abnormalities should raise the suspicion of prerenal or postrenal causes

(3) The presence of urinary eosinophils can be used to support a diagnosis of AIN or cholesterol microemboli

(4) The $F_{E_{Na}}$ is typically >3% in intrinsic ARF

(5) Serologic evaluation of patients with suspected vasculitis should include antinuclear antibody (ANA), complements factors, hepatitis B surface antigen, cryoglobulins, and rheumatoid factor

(6) More invasive studies (e.g., angiography, renal biopsy) may be appropriate depending on the clinical circumstances

e. Therapy of intrinsic ARF is largely supportive

(1) Offending drugs should be identified and withdrawn, or substituted if possible

(2) Control fluid and electrolyte balance, modify drug dosages, and consider dialysis

(3) Specific therapy directed at a particular disease process is possible in occasional circumstances. A major aspect of the management of ARF is recognizing the situations where it is likely to occur and taking appropriate measures to reduce its probability

(a) Choose medications with the least risk of nephrotoxicity for patients prone to ARF

(b) Avoid or correct volume depletion

(c) Calcium channel blockers may be helpful in ameliorating ARF if given prophylactically (i.e., before angiography or renovascular surgery)

f. Despite many advances in the diagnosis and treatment of ARF, the mortality rate remains at least 50% in critically ill patients

16.3 ELECTROLYTE ABNORMALITIES

Certain electrolyte abnormalities that occur frequently pose a serious risk to ICU patients even if the disorder has been present for a long time

Calcium

Calcium exists in three forms in the circulation: free ionized calcium (iCa^{++}); in soluble complexes with phosphate, citrate, and bicarbonate; and bound to plasma proteins (principally albumin). Of these, the iCa^{++} is physiologically the most important. The normal value for iCa^{++} is 4.0-4.9 mg/dL, 2.4-2.6 mEq/L, or 1.2-1.3 mmol/L (note difference in units)

Maintenance of normal iCa^{++} levels depends on the interaction between GI absorption, bone fluxes, and renal excretion governed by parathyroid hormone (PTH), 1,25-dihydroxyvitamin D (1,25-D_3), and calcitonin.

1. Hypercalcemia

a. Most patients with hypercalcemia are asymptomatic at the time of diagnosis. However, numerous signs and symptoms may occur depending on the severity and rate of development

These include
- (1) Nausea
- (2) Constipation
- (3) Anorexia
- (4) Pancreatitis
- (5) Peptic ulcers
- (6) Renal insufficiency
- (7) Polyuria
- (8) Urolithiasis
- (9) Bone pain
- (10) Weakness
- (11) Confusion and coma

b. Symptomatic patients require urgent treatment
c. Some causes of hypercalcemia are listed in Table 16-3
d. Hypercalcemia is a medical emergency for which acute treatment is largely independent of the cause
e. Therapy is outlined in the Box below.
- (1) Administer IV normal saline at a rate of 150-250 ml/hr
- (2) Furosemide is indicated to prevent volume overload and to decrease calcium reabsorption (a minor effect)
- (3) Calcitonin's effectiveness is limited by the phenomenon of osteoclast escape that develops within a few days of beginning treatment

Table 16-3   Disorders of calcium homeostasis

Hypercalcemia	Hypocalcemia
Hyperparathyroidism	Hypoparathyroidism
Hyperthyroidism	Pseudohypoparathyroidism
Acute renal failure	Vitamin D deficiency
Malignancy	Malignancy
Excessive vitamin A or D	Hyperphosphatemia
Granulomatous diseases	Pancreatitis
Thiazide diuretics	Neonatal tetany
Immobilization	Calcium-complex formation

Treatment of Hypercalcemia

IV fluids: Normal saline 150-250 ml/hr
 (± furosemide 40-80 mg IV q 4-6 hr)
Corticosteroids: prednisone (or equivalent) 1 mg/kg/day
Calcitonin: 4 U/kg SQ q12hr
Etidronate: 7.5 mg/kg/day IV qd × 1-4 days
Mithramycin: 25 mcg/kg IV qd × 3-4 days
Indomethacin: 25-50 mg PO q8hr
Dialysis

    (4) Diphosphonates such as etidronate reduce calcium levels to normal within 5 days in 75% of patients

    (5) Mithramycin is the most potent hypocalcemic agent available, but its use is limited by serious renal, hepatic, and bone marrow side effects

    (6) Oral NSAIDs are indicated only in patients with prostaglandin-mediated hypercalcemia

    (7) Dialysis with low-calcium dialysate may be necessary in patients with refractory hypercalcemia, particularly if renal function is impaired

2. Hypocalcemia

  a. The clinical manifestations of hypocalcemia are usually related to effects on excitable tissues

    (1) Neurologic findings include overt or latent tetany and mental status changes

    (2) Cardiovascular manifestations include dysrhythmias, hypotension, and decreased myocardial contractility

  b. Some causes of hypocalcemia are listed in Table 16-3

  c. Hypoalbuminemia can cause a lowering of the total calcium but normal iCa^{++}

  d. Treatment of hypocalcemia is summarized in the Box below

    (1) Patients with latent or overt tetany require immediate parenteral replacement. Administer IV calcium through a central catheter if possible to avoid the risk of extravasation and skin necrosis

    (2) Correction of aggravating electrolyte abnormalities (hyperphosphatemia, hypomagnesemia) should take place simultaneously

    (3) Oral calcium and vitamin D supplements are satisfactory for milder, asymptomatic cases

Magnesium

Magnesium is the second most common intracellular cation (after potassium). Most of its biologic effects depend on its role as a cofactor for intra-

---

Treatment of Hypocalcemia

Calcium bolus: 10-30 ml 10% Ca gluconate or $CaCl_2$ slow IV push over 15-30 min

Calcium infusion: 40 ml 10% Ca gluconate in 500 ml D_5W IV at 20 ml/hr, titrate to desired iCa^{++}

Hyperphosphatemia: calcium carbonate ($CaCO_3$) 650 mg 1-3 tabs PO tid with meals aluminum hydroxide ($Al(OH)_3$) gels 30-60 ml PO tid with meals

Hypomagnesemia: 2 ml 50% magnesium sulfate ($MgSO_4$) IV or IM q 4-6 hr

Oral calcium: $CaCO_3$, Ca acetate, or Ca lactate 1-3 tabs qid on an empty stomach

Vitamin D: calcitriol 0.25-0.5 mcg q 12-24 hr

cellular enzymes, particularly adenosine triphosphate (ATP) dependent systems. Magnesium balance is determined by the relationship between dietary ingestion and renal excretion. Urinary magnesium excretion is increased by sodium and calcium loading, diuretics, and PTH. It is decreased by volume depletion.

1. Hypomagnesemia
   a. Since most magnesium is intracellular, it can be difficult to estimate the magnitude of magnesium depletion from serum levels. However, hypomagnesemia and simultaneous hypomagnesiuria (U_{Mg} <1 mEq/day) strongly suggest depleted body stores
   b. Symptoms of hypomagnesemia include weakness, anorexia, and nausea. Some physical signs are latent tetany, hyperreflexia, tremors, dysrhythmias, delirium, and coma
   c. Important associated laboratory abnormalities include hypokalemia and hypocalcemia that may be refractory to treatment until magnesium stores are repleted
   d. Some common causes of hypomagnesemia are listed in Table 16-4
      (1) GI causes include steatorrhea (malabsorption), pancreatitis, dietary deficiency, and prolonged diarrhea or vomiting
      (2) Several endocrinopathies including diabetes mellitus, hyperparathyroidism, primary hyperaldosteronism, and hyperthyroidism can lead to hypomagnesemia
      (3) Excessive renal magnesium losses can occur in patients with congenital magnesium wasting, ketoacidosis, Bartter's syndrome, hyperaldosteronism, and the syndrome of inappropriate secretion of antidiuretic hormone (SIADH)
      (4) Multiple drugs cause renal magnesium loss including diuretics (except acetazolamide), *cis*-platinum, and cyclosporine
      (5) Hypomagnesemia associated with alcoholism has been attributed to urinary Mg losses, decreased dietary intake, and alcoholic or starvation ketoacidosis
   e. Many cases of hypomagnesemia can be prevented and treated by the inclusion of magnesium supplements for patients receiving parenteral nutrition and treatment for diabetic ketoacidosis
      (1) Mild cases of magnesium depletion (Mg^{++} 1.3-1.6 mg/dL) can be corrected by the intake of a high-Mg diet. Food sources of magnesium include meats and green vegetables
   f. Pharmacologic replacement is indicated in more severe cases
      (1) Oral supplementation can be provided with MgO 400-3200 mg/day. Diarrhea is a potential side effect of this treatment

Table 16-4   Disorders of magnesium homeostasis

Hypomagnesemia	Hypermagnesemia
GI disorders	Renal failure
Endocrinopathies	Massive Mg ingestion
Renal Mg losses	
Alcoholism	

  (2) Parenteral therapy with 1-2 g (2-4 ml) of 50% $MgSO_4$ repeated q 4-6 hr prn is sufficient therapy for most patients
  (3) Serum magnesium levels and deep tendon reflexes must be monitored closely during treatment since life-threatening hypermagnesemia can occur
2. Hypermagnesemia
  a. The clinical features of magnesium excess are frequently confused with those of hypercalcemia. They include
    (1) Nausea
    (2) Altered mental status
    (3) Weakness and diminished tendon reflexes
    (4) Hypotension
    (5) Dysrhythmias
    (6) Respiratory paralysis
  b. The most frequent predisposing condition to hypermagnesemia is chronic renal failure. Sustained hypermagnesemia occurs only in the setting of renal insufficiency, although acute magnesium excess can occur in the setting of the overzealous replacement of magnesium deficiency
  c. Therapy of hypermagnesemia involves discontinuing magnesium intake, infusion of Ca gluconate 15 mg/kg over 4 hr (which acts as a direct magnesium antagonist), and dialysis with an Mg-free bath in severe cases

Phosphate

Phosphate is an abundant intracellular anion that is critically important in energy metabolism and structural integrity of literally all cells. The overwhelming majority of dietary phosphate is normally absorbed, but a significant amount (approximately 200 mg/day) is secreted in the stool. Renal excretion eliminates the remainder, about 400-1500 mg/day depending on intake. Urinary phosphorus excretion is increased by PTH, volume expansion, corticosteroids, and calcitonin; it is decreased by insulin, thyroid hormone, and vitamin D. Movement of phosphate into cells is enhanced during alkalemia by glucose and other carbohydrates, and by hormones including insulin, epinephrine, and corticosteroids.

1. Hypophosphatemia
  a. Characterized by altered mental status, weakness or myopathy progressing to rhabdomyolysis, osteomalacia, dysfunction of all blood cell types, anorexia, respiratory failure, and decreased cardiac contractility. However, most cases of phosphate depletion are asymptomatic unless severe
  b. Some causes of hypophosphatemia are listed in Table 16-5
    (1) Respiratory and metabolic alkalosis is associated with intracellular uptake of phosphate
    (2) Refeeding after prolonged starvation precipitates hypophosphatemia largely due to intracellular shifts mediated by glucose and insulin
    (3) Administration or excessive activity of other hormones (epinephrine, growth hormone, steroids, gastrin, and glucagon) can cause hypophosphatemia by similar mechanisms

Table 16-5   Disorders of phosphate homeostasis

Hypophosphatemia	Hyperphosphatemia
Intracellular shifts	Massive cell lysis
Inadequate ingestion	Increased ingestion
GI losses	Renal failure
Renal losses	

  (4) Malnutrition alone does not typically cause severe hypophosphatemia. However, GI losses due to malabsorption of phosphate or use of phosphorus-binding antacids can lead to marked phosphate depletion

  (5) Excessive renal losses of phosphate are present in Fanconi's syndrome, after renal transplantation in some patients, following recovery from urinary obstruction or ATN, and with vitamin D–resistant rickets

  c. The best treatment of hypophosphatemia is prevention

   (1) Phosphate deficiency can be avoided by preemptive supplementation in patients with malnutrition undergoing hyperalimentation or refeeding; or patients who are chronic alcoholics, on long-term antacids, and with uncontrolled diabetes mellitus or ketoacidosis

   (2) Treatment of established hypophosphatemia depends on severity and cause

    (a) Patients with mild hypophosphatemia due to intracellular shifts can be followed closely without active intervention unless the serum phosphorus drops below 1.5 mg/dL

    (b) Dietary supplementation in the form of increased intake of dairy products is adequate in most asymptomatic patients

    (c) Oral supplementation can be provided with sodium and/or potassium phosphate, although diarrhea is often a dose-limiting side effect

    (d) Treat severe symptomatic hypophosphatemia with 2 mg of elemental phosphorus/kg (as sodium or potassium phosphate) IV q6hr until oral repletion can begin, usually at a phosphorus level of 2 mg/dL

    (e) Use of parenteral phosphate is relatively contraindicated in patients with oliguric renal failure

    (f) Possible complications of IV phosphorus include dysrhythmias, hyperphosphatemia, hypocalcemia, hyperkalemia, and volume overload

 2. Hyperphosphatemia

  a. Many of the symptoms of hyperphosphatemia can be attributed to the reciprocal fall in iCa^{++} that generally occurs (see above)

  b. Severe hyperphosphatemia can also cause ARF, particularly in the setting of massive cell lysis. Metastatic calcifications caused by precipitation of Ca phosphate (PO_4) crystals in essentially any tissue or organ can lead to widespread symptoms and signs

  c. The causes of hyperphosphatemia are summarized in Table 16-5

d. Treatment of hyperphosphatemia involves decreasing ingestion with phosphorus-restricted diets as well as increasing elimination via the GI tract and kidneys
   (1) Phosphate binders containing magnesium, calcium, or aluminum will accelerate stool phosphorus losses even in patients who are unable to take anything orally (NPO)
   (2) Avoid magnesium-containing agents in patients with renal failure
   (3) Renal excretion of phosphate is enhanced by acetazolamide, volume expansion, and alkaline diuresis. Unfortunately, the frequent coexistence of renal failure with hyperphosphatemia often makes this route unreliable
   (4) Hemodialysis or peritoneal dialysis is effective for acute or chronic hyperphosphatemia

Potassium

Potassium is the most abundant intracellular cation. Only about 2% of total body potassium is in the ECF. Intracellular potassium is responsible for maintaining cell volume and resting membrane potential. A number of factors regulate potassium movement into cells. These are summarized in Table 16-6.

1. Hypokalemia
   a. Abnormally low ECF $[K^+]$ can have widespread pathophysiologic effects; dominant among these are neuromuscular and cardiac events
      (1) Neuromuscular problems include GI hypomotility, skeletal muscle weakness or paralysis, and rhabdomyolysis
      (2) Cardiac manifestations include the appearance of a U wave on the electrocardiogram (ECG), ventricular and atrial dysrhythmias, predisposition to digoxin toxicity, and cardiac necrosis
      (3) Cellular metabolism and renal function may also be impaired
   b. The causes of hypokalemia are listed in Table 16-7
      (1) Pseudohypokalemia reflects in vitro K^+ uptake by leukemic cells in patients with severe leukocytosis (white blood cell count [WBC] $>10^5/mm^3$)
      (2) Intracellular shifts of K^+ occur in alkalosis, insulin overdose, use of beta$_2$ agonists, hypokalemic periodic paralysis, and barium poisoning
      (3) Patients with anorexia nervosa, alcoholism, or severe dietary restrictions may develop significant hypokalemia
      (4) Excessive GI K^+ losses occur in patients with protracted vomiting, diarrhea, and laxative abuse

Table 16-6 Factors affecting cellular potassium distribution

Increasing K^+	Decreasing K^+
Alkalosis	Acidosis
Insulin	Glucagon
Beta$_2$ agonists	Alpha agonists
	Hyperosmolarity

Table 16-7   Disorders of potassium homeostasis

Hypokalemia	Hyperkalemia
Pseudohypokalemia	Pseudohyperkalemia
Cellular K^+ uptake	Cellular K^+ loss
Poor dietary K^+ intake	Excessive K^+ intake
GI losses	Inadequate renal excretion
Renal losses	Cell lysis

    (5) Renal losses occur in patients with renal tubular acidosis, hyperaldosteronism, hypomagnesemia, metabolic acidosis, and treatment of diabetic ketoacidosis. In addition, numerous drugs cause renal K^+ wasting including diuretics and antibiotics (penicillins, cephalosporins, aminoglycosides, amphotericin)

  c. Treatment of hypokalemia is imprecise since the degree of total body K^+ depletion is usually impossible to calculate

    (1) Halt ongoing K^+ losses if possible and correct aggravating abnormalities (alkalosis, hypomagnesemia)

    (2) The particular K^+ salt employed depends on the specific clinical problem. KCl is preferred in patients with concomitant metabolic alkalosis and is effective in all forms of hypokalemia. Bicarbonate or phosphate salts of K^+ may be preferred if acidosis or hypophosphatemia is present

    (3) Oral K^+ preparations are effective but may have an unpalatable taste and cause GI irritation

    (4) K^+ can be given by slow IV infusion (10-20 mEq/hr) through a central or peripheral line; avoid concentrations >40 mEq/L in peripheral IVs to decrease the risk of phlebitis

    (5) Frequent monitoring of serum K^+ is essential during parenteral potassium repletion

    (6) Potassium-sparing diuretics are occasionally useful but should be used with caution in patients receiving K^+ supplements

2. Hyperkalemia

  a. The principal clinical abnormalities of hyperkalemia are neuromuscular and cardiac. Weakness, paresthesias, and paralysis may occur but are usually overshadowed by cardiac disturbances. These include

    (1) Progressive ECG appearance of peaked T waves

    (2) Flattened P waves

    (3) Prolonged PR interval

    (4) Widening of the QRS complex

    (5) The development of a sine wave pattern presages the onset of ventricular fibrillation or asystole

  b. Some causes of hyperkalemia are presented in Table 16-7

    (1) Pseudohyperkalemia is due to in vitro release of K^+ from red blood cells (RBC), leukocytes, or platelets

    (2) Release of K^+ from cells contributes to hyperkalemia in acidosis, poorly controlled diabetes mellitus, beta blockade, hyperkalemic periodic paralysis, hyperosmolar states, and digitalis toxicity

Therapy of Hyperkalemia

10% Calcium gluconate 10-30 ml IV
  Onset <5 min
50% dextrose 50 ml + regular insulin 5 U IV q30min
  Onset 15-30 min
NaHCO$_3$ 50 ml (50 mEq) IV q30min × 4 doses
  Onset 15-30 min
Sodium polystyrene sulfonate in sorbitol 30-60 g PO/enema q 4-6 hr
  Onset 1-2 hr
Dialysis

    (3) Potassium ingestion seldom results in hyperkalemia if renal func-
        tion is normal except when excessive parenteral K$^+$ supplements
        have been administered
    (4) Inadequate renal excretion occurs in patients with advanced renal
        failure, deficiencies of adrenal hormones, and numerous drugs.
        These include potassium sparing diuretics, NSAIDs, angiotensin
        converting enzyme (ACE) inhibitors, and cyclosporine
    (5) Severe hyperkalemia is a frequent finding in patients with mas-
        sive in vivo hemolysis or tumor lysis syndrome
  c. The treatment of hyperkalemia is outlined in the Box above
    (1) Calcium does not affect serum K$^+$ but rather antagonizes the car-
        diac toxicity of hyperkalemia
    (2) Glucose/insulin and bicarbonate infusions lower serum K$^+$ by
        stimulating cellular K$^+$ entry
    (3) Sodium polystyrene sulfonate is used to augment fecal K$^+$ excre-
        tion; it is relatively ineffective unless the patient develops diar-
        rhea or loose stools
    (4) Dialysis is extremely effective for life-threatening hyperkalemia
    (5) Diuretics and aldosterone analogs are occasionally useful adjunc-
        tive measures
    (6) The use of beta-adrenergic agents (e.g., albuterol) via nebuliza-
        tions has received considerable attention in recent years for the
        acute management of hyperkalemia in end-stage renal disease pa-
        tients

Sodium

Hyponatremia and hypernatremia are disorders of water balance. The osmolarity of a solution depends on the number of dissolved particles per liter. In
clinical practice this can be measured or calculated as:

$$P_{osm} = 2 \times Na^+ + glucose/18 + BUN/2.8$$

Solutes restricted to one side of the plasma membrane are termed *effective
osmoles;* changes in the quantity of effective osmoles in a body fluid obli-
gate transmembrane water movement to maintain balance. Freely membrane
permeable substances such as urea do not cause water movement and are

hence termed *ineffective osmoles*. The tonicity or effective osmolarity of a solution can be calculated by:

$$E_{osm} = 2 \times Na^+ + glucose/18$$

Regulation of plasma osmolarity depends on the interplay between water ingestion and renal water excretion. Renal mechanisms of water balance require the adequate delivery of salt and water to distal nephron sites as well as manipulation of tubular water permeability under the influence of antidiuretic hormone (ADH). ADH is secreted by the posterior pituitary in response to hypertonicity as well as other nonosmotic stimuli including hypovolemia, nausea, pain, and several drugs (i.e., nicotine, narcotics, vincristine, cyclophosphamide, chlorpropamide, and clofibrate). ADH increases renal water permeability, leading to increased water reabsorption and hypertonic urine. Normal thirst is even more responsive to changes in osmolarity than ADH is; consequently, thirst should be considered the primary guardian of plasma tonicity.

1. Hyponatremia
   a. Symptoms of hyponatremia are caused by osmotic movement of water from ECF into cells
      (1) Conditions characterized by hyponatremia with normal or elevated osmolarity (due to accumulation of unmeasured osmotically active solutes) are not symptomatic
      (2) Brain cells are most sensitive to changes in volume; hence, most symptoms of hyponatremia are neurologic. They include nausea, neuromuscular irritability, altered mental status, and seizures
      (3) The likelihood of symptomatic hyponatremia depends on its severity and the rapidity with which it develops
   b. Some causes of hyponatremia are listed in the Box below
      (1) Pseudohyponatremia is defined as a low measured serum sodium despite a normal or elevated plasma osmolarity. Causes include

---

Causes of Hyponatremia

Pseudohyponatremia
Pure water intoxication
Hyponatremia with appropriate ADH secretion
   Hypovolemia
   Congestive heart failure
   Endocrinopathies
   Renal disease
   Cirrhosis
Syndrome of inappropriate secretion of antidiuretic hormone
   Idiopathic
   Drug-induced
   Pulmonary diseases
   CNS diseases
   Malignancy

hyperlipidemia, hyperproteinemia, hyperglycemia, mannitol infusion, and radiographic contrast agents. Measurement of plasma osmolarity prior to initiation of therapy for hyponatremia is vital to exclude pseudohyponatremia

(2) Hyponatremia due to pure water intoxication is extremely rare due to the efficiency with which the kidneys can excrete even massive water loads

(3) Most cases of true hyponatremia are associated with elevated ADH activity that is provoked by some nonosmotic stimulus

(4) Volume depletion of any cause is a major stimulus for ADH release. This includes states of relative volume depletion such as CHF

(5) Hypothyroidism and adrenal insufficiency are also causes of hyponatremia (see also Chapter 6)

(6) Many renal diseases, including nephrotic syndrome, predispose to hyponatremia due to inadequate delivery of solute to the distal nephron

(7) Hyponatremia in untreated cirrhosis is caused by excessive ADH secretion and impaired distal sodium delivery

(8) SIADH has multiple causes including drugs, pulmonary diseases, CNS diseases, and cancer (See also Chapter 6)

c. Symptomatic hyponatremia is a medical emergency regardless of duration

d. After the plasma osmolarity has been determined, institute therapy with 3% NaCl. The amount of NaCl required to correct hyponatremia to a specified target level is

$$mEq\ NaCl = 0.6 \times (weight\ [kg]) \times (target\ Na^+ - plasma\ Na^+)$$

The amount of 3% saline required to achieve this goal is

$$3\%\ NaCl\ (ml) = (1000) \times (mEq\ NaCl)/513$$

The target Na^+ is an increase of 20 mEq/L above the actual Na^+ or 130 mEq/L, whichever is lower. The rate of correction is 1-1.5 mEq/L/hr. These calculations often underestimate the actual rate of correction due to ongoing urinary sodium losses

e. In addition to hypertonic saline infusion, give all IV fluids (including medications) in 0.9% NaCl and a fluid restriction of 1000-1500 ml/day instituted if possible

f. Demeclocycline 150-300 mg PO q12hr has been used successfully in the treatment of SIADH but is contraindicated in cirrhosis

g. Central pontine myelinolysis is a rare complication occurring after correction of chronic (but not acute) hyponatremia if the serum Na^+ is raised by >25 mEq/L during the first 48 hr of therapy

2. Hypernatremia

a. Symptoms of hypernatremia are caused by cellular dehydration, particularly of neurons. They include altered mental status, nausea, seizures, and intracranial hemorrhage. Myoclonus, metabolic acidosis, and hyperglycemia due to peripheral insulin resistance are also common

b. Most hypernatremic patients are volume-depleted; the finding of volume overload suggests the possibility of acute salt poisoning

c. Causes of hypernatremia are listed in the Box on p. 314

Causes of Hypernatremia

Diabetes insipidus
H_2O losses
   Renal
   GI
   Insensible
Salt poisoning
H_2O deprivation
Primary hypodipsia
Mineralocorticoid excess

---

  (1) Diabetes insipidus (DI) can be of central or nephrogenic origin (see also Chapter 6)
  (2) The most common cause of hypernatremia is excessive water loss
    (a) Excessive renal water loss with hypernatremia has been reported in patients with renal failure, hypercalcemia, hypokalemia, sickle-cell disease, osmotic diuresis, postobstructive diuresis, and drugs (including alcohol, lithium, demeclocycline, oral hypoglycemics, and others)
    (b) GI water losses due to gastroenteritis are an especially common cause of hypernatremia in children
    (c) Insensible water losses via the skin or respiratory tract occur with prolonged exposure to hot climates, thermal burns, and fever
  (3) Salt poisoning is a rare cause of outpatient hypernatremia; it is more common in hospitalized patients as a complication of hypertonic $NaHCO_3$ therapy for severe acidosis
  (4) Water deprivation is a fundamental feature of practically all cases of hypernatremia but is rarely the sole cause of the problem
  (5) Entities characterized by increased mineralocorticoid activity (Conn's syndrome and Cushing's syndrome) are sometimes accompanied by mild to moderate hypernatremia
 d. The treatment of hypernatremia is to replace free water deficits, and correct contributing electrolyte problems and hypovolemia (if present)
  (1) The water deficit is calculated as

$$H_2O \text{ deficit (L)} = 0.6 \times \text{weight(kg)} \times [(\text{target } Na^+)/(\text{actual } Na^+) - 1]$$

    The target Na^+ is either 148 mEq/L or a decrease of 20-25 mEq/L in the plasma Na^+ from its initial value, whichever is higher. The goal of therapy is to reduce the plasma Na^+ by 1-1.5 mEq/L/hr
  (2) Faster rates of correction of chronic hypernatremia may precipitate rehydration seizures
  (3) The choice of fluid and route of administration depend on the clinical circumstances. Distilled or tap water given PO or via NG tube is preferred when feasible. If the enteral route is unavailable 0.45% NaCl can be administered by peripheral vein without significant risk of hemolysis

(4) Patients with clinical evidence of volume overload who cannot tolerate the sodium load of 0.45% NaCl should be given distilled water IV through a central catheter

(5) D_5W is at least relatively contraindicated in many patients because of the coexistence of insulin resistance and the consequent risk of worsening hyperosmolarity due to unmetabolized dextrose

(6) Diuretics or dialysis can be employed for patients with salt poisoning

(7) Vasopressin analogs are useful in the long-term management of central DI

16.4   FLUID AND ELECTROLYTE THERAPY

In addition to the more specific treatments outlined above, some general guidelines regarding fluid and electrolyte therapy are useful. Administration of fluids and nutrition is essential but a frequently overlooked consideration in the care of the ICU patient. Special care must be exercised in the selection and administration of IV fluids to the critically ill with ongoing renal or extrarenal fluid and electrolyte losses. IV fluids are potentially the most dangerous drugs used in the hospital; constant vigilance is required.

1. Some form of IV access is necessary for all ICU patients
2. Whenever possible, employ the GI tract for maintenance fluids, nutrition, and medications
3. The type of fluid used depends on the clinical situation. Some general comments can be made
   a. Crystalloid solutions are employed for routine maintenance
      (1) In an otherwise well NPO patient, obligatory water losses amount to about 1000 ml/day
      (2) Na^+ losses are minimized by virtually complete renal Na^+ reclamation, but some urinary K^+ excretion continues (30-60 mEq/day) and must be replaced
      (3) Excessive protein catabolism and starvation ketosis can be prevented by inclusion of glucose 150-200 g qd in maintenance fluids
      (4) Supplements of other vitamins and minerals may be necessary if parenteral therapy lasts a week or more
   b. Colloid solutions such as blood products, albumin, and plasma are indicated for the rapid expansion of intravascular volume with minimal effects on other components of ECF

16.5   DIALYSIS

ICU patients frequently develop homeostatic abnormalities that cannot be managed conservatively. In such cases, dialysis or a related modality becomes necessary.

1. Dialysis is indicated in many different situations
   a. Volume overload manifested by pulmonary edema or severe hypertension that is unresponsive to diuretics can be effectively treated with dialysis or ultrafiltration

   b. Dialysis is useful for the treatment of several electrolyte abnormalities including severe acidosis or alkalosis, hyperkalemia, hyponatremia or hypernatremia, hypercalcemia, hyperphosphatemia, and hypermagnesemia

   c. Symptoms caused by the accumulation of uremic toxins are best treated with dialysis

   d. Poisonings with ethylene glycol, methanol, salicylates, and others can be effectively treated with dialysis

2. The most frequently used dialysis modality in the ICU is hemodialysis (HD) or one of its variants. The choice between HD and peritoneal dialysis (PD) is usually a matter of the physician's preference, but in some cases a clear preference is evident

   a. HD is the therapy of choice for severely catabolic patients due to more efficient removal of urea and other low molecular weight nitrogenous wastes

     (1) A large-bore, dual-lumen central venous catheter is required for vascular access

     (2) For standard hemodialysis orders, the physician specifies the type of membrane to be used (more biocompatible membranes such as cellulose acetate are preferred in the ICU), the duration of therapy, blood flow speed, type of anticoagulation, composition of the dialysate with respect to Na^+, K^+, Ca^{++}, and HCO_3^-, the desired amount of fluid removal, and any additional medications or treatments required (e.g., blood products, antibiotics, or erythropoietin)

     (3) The most common complication of HD is hypotension, generally treated with fluid boluses of normal saline or albumin. In some cases, alternate treatments must be considered if hypotension is severe. Other serious potential complications of dialysis include dysrhythmias (presumably due to acute electrolyte fluxes) and hypoxemia (caused by membrane-induced complement activation and leukocyte sequestration in pulmonary capillaries, as well as a decrease in minute ventilation due to removal of CO_2 by dialysis)

   b. Several variants of hemodialysis have been developed to accomplish fluid and solute removal in hypotensive patients

     (1) *Continuous arteriovenous hemofiltration* (CAVH) with or without dialysis is used in many ICUs. It has the specific advantage of allowing removal of large amounts of fluid even in patients with serious hemodynamic compromise. The patient's own arterial pressure is used to drive ultrafiltration across a highly permeable membrane. Fluid removal may exceed 500 ml/hr with CAVH, so the provision must be made for a pump to limit ultrafiltration or replacement with an adequate amount of a balanced salt solution. Solute removal can be accelerated by the passing peritoneal dialysate across the ultrafiltrate side of the membrane. CAVH generally requires femoral arterial access; thus, it may not be possible in patients with severe vascular disease

     (2) A modification of this technique known as *continuous venovenous hemofiltration* (CVVH) has recently been introduced and is gaining favor. Vascular access is simplified since arterial access is not

required, but CVVH does require additional equipment in the form of pumps and alarms
c. PD has less efficient clearance of low molecular weight solutes than HD, so it is not generally first-line therapy in hypercatabolic ICU patients
  (1) PD is much better tolerated from a hemodynamic standpoint and may be preferred in unstable patients
  (2) PD is technically easier than HD for small children. Access to the peritoneal cavity is obtained with a flexible catheter that can be placed at the bedside
  (3) PD can be done continuously or intermittently with a minimum of equipment and staff. Ultrafiltration is controlled by changing the glucose concentration (and hence osmolarity) of the dialysate
  (4) PD orders should include the number and duration of exchanges; the composition of the dialysate with respect to glucose, sodium, and calcium; and whether any additives such as antibiotics, heparin, insulin, or K^+ are to be included
  (5) The most common complication of PD is peritonitis. Parenteral or intraperitoneal antibiotics should result in clinical improvement within 24-48 hr; if not, consider catheter removal
  (6) Hyperglycemia resulting from absorption of dialysate glucose can be managed by intraperitoneal or subcutaneous insulin administration

16.6 RHABDOMYOLYSIS

Definition

Rhabdomyolysis is a condition characterized by the release of muscle cell contents into the circulation due to skeletal muscle necrosis.
1. Signs and symptoms occur due to toxicity of pigment globin proteins and accompanying fluid and electrolyte shifts
2. Some causes of rhabdomyolysis are listed in the Box below
   a. Trauma causes muscle injury both by direct pressure and muscle hypoperfusion due to shock and vasospasm
   b. Ischemic events such as arterial thrombosis and compartment syndromes can lead to muscle necrosis

Causes of Rhabdomyolysis

Trauma
Ischemia
Drugs/toxins
Infections
Excessive muscle activity
Heatstroke

   c. Numerous drugs and toxins including heroin, phencyclidine, cocaine, succinylcholine, and lipid-lowering agents have also been associated with rhabdomyolysis

   d. Infections due to Coxsackie, influenza, and measles viruses, as well as bacterial infections with *Clostridium, Staphylococcus,* and *Legionella* can cause skeletal muscle injury

   e. Excessive muscle activity (seizures, status asthmaticus, marathon running) has been reported as an infrequent cause of rhabdomyolysis. In cases of heatstroke some degree of muscle injury is invariably present

3. The diagnosis of rhabdomyolysis depends on a thorough history and physical examination

   a. Muscle pain is present in about half the cases

   b. Symptoms or signs related to various electrolyte abnormalities may be present

   c. Fever and evidence of ECF volume depletion can frequently be documented

   d. U/A reveals urine that appears to be bloody with a positive dipstick test for blood *in the absence of* apparent red blood cells on microscopic examination of the sediment

   e. Common early electrolyte abnormalities include hyponatremia, hyperkalemia, hypocalcemia, hyperphosphatemia, hypermagnesemia, hyperuricemia, and metabolic acidosis. Hypercalcemia may be a later finding

   f. ARF occurs in about 30% of patients

   g. Intracellular muscle enzymes (creatine kinase and aldolase) are invariably elevated, often to astronomic levels

   h. Low-grade DIC is present in the overwhelming majority of cases; its absence should prompt consideration of other diagnoses

   i. As muscle groups swell in response to injury, persistent or recurrent muscle injury can occur leading to clinical exacerbation 48-72 hr after the initial injury (second-wave phenomenon)

4. Principles of treatment are outlined in Table 16-8

   a. Vigorous volume expansion is essential, especially in the initial stages when 2-3 L/hr is frequently necessary. After the patient has stabilized, fluid administration is reduced to 300-500 ml/hr to maintain brisk urine output (>200 ml/hr)

Table 16-8   Treatment of rhabdomyolysis

IV fluids

Normal saline volume expansion
Bicarbonate infusions

Diuretics

Mannitol
Furosemide

Treatment of electrolyte disorders

Dialysis

b. Producing an alkaline diuresis (urine pH >8) by IV infusion of isotonic $NaHCO_3$ (3 amps $NaHCO_3$/L D_5W) has been suggested as a possible means of increasing urine myoglobin solubility, but this has not been tested in well-controlled clinical trials. The use of diuretics to prevent tubular obstruction has some experimental support but has not been validated in practice

c. Treatment of electrolyte abnormalities as discussed previously is of paramount importance

d. Dialysis is indicated for the treatment of severe ARF and resistant electrolyte problems

5. Survival of patients with rhabdomyolysis who have been given appropriate intensive care is 80%-90%

Suggested readings

Ayus JC, Krothapalli RK, Arieff AI: Changing concepts in the treatment of severe symptomatic hyponatremia: rapid correction and possible relation to central pontine myelinolysis. *Am J Med* 1985; 79:897-902.

Barnett VT, Schmidt GA: *Acid-base disorders.* In Hall JB, Schmidt GA, Wood LDH, editors: *Principles of critical care,* New York, 1992, McGraw-Hill.

Billhardt RA, Rosenbush SW: Cardiogenic and hypovolemic shock. *Med Clin North Am* 1986; 70:853-76.

Bourgoignie JJ, Oster JR, Perez GO, et al: *Disorders of potassium metabolism.* In Suki WN, Massry SG, editors: *Therapy of renal diseases and related disorders,* ed 2, Boston, 1991, Kluwer Academic Publishers.

Brennan S, Ayus JC: Acute versus chronic hypernatremia: how fast to correct ECF volume? *J Crit Illness* 1990; 5:330-3.

Brennan S, Ayus JC: *Systemic disorders and cerebral demyelinating lesions.* In Arieff AI, Griggs RC, editors: *Metabolic brain dysfunction in systemic disorders,* Boston, 1992, Little, Brown.

Brennan S, Ayus JC: *Treatment of hypo-osmolar and hyperosmolar states.* In Suki WN, Massry SG, editors: *Therapy of renal diseases and related disorders,* ed 2, Boston, 1991, Kluwer Academic Publishers.

Brennan S, Lederer ED: *Severe electrolyte disturbances.* In Hall JB, Schmidt GA, Wood LDH, editors: *Principles of critical care,* New York, 1992, McGraw-Hill.

Conger JD, Briner VA, Schrier RW: *Acute renal failure: pathogenesis, diagnosis, and management.* In Schrier RW, editor: *Renal and electrolyte disorders,* Boston, 1992, Little, Brown.

Corwin HL, Teplick RS, Schreiber MJ, et al: Prediction of outcome in acute renal failure. *Am J Nephrol* 1987; 7:8-12.

Dyckner T: *Disorders of magnesium metabolism.* In Suki WN, Massry SG, editors: *Therapy of renal diseases and related disorders,* ed 2, Boston, 1991, Kluwer Academic Publishers.

Ferri FE: *Acid-base disturbances.* In Ferri FE, editor: *Practical guide to the care of the medical patient,* ed 2, St. Louis, 1991, Mosby–Year Book.

Gabow PA: Disorders associated with an altered anion gap. *Kidney Int* 1984; 27:472-83.

Gabow PA, Kaehny WD, Kelleher SP: The spectrum of rhabdomyolysis. *Baltimore* 1982; 61:141-52.

Gillum DM, Brennan S: *Acute renal failure.* In Hall JB, Schmidt GA, Wood LDH, editors: *Principles of critical care,* New York, 1992, McGraw-Hill.

Gums JG: Clinical significance of magnesium: a review. *Drug Intell Clin Pharm* 1987; 21:240-6.

Halabe A, Sutton RAL: *Disorders of calcium metabolism.* In Suki WN, Massry SG, editors: *Therapy of renal diseases and related disorders,* ed 2, Boston, 1991, Kluwer Academic Publishers.

Hou SH, Bushinsky DA, Wish JB et al: Hospital-acquired renal insufficiency: a prospective study. *Am J Med* 1983; 74:243-8.

Kunis KL, Lowenstein J: The emergency treatment of hyperkalemia. *Med Clin North Am* 1981; 65:165-76.

Lau K: *Phosphate disorders.* In Kokko JP, Tannen RL, editors: *Fluids and electrolytes,* Philadelphia, 1986,WB Saunders.

Lederer ED, Gillum DM: *Dialysis in the critical care patient.* In Hall JB, Schmidt GA, Wood LDH, editors: *Principles of critical care,* New York, 1992, McGraw-Hill.

Lentz DR, Brown DM, Kjellstrand CM: Treatment of severe hypophosphatemia. *Ann Intern Med* 1978; 89:941-4.

Snyder NA, Feigal DW, Arieff AI: Hypernatremia in elderly patients: a heterogeneous, morbid, and iatrogenic entity. *Ann Intern Med* 1987; 107:309-19.

Stacpoole PW: Lactic acidosis: the case against bicarbonate therapy. *Ann Intern Med* 1986; 105:276-9.

Toto RD: *Metabolic acid-base disorders.* In Kokko JP, Tannen RL, editors: *Fluids and electrolytes,* Philadelphia, 1986, WB Saunders.

Varon J, Jacobs MB, Mahoney CA: Reflections on the anion gap in hyperglycemia. *West J Med* 1992; 157:670-2.

Special Techniques

17

Joseph Varon and Robert E Fromm, Jr.

AIRWAY MANAGEMENT

1. The first technique in the management of patients with airway problems is manual opening of the airway (i.e., head-tilt, chin-lift). (See Chapter 4.)
2. Adjuncts for artificial airway
   a. Oropharyngeal airways
      (1) Available in a number of different sizes and styles
      (2) These devices routinely should be sized from the angle of the jaw to the central incisors
      (3) Techniques for insertion include
         (a) The inverted technique: the oral airway is placed upside down and rotated to the appropriate position
         (b) Tongue depressor technique: a tongue depressor is used to manipulate the base of the tongue to prevent occlusion of the airway by impinchment of the tongue on the end of the oral airway
   b. Nasopharyngeal airways
      (1) Also available in a number of sizes; measure from the tragus of the ear to the tip of the nose
         (a) Exercise great care to ensure that the angled opening of the distal portion of the airway does not traumatize nasal passages and result in epistaxis
         (b) Well-lubricated nasopharyngeal airways appear to be better tolerated than oropharyngeal airways in the alert patient
3. Endotracheal intubation
   a. Common indications for endotracheal intubation are depicted in the Box on p. 322
   b. Orotracheal intubation
      (1) The oral route is the most common and easily mastered approach for tracheal intubation
      (2) This technique routinely involves visualization of the glottis, the use of a laryngoscope, and passage of the endotracheal tube into the trachea under direct vision. The Box on p. 322 lists the essential equipment that should be available for orotracheal intubation

---

Indications for Intubation

1. Ventilation of the patient
2. Airway obstruction
3. Tracheobronchial toilet
4. Airway protection
5. Impending respiratory failure

Equipment Necessary for Endotracheal Intubation

Oxygenation Equipment

Oxygen source
Regulators and tubing

Endotracheal Tubes

Appropriate numbers and sizes of endotracheal tubes should be available
A malleable stylet to stiffen the tube for insertion
Silicon jelly as a lubricant
Appropriate volume syringe(s) for cuff inflation

Laryngoscope

Laryngoscope handle with functioning batteries
Straight and curved blades in the sizes necessary for the proposed intubation with functioning light bulbs or fiberoptic tracks

Fixation Device for the Endotracheal Tube

Adhesive tape or commercially available tube-fixation devices

Means of Assessment for Appropriate Position of Endotracheal Tube

Stethoscope
End-tidal CO_2 monitoring device
Pulse oximeter

---

(3) Intubation technique
    (a) Positioning of the patient: it is important to align the axis of the trachea, pharynx, and oral cavity in order to effect endotracheal intubation. This requires that the axis be aligned by placing the patient's head in the "sniffing" position. A small pad or folded towel may be used to raise the occiput for proper alignment (see Fig. 17-1)
    (b) After proper positioning and ensuring that all the necessary equipment is available, laryngoscopy may be performed by

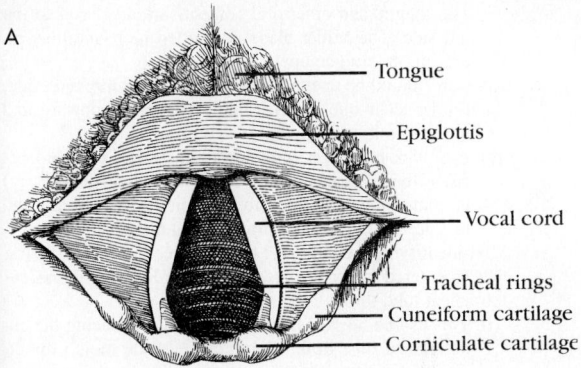

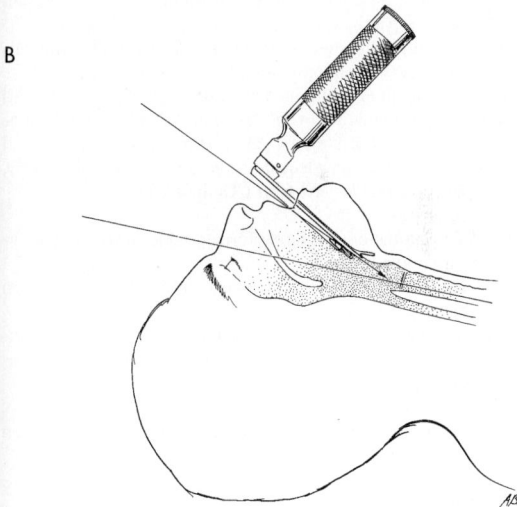

Figure 17-1
Endotracheal intubation. **A,** View. **B,** Proper insertion. (From Allison EJ Jr: Advanced life support skills, St. Louis, 1994, Mosby–Year Book.)

inserting the laryngoscope into the oropharyngeal and examining the airway. Two types of blades are commonly used:
  (i) The Miller blade is used to lift the epiglottis to obtain visualization of the tracheal opening (see Figure 17-1)
  (ii) The Mackintosh blade fits into the vallecula resulting in adherence of the epiglottis to the back of the blade

The tongue and other oral contents are displaced to the left side. The Miller blade is inserted more midline, elevating the tongue upward

(iii) Care should be exercised in the use of the laryngoscope. Proper technique is to lift the laryngoscope upward and not to use it as a fulcrum

(iv) A Sellick maneuver (pressure on the cricoid to help occlude the epiglottis during manipulation of the airway) is commonly performed to help prevent aspiration and to stabilize the glottis during the intubation procedure

(c) After identifying the laryngeal opening (see Fig. 17-1) the trachea is entered under direct visualization by placing the endotracheal tube through the vocal cords

(i) This can be most easily accomplished by placing the endotracheal tube in the right corner of the mouth directing the tip into the glottic opening. This technique does not require interruption of the view of the vocal cords during intubation

(ii) Stop insertion when the cuff is displaced 2 cm from the glottic opening (external markings are typically 21 or 23 cm from the central incisors of average size women and men, respectively)

(iii) The cuff is inflated to a moderate tension of the pilot balloon and ventilation with 100% oxygen begins

(d) Tube placement is ascertained by auscultation of the chest and abdomen, examination of the rise and fall of the chest, condensation of the respiratory gas mixture in the endotracheal tube, maintenance of adequate saturation on pulse oximetry, and (when available) end-tidal CO_2 indicators

c. Nasotracheal intubation

(1) Nasotracheal intubation can be performed under direct visualization using the laryngoscope

(a) The tube is placed through the nares and the tip visualized in the pharynx

(b) Magill forceps can be used to manipulate the end of the endotracheal tube through the vocal cords to achieve proper positioning

(2) Blind nasal insertion

(a) The location of the endotracheal tube is ascertained through auscultation

(b) This technique is reserved for those patients who have spontaneous ventilations

(c) An endotracheal tube of appropriate size is inserted through the naris and advanced to the pharynx

(d) Auscultation using the unaided ear and listening at the nasal end is used as the endotracheal tube is advanced

(e) The tube is inserted through the glottic opening during inspiration and appropriate position confirmed as noted above

      (f) Nasal intubation may result in severe epistaxis in patients with coagulopathy or if performed with excessive force

      (g) Patients with midface fractures should *not* be nasally intubated

      (h) Sinusitis is a recognized complication of nasal intubation and should be considered when determining the route of intubation

  d. No matter the route of intubation of the trachea, secure all endotracheal tubes with adhesive tape or other securing devices to prevent dislodgement

  e. Common complications of endotracheal intubation

    (1) During laryngoscopy and intubation

      (a) Dental and/or oral soft-tissue trauma

      (b) Dysrhythmias and hypertension/hypotension

      (c) Aspiration of gastric contents

    (2) While endotracheal tube is in place

      (a) Tube obstruction

      (b) Esophageal intubation

      (c) Accidental extubation

      (d) Tracheal mucosa ischemia

    (3) Delayed complications

      (a) Tracheal stenosis

      (b) Vocal-cord paralysis

      (c) Laryngeal edema

4. Cricothyroidotomy

  a. The cricothyroid membrane can be identified by palpation below thyroid cartilage

  b. A large-bore (14- or 16-gauge) catheter may be placed through the cricothyroid membrane into the trachea and used to ventilate and oxygenate patients in whom other airway maneuvers are unsuccessful

  c. Free release of air from the catheter will confirm tracheal position

  d. Angle the tip of the catheter inferiorly and advance after tracheal penetration with the plastic cannula

  e. The cannula may be adapted to fit the 15 mm opening of a standard *Ambu* bag or alternatively, a portable high-frequency jet ventilator device may be used to provide oxygenation

  f. Surgical cricothyroidotomy

    (1) Percutaneous technique: a needle is used to pass into the trachea and a guide-wire positioned in the trachea through the needle. A dilator is then passed and a cricothyroidotomy tube with an internal obturator is inserted

    (2) Surgical technique: a small midline incision is made over the cricothyroid membrane that is then opened and an appropriate cannula is placed in the trachea

| 17.2 | CARDIOVERSION/DEFIBRILLATION |

1. The major indications for utilizing these techniques are covered in Chapters 4 and 5.

2. Preparation
An appropriately functioning monitor/defibrillator and conductive pads or gel must be available

3. Procedure for defibrillation
   a. Institute basic life support if not already begun
   b. Determine cardiac rhythm. If the patient has not been placed on a cardiac monitor, then the "quick-look" capabilities of the monitor/defibrillator may be used
   c. Turn on the monitor section of monitor/defibrillator
   d. Select a paddle lead for the monitor/defibrillator
   e. Place paddles on the right upper sternal and left lateral position or anteroposteriorly (see Fig. 17-2)
   f. Observe rhythm
      (1) If ventricular fibrillation is observed
         (a) Turn power to defibrillator unit on and make sure that the unit is in the defibrillation ("defib") mode
         (b) Select appropriate energy level. See Chapters 4 and 5
         (c) Place electrode gel or other conductive media and position the paddles as mentioned above. Apply firm pressure
         (d) Perform discharge of the defibrillator by simultaneously depressing both discharge buttons located on the defibrillator paddles
4. Procedure for synchronized cardioversion after determining cardioversion is appropriate:
   a. Turn power to defibrillator unit on
   b. Make sure that the defibrillator unit is in the synchronized ("sync") mode
   c. Apply conductive gel or other material to paddles and position them as noted above

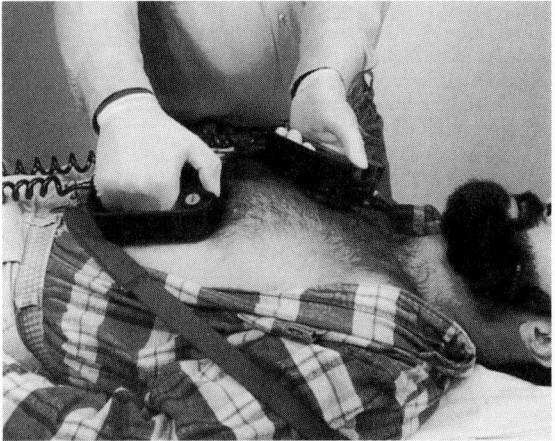

Figure 17-2
Standard positioning of cardioversion/defibrillation electrodes. (From Allison EJ Jr: *Advanced life support skills,* St. Louis, 1994, Mosby–Year Book.)

d. Confirm that an acceptable electrocardiogram (ECG) signal is being received from the monitor/defibrillator unit

e. Discharge the energy by depressing both discharge buttons located on the defibrillator paddles and observe the unit to ensure that the shock is delivered

5. Avoid administering counter-shocks directly over implanted pacemakers, defibrillators, or over nitroglycerin patches on the surface of the patient's skin. The potential exists for serious injury with this device. Make sure that other rescuers/health-care providers are clear of the victim prior to delivering shocks.

6. Complications

   a. An adverse rhythm may be produced by administering electrical counter-shocks

   b. Burns of the skin may result, particularly when poor electrical conduction has been established. The use of gel or other conductive material is mandatory and firm pressure (approximately 25 pounds) should be applied to the paddles

   c. Myocardial injury

   d. Systemic embolization

17.3 VASCULAR ACCESS

1. Modified Seldinger technique

   This technique is a simple method of obtaining access to vascular spaces.

   a. After appropriate preparation, draping, and positioning, a needle is percutaneously placed into the vascular structure. A guide-wire with a flexible end (either J or straight) is inserted through the needle and into the lumen of the vessel (see Fig. 17-3)

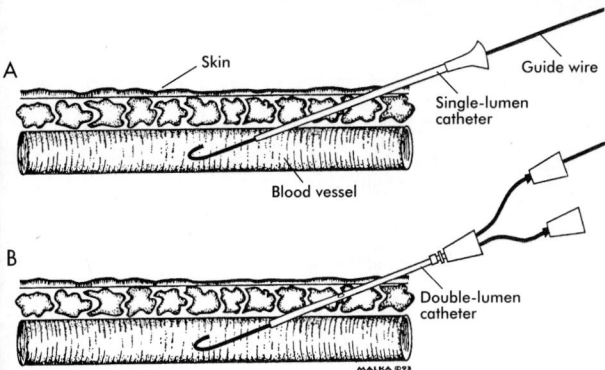

Figure 17-3
Modified Seldinger technique for vascular access. **A,** Single-lumen catheter. **B,** Double-lumen catheter.

    b. The needle is subsequently removed and the catheter inserted over the extraluminal end of the guide-wire and subsequently passed over the wire into the vessel

    c. The catheter is advanced and the guide-wire is removed. When appropriately positioned, the catheter is secured with suture or tape

2. Central venous access

    a. The major indications for central venous access are depicted in the first Box

    b. No absolute contraindications to central venous access exist. Relative contraindications may include bleeding diathesis and central venous thrombosis

    c. Choice of central cannulation route

        (1) Subclavian, internal jugular, and femoral routes have all been used extensively for central cannulation

        (2) The specific site chosen is dependent on the clinical circumstances and the skill of the operator

        (3) Subclavian insertion has a higher risk of pneumothorax. It also presents a noncompressible vascular puncture site

        (4) There is a small but significant incidence of carotid puncture during internal jugular cannulation

    d. The second Box below displays the equipment necessary for central venous cannulation

---

Indications for Central Venous Cannulation

Difficult peripheral venous cannulation
Drug administration
Emergency dialysis
Total parental nutrition
Hemodynamic monitoring

Equipment Necessary for Central Venous Cannulation

Appropriate intravenous fluid with administration tubing
Prep solution (routinely Iodophor)
Sterile towels
10 ml syringe with Luer-Lok
25-gauge needle for local anesthesia
1% lidocaine
Appropriate size and gauge introducer needle
Spring guide-wire
Number 11 blade
Vessel dilator
Selected catheter
Suture material

e. Internal jugular catheterization (anterior approach)
    (1) In the nonemergent setting, obtain informed consent
    (2) Position the patient in 15°-20° Trendelenburg position and remove the headboard of the bed
    (3) Wash, gown, and glove
    (4) Prep the operative site gently with iodophor solution and drape with sterile towels
    (5) The internal jugular vein lies beneath the sternocleidomastoid muscle and slightly in front of the carotid artery as shown in Fig. 17-4
    (6) In the anterior approach, the carotid artery is palpated (left index and middle finger), the puncture site is infiltrated with 1% lidocaine, and a finding needle is passed immediately lateral to the carotid pulsation beneath the medial edge of the sternocleidomastoid muscle at the level of the thyroid cartilage. The needle is advanced at an angle of approximately 30° to the skin (directed toward the ipsilateral nipple). The vessel should be encountered within 3 cm. When gentle suction on the syringe produces a rush of venous blood, the needle is removed and the procedure is repeated with the larger gauge introducer needle on a 5- or 10-ml Luer-Lok syringe. Once the venous puncture has been achieved, a guide-wire is passed into the vessel (a vessel dilator can be used) and the venous catheter is inserted over the wire through a very small skin incision made over the wire. The wire is subsequently removed and IV extension tubing attached

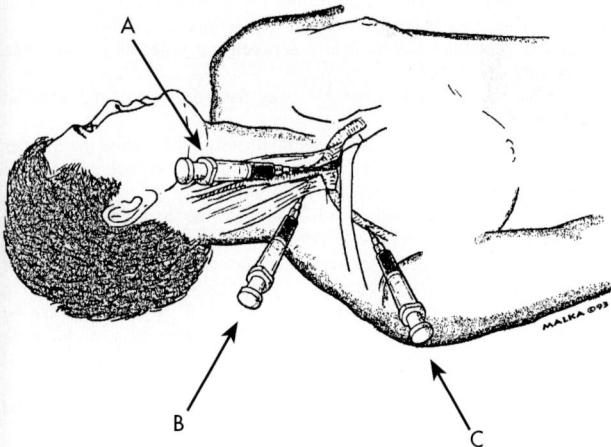

Figure 17-4
Central venous cannulation. **A,** internal jugular, middle approach. **B,** internal jugular, posterior approach. **C,** subclavian vein cannulation.

    f. Internal jugular catheterization (middle approach)
      (1) With the patient supine in 20° Trendelenburg position and the head slightly turned to the contralateral side, local anesthetic is infiltrated at the junction of the sternal and clavicular heads of the sternocleidomastoid muscle. The needle is inserted with an angle of approximately 30° to the skin and again directed toward the ipsilateral nipple. The vessel should be entered within 2-3 cm of insertion (see Fig. 17-4, A). Once vascular access has been obtained, the procedure is repeated with the introducer needle; the guide-wire is passed through the needle and cannulation is completed as noted above
    g. Internal jugular catheterization (the posterior approach)
      (1) The patient is positioned in the 20° degree Trendelenburg position with the head facing the contralateral shoulder. After skin preparation and local anesthesic as noted above, the needle is inserted through the skin at the posterolateral margin of the sternocleidomastoid muscle (approximately 4 cm above the sternoclavicular junction). This is the approximate point where the external jugular vein crosses the posterior margin of the sternocleidomastoid muscle, a commonly used landmark. The needle is advanced in a caudal and medial direction aiming at the contralateral nipple (see Fig. 17-4, B). Once venous access with the introducer needle has been obtained, a guide-wire is placed into the catheter and cannulation proceeds as noted above
3. Subclavian vein cannulation
    a. The patient is prepped and positioned in a manner analogous to that for internal jugular vein cannulation; however, a rolled-up towel should be placed longitudinally between the scapulas to allow the shoulders to drop back
    b. The patient's head is turned 45° away from the side of the intended placement
    c. The puncture site is identified approximately 1 cm below the inferior margin of the clavicle at the junction of the medial and middle two-thirds (see Fig. 17-4, C)
    d. Infiltration of the region with 1% lidocaine is accomplished. In addition, lidocaine is injected into the periosteum of the clavicle
    e. The anesthesia needle is removed and the introducer needle is inserted into the skin. The tip is aimed at the suprasternal notch, passing just beneath the clavicle. The bevel of the needle should be pointed toward the head (cephalad). When free flow of blood is obtained from the introducer needle, the bevel can be rotated 180° helping to facilitate thoracic placement of the guide-wire. The catheter is threaded, the wire removed, fluid flow is established, and the catheter is then secured
4. Femoral vein
    a. This approach is easily performed in most patients
    b. The patient is placed supine, knees extended, and the foot of the anticipated cannulation site rotated outward 15-30°

c. The site of insertion is cleaned and prepped, as noted previously, and the region draped

d. The insertion point is identified, lying 2-3 cm inferior to the inguinal ligament (1-2 cm medial to the femoral pulse.) (The reader is reminded of the *navl* mnemonic of the structures in this region: nerve, artery, vein, lymphatics)

e. As for internal jugular cannulation, a 22-gauge finder needle is commonly used for local anesthesia infiltration as well as for localization of the vessel

f. After the femoral vein has been found, the introducer needle is placed on a syringe and inserted into the femoral vein

g. A flexible guide-wire is then placed and the needle exchanged for the vascular cannula. The catheter is then secured

5. Complications of central venous access
Infection, pneumothorax (more common with subclavian approach), hemothorax, chylothorax, intrapleural infusion of IV fluids, dysrhythmias, thrombosis, air embolism, pericardial tamponade, neurologic injuries, and hematomas.

17.4 ARTERIAL LINE

1. Common sites for arterial cannulation include radial, femoral, dorsalis pedis, and axillary; the radial artery is most frequently used

2. Before radial artery cannulation, many authorities believe Allen's test should be performed. This test is done by occluding both radial and ulnar arteries immediately proximal to the palmar crest. Opening and closing the hands produces blanching of the hands and digits. The tester removes pressure over the ulnar artery and notes the time it takes to return to normal color. Seven seconds is reported as normal, 7-14 seconds indeterminate, >14 seconds is abnormal. However, this may be quite difficult to perform in the ICU with an uncooperative patient and a normal Allen's test does not ensure that a vascular complication will not occur

3. Preparation after informed consent is obtained

a. Extend the patient's arm with the volar side upward on an arm-board or bedside table

b. Place a small towel at the level of the wrist. Placing the hand in dorsiflexion will facilitate cannulation (see Fig. 17-5)

c. Cleanse the region of insertion as noted above, place sterile drapes, and use a fine-gauge needle to infiltrate a small quantity of 1% lidocaine at the site of insertion

4. The authors find a typical 20- or 22-gauge catheter-over-needle technique to be acceptable for radial artery cannulation. Catheter-over-needle techniques with guide-wire devices are also available, and a traditional Seldinger technique may also be used

a. The over-needle catheter (usually without syringe) is inserted parallel to the projected course of the radial artery at an angle of 30° -45° with the skin

b. The needle is advanced slowly until pulsatile blood is obtained

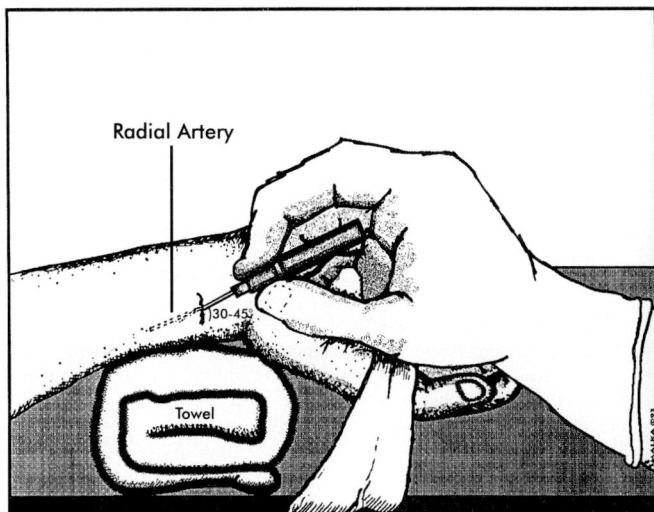

Figure 17-5
Radial arterial cannulation.

    c. The plastic catheter is then advanced into the artery; if a guide-wire is being used, this is placed through the needle into the vessel and subsequently the catheter is advanced
    d. The needle is removed and appropriate tubing is attached. The catheter is then secured in place
5. Complications include thrombosis, infection, and aneurysm formation (especially in femoral arterial lines)

17.5   PULMONARY ARTERY (PA) CATHETERIZATION

1. IV access must be obtained using one of the techniques described above and placing the introducer sheath into the desired vessel.
2. The appropriate monitoring system must be in place, including pressure transducers for all ports that will be monitored.
    a. Flush high-pressure tubing with appropriate solution
    b. Observe and test the dynamic response by watching the pressure wave on the bedside monitor while activating and quickly releasing the flush device
    c. Flush each lumen of the catheter and connect each one to the appropriate monitoring line. Inflate the balloon to ensure that it is intact and symmetric
    d. Rapid whipping of the catheter tip will convince the operator that the monitoring system is functioning properly when the catheter is inserted into the introducer

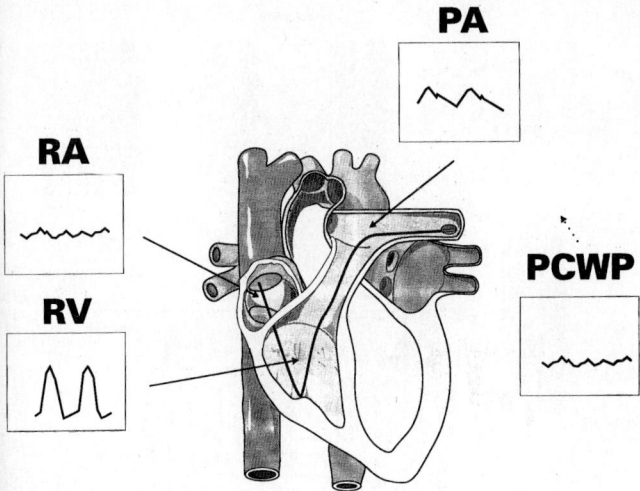

Figure 17-6
Pulmonary artery catheterization and wave forms. RA: right atrium, RV: right ventricle, PA: pulmonary artery, PCWP: pulmonary capillary wedge pressure.

3. Institute continuous recording of the distal port.
4. Advance the catheter approximately 20 cm (in the adult patient) for either subclavian or internal jugular insertions; at this point a central venous pressure wave form should be seen (see Fig. 17-6).
5. Inflate the balloon with 1-1.5 cc of air and further advance the catheter into the vascular system.
6. Within 30-40 cm of catheter insertion, the right ventricle (RV) pressure wave form is usually seen (see Fig. 17-6). This is easily identified by the steep upstroke, typically 2-3 × larger than the Right atrium (RA) pressure.
7. Passage in the PA generally occurs at 40-50 cm of catheter insertion and may be identified by the dicrotic notch of the down-slope.
8. A pulmonary artery wedge pressure is usually noted at 50-60 cm of catheter insertion and looks much like an RA wave form.
9. Complications include dysrhythmias, valvular damage, knotting of the catheter, atrial or ventricular perforation, air embolism, pulmonary embolism, pulmonary arterial injury, and catheter-related sepsis.

17.6 TUBE THORACOSTOMY

1. Prepare the drainage system before the chest tube is placed
   a. Inspect all the couplings and tubing, and maintain appropriate fluid levels
   b. A "three-bottle system" (all of the bottles that may be maintained in a single commercial thoracostomy drainage system) is depicted in

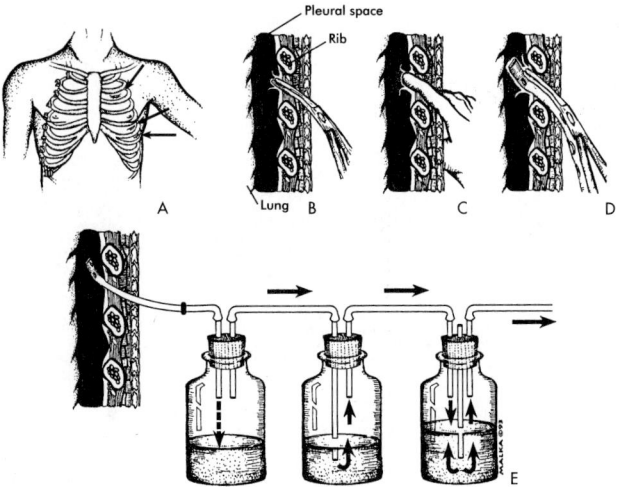

Figure 17-7
Tube thoracostomy.

Fig. 17-7. The first bottle is the trap bottle which collects the fluid emanating from the chest tube itself. The second bottle represents the water seal bottle. Air is precluded from entering the pleural space through the system by the water in the water seal bottle. The third bottle represents the manometer bottle. Suction applied to the manometer bottle is regulated by the distance of the center tube from below the surface of the water. For example, if the central tube lies 20 cm below the surface of the water, suction levels producing pressure in excess of -20 cm of water simply result in bubbling of ambient air in the manometer bottle, thus maintaining the −20 cm water pressure limit

2. Surgical technique
   a. The contents of a chest tube tray are depicted in the Box on p. 335
   b. Position the patient so that the side for tube insertion is uppermost
   c. The operator should be gowned and gloved
   d. The chest tube is usually inserted in the anterior axillary line in the fifth or sixth intercostal space (see Fig 17-7, A)
   e. Prep and drape the incision site and infiltrate lidocaine one intercostal space below the rib of the selected intercostal space of insertion. Infiltrate the periosteum, subcutaneous tissue, and pleural space. Aspiration of fluid or air will confirm infiltrated pleural space
   f. Using a scalpel over the anesthetized rib, make a small skin incision appropriate to the size of the chest tube (see Fig. 17-7, A)
   g. Extend the incision into the subcutaneous tissue and muscle at the intercostal space, preferably using the blunt side of the scalpel or trocar

Contents of the Chest Tube Tray

- Sterile towels and drapes
- 1% or 2% lidocaine
- 10 ml syringe
- 22- and 25-gauge needles
- 1-0 silk suture with cutting needle (2 packages)
- 2 large Kelly clamps
- 2 medium Kelly clamps
- Suture scissors
- 4″ square gauze pads
- Chest drainage, suction system, and appropriate chest tube

h. Employ a large clamp with an open end using spreading maneuvers until the pleural space is reached (see Fig. 17-7, *B*)

i. The operator's index finger is used to explore the pleural space to ensure that the lung, diaphragm, or another structure is not adherent (see Fig. 17-7, *C*)

j. Insert the tube generally toward the apex of the pleural space for treatment of pneumothoraces, grasping the tube with a medium clamp and maneuvering it through the dissected tunnel (see Fig. 17-7, *D*). Assure that the last hole of the thoracostomy tube lies within the pleural space. Fix the tube at the insertion site with 1-0 silk suture

    (1) A number of techniques are used; commonly the suture ends are not cut but wrapped around the tube and secured with tape. These may be used to close the wound when the tube is pulled out

k. Then attach the external end of the chest tube to the system and tape over the connections

l. Apply a sterile dressing with tape to the skin

3. Complications include tube malposition, empyema or wound infection, blockage of the tube by blood or fibrin clot, and lung injuries

17.7   INTRAAORTIC BALLOON PUMP (IABP)

1. Indications for the use of IABP include:
   a. Pump failure
       (1) After an acute myocardial ischemic event
       (2) Cardiogenic shock
       (3) Post-cardiac transplant patient
       (4) In the pre- or postoperative period of cardiac surgery
   b. Acute mitral valvular regurgitation
   c. Unstable angina pectoris
   d. Other

2. Insertion should normally be accomplished by those with experience. The technique is also dependent on the particular catheter and approach to be used.

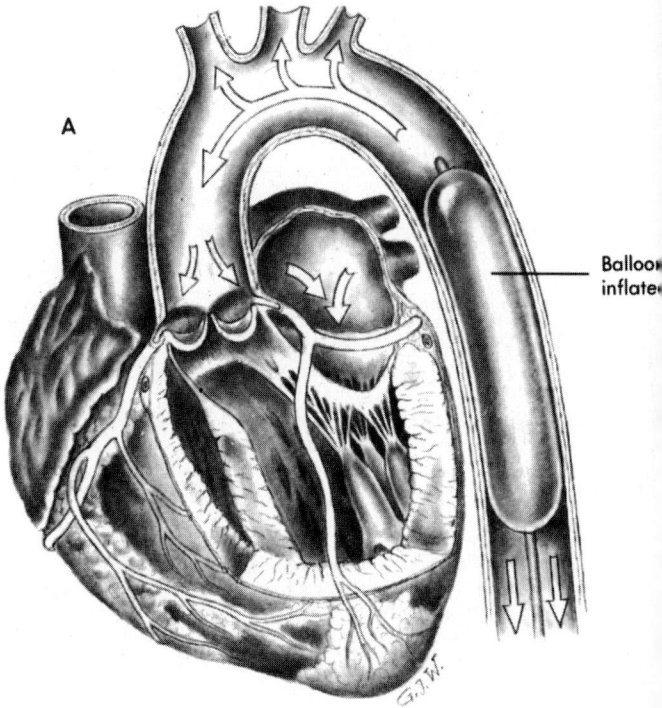

A

Balloon
inflated

Figure 17-8
Mechanisms of action of intraaortic balloon pump. **A,** Diastolic inflation augments coronary blood flow. **B,** Systolic balloon deflation decreases afterload. (From Thelan LA et al: *critical care nursing,* ed 2, St. Louis, 1994, Mosby–Year Book.)

  a. Once the catheter is in place, its function is rather easy to visualize (see Fig. 17-8)
  b. During ventricular systole the balloon (present in the proximal aorta) deflates, decreasing afterload on the heart and improving ventricular performance
  c. During diastole the inflated balloon occludes 75-90% of the cross-sectional area of the descending aorta, thereby increasing coronary perfusion
  d. Helium is most commonly used for inflation and deflation of the balloon
3. Complications include balloon membrane rupture or perforation, limb ischemia, aortic dissection, renal failure, thrombocytopenia, and infection.

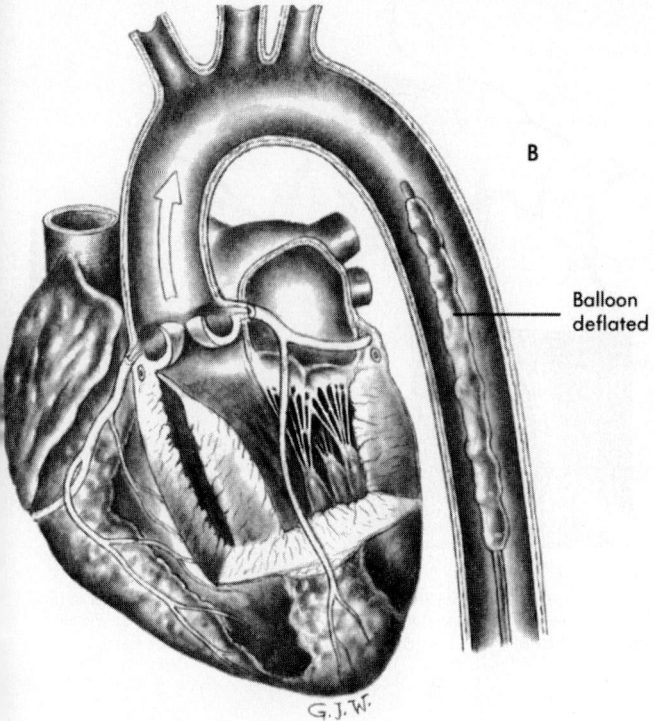

Figure 17-8, cont'd For legend see opposite page.

17-8   PERICARDIOCENTESIS

1. Blind pericardiocentesis should be performed in life-threatening situations (e.g., decompensated cardiac tamponade).
   a. The authors prefer the subxiphoid approach
      (1) If possible, place the patient upright or if necessary in a semireclining position
      (2) Venous access, continuous ECG monitoring, and BP monitoring should have been established. Personnel and equipment necessary for cardiac resuscitation must be on hand
      (3) Provide sedation and analgesia as appropriate to the setting
      (4) Prep and drape the region
      (5) Provide 1% lidocaine local and prepare an 18- or 20-gauge cardiac or spinal needle attached to a syringe with local anesthetic
      (6) For ECG monitoring, an alligator clip connected to the "v" lead of an ECG monitor may be placed on the needle (see Fig. 17-9)

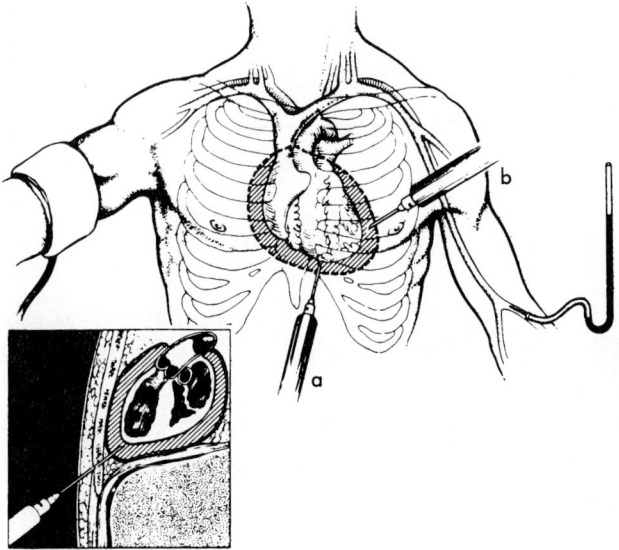

Figure 17-9
Pericardiocentesis may be performed using either *A,* via subxiphoid approach (also seen in insert) or *B,* at lateral heart border. (From McKenna RJ Jr et al: Pleural and pericardial effusions in cancer patients. *Curr Prob Cancer* 1985; 9:1.)

    (7) Introduce the needle tip between the xiphoid and left costal margin directed toward the left shoulder
    (8) Apply continuous gentle suction to the syringe. Intermittently, local anesthetic may be injected, which helps to clear the needle and anesthetize the deeper tissues
    (9) The operator will usually feel the sensation of pericardial passage
    (10) The ECG tracing showing injury current recognizes epicardial contact. If this should occur, slightly withdraw the needle
  b. After entrance into the pericardial cavity, removal of 50 ml of pericardial fluid is usually enough
  c. A pliable soft catheter may be inserted into the pericardial space using a guide-wire, allowing the needle to be withdrawn. Real-time transthoracic echocardiography allows tracking of the needle tip to ensure correct location throughout the aspiration procedure
  d. In an alternative approach, the needle is angled toward the right shoulder rather than the left shoulder
2. Complications include cardiac chamber puncture, dysrhythmias, pneumothorax, vasovagal reactions, and cardiac arrest.

Selected readings

Agee KR, Balk RA: Central venous catheterization in the critically ill patient. *Crit Care Clin* 1992; 8:677-86.

Amin DK, Shah PK, Swan HJC: The technique of inserting a Swan-Ganz catheter. *J Crit Illness* 1993; 8:1147-56.

Colvin MP, Curran JP, O'Shea PJ: Femoral artery pressure monitoring: use of Seldinger technique. *Anaesthesia* 1977; 32:451-5.

Ermakov S, Hoyt JW: Pulmonary artery catheterization. *Crit Care Clin* 1992; 8:773-806.

Gallagher TJ: Endotracheal intubation. *Crit Care Clin* 1992; 8:665-76.

Gurman GM, Kriemerman S: Cannulation of big arteries in critically ill patients. *Crit Care Med* 1985; 13:217-20.

Hauser AM, Gordon S, Gangadharan V et al: Percutaneous intraaortic balloon counterpulsation: clinical effectiveness and hazards. *Chest* 1982; 82:422-5.

Iberti TJ, Stern PM: Chest tube thoracostomy. *Crit Care Clin* 1992; 8:879-95.

Ivatury R, Siegel JH, Stahl WM, et al: Percutaneous tracheostomy after trauma and critical illness. *J Trauma* 1992; 32:133-40.

Kerber RE: External defibrillation: New technologies. *Ann Emerg Med* 1984; 13:794-7.

Kirkland LL, Taylor RW: Pericardiocentesis. *Crit Care Clin* 1992; 8:699-712.

Miller KS, Sahn SA: Chest tubes: indications, technique, management and complications. *Chest* 1987; 91:258-64.

Natanson C, Shelhamer JH, Parrillo JE: Intubation of the trachea in the critical care setting. *JAMA* 1985; 253:1160-5.

Patel AK, Kosolcharoen PK, Nallasivan M, et al: Catheter drainage of the pericardium: practical method to maintain long-term patency. *Chest* 1987; 92:1018-21.

Shah KB, Rao TLK, Laughlin S, et al: A review of pulmonary artery catheterization in 6245 patients. *Anesthesiology* 1984; 61:271-5.

Stone DJ, Bogdonoff DL: Airway considerations in the management of patients requiring long-term endotracheal intubation. *Anesth Analg* 1992; 74:276-87.

Wilson GL, McGregor PJ, Thompson GR: Long-term complications of intravascular cannulation. *Prob Crit Care* 1988; 2:296-305.

Toxicology

George L. Sternbach

18.1 GENERAL MANAGEMENT

History

Obtain a history as accurately as possible, including the substance ingested or inhaled, the amount, and time of ingestion. Always consider possible ingestion or inhalation of multiple substances.

Cardiorespiratory care

The most important aspects of initial management are basic care of respiratory and cardiovascular function. Maintain a patent airway, assure adequate respiration (support ventilation when necessary), and treat shock if present. (see Chapter 4).

Airway

1. Loss of airway patency and reflexes may lead to obstruction, aspiration, or respiratory arrest
2. Maintain proper airway position, suction, and use oropharyngeal or nasopharyngeal adjuncts as needed
3. Absent or depressed gag reflex in an unconscious or obtunded patient indicates the inability to protect the airway and endotracheal intubation is indicated

Respirations

1. Respiratory failure is the most frequent cause of death in poisoned patients, usually as the result of central nervous system (CNS) depression
2. Assist ventilation and perform endotracheal intubation as required
3. Obtain and follow arterial blood gases (ABGs)

Circulation

1. Monitor blood pressure (BP), pulse, and cardiac rhythm
2. Initiate intravenous (IV) line
3. If hypotension is present, administer fluid challenge with normal saline 10-20 ml/kg
4. If hypotension persists, administer dopamine 5-15 mcg/kg/min

5. With intractable hypotension, insert a pulmonary artery catheter, if possible
   a. If central venous pressure or pulmonary artery occlusion (wedge) pressure is low, administer fluids
   b. If cardiac output is low, consider increasing the dosage of dopamine or administering dobutamine (begin dopamine at 1-5 mcg/kg/min IV and adjust as required)
   c. If systemic vascular resistance is low, administer norepinephrine. Begin at 0.1 mcg/kg/min IV and increase as required. Once norepinephrine is initiated, decrease the dopamine dosage to 1-3 mcg/kg/min

Gastrointestinal (GI) decontamination

Traditional sequence is emptying the stomach by induced emesis or gastric lavage followed by administration; of activated charcoal however, there is controversy regarding this. Activated charcoal administration may be as effective as gastric emptying if 60 min or longer has elapsed since ingestion. This portion of treatment of the poisoned patient will generally be performed prior to admission to the intensive care unit (ICU). However, it will occasionally be necessary in the intensive care area, especially if the diagnosis of poisoning is delayed.

Induced emesis

1. Useful in early management of oral poisoning and for removal of material poorly adsorbed by activated charcoal (alcohols, ethylene glycol, iron, lithium)
2. Of relatively rare usefulness for the ICU patient, who is likely to have a diminished level of consciousness or decreased capacity to protect the airway
3. Administer syrup of ipecac (30 ml for adults, 15 ml for children <5 years old, 10 ml for children <1 year old). Repeat if no emesis in 20 min
   a. Not recommended in children <9 months old
   b. If the second dose does not produce vomiting, perform gastric lavage
4. Contraindications
   a. Comatose or patient experiencing seizures
   b. Ingestion of corrosive agents or petroleum distillates
   c. Ingestion of a substance likely to produce coma or seizures rapidly

Gastric lavage

Contraindicated if the patient is obtunded or comatose until endotracheal intubation is performed to protect the airway. Performance in an obtunded patient may lead to vomiting and aspiration of gastric contents. Other complications include perforation of the nasal mucosa, production of epistaxis, inadvertant (rather than gastric) tracheal intubation, and stimulation of ventricular dysrhythmias. Lavage is controversial in corrosive ingestion.

   Utilize a 36-40 Fr tube in adults, 24-26 Fr tube in children. Check for the position of the tube by injecting air and auscultating the stomach. Administer lavage fluid in aliquots of 200-300 ml, then allow the return of fluid by gravity drainage. Continue until the lavage fluid is clear of ingested fragments or substance color (or longer if the circumstances of the ingestion dictate).

Activated charcoal

1. Limits absorption of virtually all ingested substances. Administer 1 g/kg PO or via gastric tube after emesis or lavage is completed
2. Repeat doses of 15-20 g at 1- or 2-hr intervals; alternatively, continuous activated charcoal instillation may be useful in some instances (e.g., theophylline overdose)
3. Contraindicated in corrosive ingestion, ileus, or intestinal obstruction

Cathartics

1. Frequently used but effectiveness is not well established
2. Administer along with activated charcoal
3. Magnesium citrate 10% 3-4 ml/kg or sorbitol 70% 1-2 ml/kg. If there is no charcoal in the stool after 6 hr, repeat a half-dose

Whole bowel irrigation

1. Effectiveness is not fully studied. It may be useful in substantial ingestion of substances that are poorly adsorbed by activated charcoal or enteric-coated tablets
2. Administer polyethylene glycol electrolyte solution 2 L/hr by gastric tube until the stool is free of particulate material
3. Do not use in unconscious or obtunded patients

Forced diuresis and control of urine pH

May increase urinary excretion of some agents for which renal excretion is the major route of elimination. Do not use in renal failure or congestive heart failure (CHF).

Alkalinization

1. May be useful in overdose with salicylates and phenobarbital
2. Administer sodium bicarbonate 1-2 mEq/kg IV to achieve a urinary pH ≥7
3. Monitor serum pH

Acidification

1. May be useful in overdose with phencyclidine, amphetamines, quinine, quinidine, strychnine, and cyclic antidepressants
2. Administer ammonium chloride 75 mg/kg IV in 4-6 divided doses to achieve a urinary pH ≤6
3. Do not use in the presence of rhabdomyolysis, myoglobinuria, or hepatic failure
4. Monitor serum pH

Hemodialysis

May be useful in severe intoxication with amphetamines, methanol, ethylene glycol, isopropyl alcohol, lithium, and salicylates. If fluid or acid-base abnormalities are present, these can also be corrected.

Charcoal hemoperfusion

1. Utilizes an extracorporeal circuit through an activated charcoal column
2. May be useful in severe intoxication with barbiturates, some beta-

Table 18-1 Telephone numbers for U.S. regional poison control centers

State	City	800 Number (in State Only)	Telephone Number
Alabama	Birmingham	(800) 292-6678	(205) 939-9201
	Tuscaloosa	(800) 462-0800	(205) 345-0600
Arizona	Phoenix		(602) 253-3334
	Tucson	(800) 362-0101	(602) 626-6016
California	Fresno	(800) 346-5922	(209) 445-1222
	Los Angeles	(800) 825-2722	(213) 484-5151
	Sacramento	(800) 342-9293	(916) 453-3692
	San Diego	(800) 876-4766	(619) 543-6000
	San Francisco	(800) 523-2222	(415) 476-6600
Colorado	Denver	(800) 332-3073	(303) 629-1123
District of Columbia	Washington		(202) 625-3333
Florida	Tampa	(800) 282-3171	(813) 253-4444
Georgia	Atlanta	(800) 282-5846	(404) 589-4400
Kentucky	Louisville	(800) 722-5725	(502) 589-8222
Maryland	Baltimore	(800) 492-2414	(301) 528-7701
Massachusetts	Boston	(800) 682-9211	(617) 232-2120
Michigan	Detroit	(800) 462-6642	(313) 745-5711
	Grand Rapids	(800) 632-2727	(616) 774-7851
Minnesota	Minneapolis		(612) 347-3141
	St. Paul	(800) 222-1222	(612) 221-2113
Missouri	St. Louis	(800) 392-9111	(314) 772-5200
Montana		(800) 332-3073	
Nebraska	Omaha	(800) 642-9999	(402) 390-5400
New Jersey	Newark	(800) 962-1253	(201) 923-0764
New Mexico	Albuquerque	(800) 432-6866	(505) 843-2551
New York	New York City		(212) 340-4494
Ohio	Cincinnati	(800) 872-5111	(513) 558-5111
	Columbus	(800) 682-7625	(614) 228-1323
Oregon	Portland	(800) 452-7165	(503) 279-8968
Pennsylvania	Pittsburgh		(412) 681-6669
	Philadelphia		(215) 386-2100
Rhode Island	Providence		(401) 277-5727
Texas	Austin		(512) 478-4490
	Dallas	(800) 441-0040	(214) 590-5000
	Galveston		(409) 765-9728
	Houston	(800) 392-8548	(713) 654-1701
Utah	Salt Lake City	(800) 456-7707	(801) 581-2151
West Virginia	Charleston	(800) 642-3625	(304) 348-4211
Wyoming		(800) 332-3073	

blockers, ethchlorvynol, meprobamate, phenytoin, salicylates, and the-ophylline
2. Potential complications are hypotension and thrombocytopenia

Toxicology screen

1. Should be used to confirm diagnosis in all cases
2. Specific levels may be necessary in overdose with certain substances to guide therapy (i.e., acetaminophen, iron, lithium, methanol, salicylates, and theophylline)

Poison control centers

Notify poison control centers with management questions, or complicated or unusual poisonings. Telephone numbers for these centers are listed in Table 18-1.

| 18.2 | ACETAMINOPHEN

Acetaminophen is a widely used analgesic and antipyretic that is found in combination with other analgesics and in various cold remedies (e.g., Comtrex, Congespirin, Excedrin PM, 4-Way Cold Tablets). Toxicity of significant overdose lies in the production of hepatic necrosis. This is probably related to the overwhelmed capacity of hepatic glutathione to detoxify acetaminophen metabolic products. The diagnosis may be overlooked, especially in patients with alcoholic liver disease.

Clinical effects

1. With the exception of GI distress, there are minimal symptoms in the 16-24 hr following ingestion
2. The patient may be asymptomatic for the next 4 days. Liver function abnormalities peak at 72-96 hr after ingestion
3. Resolution or hepatic failure may result; renal failure occasionally occurs

Diagnostic studies

1. Obtain serum acetaminophen as soon as 4 hr and as late as 24 hr following ingestion and plot the level on a nomogram (see Fig. 18-1). The nomogram is useful only for acute ingestion
2. There is good correlation between timed serum level and subsequent hepatotoxicity. If the level is in the hepatotoxic range, administer acetyl-cysteine
3. Obtain prothrombin time (PT), transaminase levels, blood urea nitrogen (BUN), and creatinine

Management

1. Induce emesis or perform gastric lavage
2. Antidote: acetylcysteine
   a. Prevents liver injury when administered early following intoxication
   b. Only oral administration is approved in United States. However, IV formulation may be available at participating study centers. Contact poison control center or toxicologic consultant if IV administration is necessary

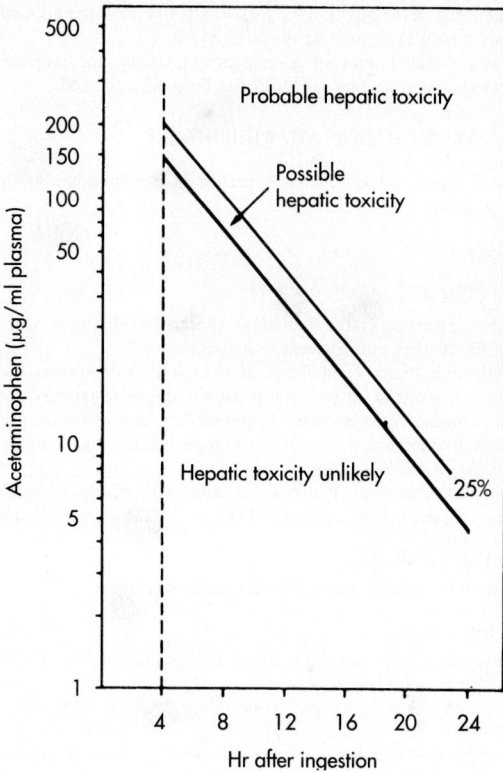

Figure 18-1
Rumack-Matthew nomogram for acetaminophen poisoning. (From Rumack BH, Matthew H: Acetaminophen poisoning and toxicity. *Pediatrics* 1975, 55:871-6.)

3. Cimetidine may be an adjunctive agent in treatment because of its ability to inhibit cytochrome P-450, preventing the formation of toxic metabolites. The dosage is not determined; it may be administered 300 mg q6hr

Adverse effects of acetylcysteine

1. Nausea and vomiting. If the dose is vomited, repeat administration
2. Antiemetic medication (i.e., metoclopramide 10-20 mg IV q4hr prn) may be necessary for persistent vomiting

Antidote administration

1. Loading dose of 140 mg/kg (1.4 ml/kg of 10% solution or 0.7 ml/kg of 20% solution) diluted to 5% solution in grapefruit juice

2. Maintenance of 70 mg/kg q4hr for 17 doses or until the acetaminophen level is zero. Levels may be obtained q12hr
3. Because activated charcoal adsorbs acetylcysteine, increase the acetylcysteine loading dose by 30% if it has been administered

18.3 ALCOHOL OVERDOSE AND WITHDRAWAL

Ethyl alcohol is found in beverages, perfumes, mouthwashes, and pharmaceutical preparations.

Overdose

Clinical effects

1. Variable depending on the individual: slurred speech, impaired judgment, behavior changes, combativeness, and ataxia
2. At very high levels: somnolence and respiratory depression. Death occuring as a result of intoxication is usually due to respiratory depression
3. Other: cardiac dysrhythmias, hypertension, hypoglycemia, hypomagnesemia, hypophosphatemia, seizures, hypothermia, rhabdomyolysis, and Wernicke's encephalopathy
4. Alcoholic ketoacidosis: metabolic acidosis with increased anion and osmolar gaps, and ketosis. Associated nausea, vomiting, and abdominal pain

Metabolism of alcohol

Rate is 12-50 mg/dL/hr (average of 20 mg/dL/hr)

Admission criteria

Admission to the ICU may be required for trauma, seizures, hypothermia, and severe metabolic abnormalities.

Management

1. Management is mainly supportive and predominantly observational. Intubate and ventilate if necessary
2. Administer IV glucose 50 g and thiamine 100 mg to all obtunded patients after serum glucose level is drawn
3. Correct volume depletion as needed
4. If the patient is violent or very agitated, use physical restraints as needed. Sedation with haloperidol may be necessary
5. Treatment of alcoholic ketoacidosis: fluid replacement with Dextrose 5%/ normal saline. Observe for the appearance of hypoglycemia, hypophosphatemia, and hypokalemia

Withdrawal

1. Withdrawal following chronic use produces a number of signs and symptoms including anxiety, insomnia, tremulousness, nausea, vomiting, tachycardia, hyperthermia, delirium, hallucinations, and seizures. The typical time of appearance of withdrawal findings are listed in Table 18-2
2. The hallmark of *delirium tremens* is significant alteration of the sensorium (global confusion, hallucinations, delusions, disorientation) accompanied by autonomic CNS hyperreactivity

Table 18-2   Appearance of findings of alcohol withdrawl

Findings	Hours Elapsed Since Cessation of Alcohol Intake
Tremor, agitation, sleep disturbance, hyperexcitability	6-8
Hallucinations	24-36
Seizures	7-48
Confusion, delusions, autonomic hyperreactivity, disorientation	72-120

Management

1. Sedation
   a. Benzodiazepines: administer diazepam 2-5 mg IV, repeat q5min prn, then 5-20 mg IV or PO q6hr, or chlordiazepoxide 25-100 mg IV or PO q6hr, or lorazepam 1-2 mg IV, IM, or PO, or
   b. Phenobarbital 260 mg slow IV, repeat prn to produce light sedation, or
   c. Haloperidol: begin with 0.5-1 mg IV or IM q 1-6 hr, though much larger doses may be required
2. Thiamine 100 mg IV
3. If severe hypertension or tachycardia are present, administer clonidine 0.1-0.2 mg q6hr

Other alcohols

Methanol

1. Methanol (methyl alcohol) is widely used as a solvent. It is found in windshield washer solution, antifreeze, and is used as a solid canned fuel
2. Produces CNS intoxication similar to that of ethanol. Other toxic effects include acidosis and retinal cell toxicity
3. Ethanol acts as a competitive substrate for alcohol dehydrogenase, the enzyme that produces toxic metabolites from methanol
4. Treatment
   a. Hemodialysis
   b. Administration of IV ethanol 0.6 mg/kg initially and infusion of 66 mg/kg/hr to maintain a blood alcohol of 100 mg/dL. Administer as 10% ethanol diluted in D_5W
   c. Hemodialysis and treatment with ethyl alcohol are indicated with serum methanol levels >50 mg/dL

Isopropyl alcohol

1. Isopropyl alcohol is used as a solvent and, medicinally, as a rubbing alcohol and a sterilizing agent
2. More toxic than ethyl alcohol but less toxic than methyl alcohol
3. Toxicity may be produced by ingestion of isopropyl alcohol or by inhalation of its vapor

4. Signs and symptoms of intoxication are similar to methanol but there is no retinal toxicity. Additional complications are dehydration and hemorrhagic gastritis
5. Treatment: gastric lavage, activated charcoal, and maintenance of fluid balance and BP. Hemodialysis may be used in severe cases

18.4   ANGIOTENSIN CONVERTING ENZYME (ACE) INHIBITORS

These antihypertensive agents are in common use either as individual agents or in combination with a diuretic (see Box below)

Toxic effects

The most common finding is hypotension. Fluid disturbances and electrolyte abnormalities may occur with agents when combined with diuretics.

Clinical effects

Dizziness, light-headedness, syncope, and cough.

Management

1. Perform gastric lavage or induce emesis
2. Administer activated charcoal and cathartic
3. Monitor BP continuously
4. Treatment is largely supportive. If hypotension is present, administer normal saline fluid infusion. Administer dopamine infusion if this does not correct hypotension. Naloxone has been reported to reverse hypotension
5. Consider hemodialysis in severe overdose with captopril, enalapril, or lisinopril

18.5   BETA-BLOCKERS

Common beta-blockers in use include propranolol, atenolol, metoprolol, pindolol, and nadolol (see the Box on p. 349). Agents are used for a variety of

---

Angiotensin Converting Enzyme Inhibitors

Benazepril (Lotensin)
Captopril (Capoten)
Enalapril (Vasotec)
Fosinopril (Monopril)
Lisinopril (Prinivil, Zestril)
Quinapril (Accupril)
Ramipril (Altace)
Combined with hydrochlorothiazide:
Captopril (Capozide)
Enalapril (Vaseretic)
Lisinopril (Prinzide, Zestoretic)

Beta-Adrenergic Blockers

Acebutolol (Sectral)
Atenolol (Tenormin)
Betaxolol (Kerlone)
Carteolol (Cartrol)
Labetalol (Normodyne)
Metoprolol (Lopressor, Toprol)
Nadolol (Corgard)
Penbutolol (Levatol)
Pindolol (Visken)
Propranolol (Inderal)
Timolol (Blocarden)
Combined with a diuretic
Bendroflumethazide
  Nadolol (Corzide)
Chlorthalidone
  Atenolol (Tenoretic)
Hydrochlorothiazide
  Metoprolol (Lopressor HCT)
  Propranolol (Inderide)
  Timolol (Timolide)

medical indications including hypertension, control of cardiac dysrhythmias, angina pectoris, and glaucoma. Duration of toxicity varies greatly depending on the agent ingested.

Clinical effects

1. Toxic effects include beta-adrenergic blockade, producing bradycardia, hypotension, and bronchospasm
2. Effects resulting from sodium-dependent membrane depression are seen primarily with lipid-soluble agents (e.g., propranolol, metoprolol) and include hypotension, atrioventricular (AV) block, and QRS widening
3. Seizures and coma may also occur
4. Metabolic effects include hyperkalemia and hypoglycemia

Management

1. Perform gastric lavage; *do not induce emesis*
2. Administer activated charcoal and cathartic
3. Monitor cardiac rhythm
4. If patient is hypotensive, administer fluids and pressor agents as required
5. Administer atropine (0.01-0.03 mg/kg IV) and isoproterenol (start at 4 mcg/min) for bradycardia
6. In unresponsive hypotension and bradycardia, administer glucagon, 5-10 mg IV. Follow with 1-5 mg/min IV infusion
7. Hemoperfusion may be useful for atenolol and nadolol overdose
8. Monitor serum glucose and electrolytes, particularly potassium

| 18.6 | COCAINE

Cocaine produces clinical symptoms on the basis of adrenergic stimulation, CNS stimulation, and increased metabolic rate. It is most commonly inhaled or injected parenterally. Free-base "crack" cocaine is very prevalent used concomitantly with other drugs. Complications of cocaine abuse include hypertension with resulting intracerebral hemorrhage or aortic dissection, myocardial infarction (MI), cerebrovascular accidents, hyperthermia, and rhabdomyolysis.

Clinical effects

1. Onset of toxic symptoms is within 30-60 min of injection or inhalation
2. The most common presentation is with hypertension, dysrhythmias, pupillary dilatation, agitation, anxiety, or psychosis
3. Seizures, hyperthermia, and rhabdomyolysis may occur
4. Hypertension may produce intracranial hemorrhage or thoracic aortic rupture
5. Chest pain may occur and is sometimes of myocardial origin. MI may occur. Cocaine is dysrhythmogenic and may produce sinus tachycardia, premature ventricular contractions, ventricular tachycardia, and ventricular fibrillation

Management

1. For oral ingestion perform gastric lavage and administer activated charcoal
2. Sedate with IV benzodiazepines or haloperidol
3. For hypertension treat with phentolamine 0.02-0.2 mg/kg or nitroprusside 2-10 mcg/kg/min IV. If tachycardia is also present, administer esmolol (0.5 mg/kg loading, then 0.05 mg/kg/min) IV or labetalol 10-20 mg IV. Clonidine 0.1-0.2 mg q6hr may also be used
   a. Avoid isolated use of beta-blockers
   b. Consider head computed tomography (CT) in case of possible intracerebral hemorrhage
4. Urine toxicology screen will confirm the diagnosis

| 18.7 | CYANIDE

Cyanide is a chemical with a variety of industrial uses. Sodium nitroprusside contains cyanide, which is released into the solution in increased quantities by exposure to light. Gas hydrogen cyanide is a product of combustion of plastics and a variety of other materials. A third of all smoke inhalation victims have increased cyanide levels.

Mechanism

Toxicity is via chemical asphyxia (i.e., cyanide blockade of cellular oxygen utilization). Exposure to small amounts of hydrogen cyanide gas or ingestion of a small quantity of cyanide salt can be rapidly fatal.

Clinical effects

1. Respiratory failure and cardiovascular collapse. Rapidly developing coma and severe lactic acidosis

2. Syncope, seizures, headache, nausea, and confusion
3. Cyanide poisoning may occur with prolonged IV administration of sodium nitroprusside. Consider this if such patients develop CNS depression, seizures, lactic acidosis, or cardiovascular instability
   a. May occur with infusion rate >2 mcg/kg/min
   b. Infusion rates of >10 mcg/kg/min should not be continued for prolonged periods of time because of this hazard
   c. If cyanide intoxication is suspected, discontinue infusion and treat as below
   d. Onset is usually at least several days after institution of sodium nitroprusside treatment, but it may occur within 6 hr of high-dose administration

Management

1. Administer oxygen, maintain airway, and assist respirations
2. Treat hypotension and seizures in standard fashion
3. Administer cyanide antidote kit
   a. Have the patient inhale an amyl nitrite capsule
   b. Administer sodium nitrite 300 mg IV
   c. Both of these produce methemoglobinemia, which may itself be toxic
   d. Administer sodium thiosulfate, which converts cyanide to thiocyanate, 150 mg/kg of a 25% solution IV (relatively contraindicated in renal failure)
4. If cyanide salt is ingested, lavage stomach and administer activated charcoal
5. Hydroxocobalamin, a form of vitamin B_{12}, is also used as an antidote
   a. Administer 4 g IM
   b. IV formulation is not available in the United States
6. Other cyanide antidotes, dicobalt-EDTA and 4-dimethylamineophenol, are not currently available in the United States

18.8   CYCLIC ANTIDEPRESSANTS

There is an estimated annual incidence of 500,000 cases of overdose with these medications. Many agents are in common use, including amitriptyline, desipramine, nortriptyline, doxepin, and imipramine (see Box on p.352). These may be found in medication combinations with other psychotropic agents.

Toxicity occurs via anticholinergic effects, alpha-adrenergic blockade, inhibition of norepinephrine reuptake, and inhibition of the fast sodium channel. Some drugs, such as haloperidol, morphine, and disulfiram, may prolong cyclic antidepressant toxicity by interfering with hydroxylation.

Clinical effects

1. Tachycardia, myoclonus, delirium, coma, hyperthermia, pupillary dilatation, hypertension or hypotension, prolongation of QRS and QT, AV block, and myocardial depression
2. The most important toxic effects are cardiovascular. QRS duration >0.12 indicates serious toxicity. Sinus tachycardia is typical; supraventricular tachycardia, ventricular tachycardia, torsades de pointes, and ventricular tachycardia may occur. Bradycardia is a poor prognostic sign

Cyclic Antidepressants

Tricyclic

Amitriptyline (Elavil, Endep, Etrafon, Limbitrol, Triavil)
Amoxapine (Asendin)
Desipramine (Norpramin)
Doxepin (Sinequan)
Imipramine (Tofranil)
Nortriptyline (Pamelor)
Protriptyline (Vivactil)
Trimipramine (Surmontil)

Tetracyclic

Maprotiline (Ludiomil)

3. Rapid deterioration with development of cardiovascular collapse, coma, or seizures may occur. Persistent seizures may produce hypothermia or rhabdomyolysis

Management

1. Perform gastric lavage and administer activated charcoal 100 g. Do not administer syrup of ipecac. Repeat doses of activated charcoal may be useful, and some have advocated continuous nasogastric instillation
2. Continuous electrocardiographic (ECG) monitoring is essential
3. Treat hyperthermia (see Chapter 7) and seizures in the usual fashion (diazepam 0.1 mg/kg IV per dose as needed or phenytoin 15 mg/kg IV over 30 min)
4. Do not give physostigmine as an antidote as it may produce seizures
5. Administer sodium bicarbonate 50-100 mEq IV bolus for widened QRS, hypotension, or metabolic acidosis. Monitor serum pH and electrolytes. Do not administer for metabolic alkalosis or pulmonary edema
6. Beta-blockers have been used, but caution must be utilized as patients may develop hypotension and cardiac arrest
7. For ventricular dysrhythmias, administer lidocaine or phenytoin
8. For torsades de pointes, administer magnesium 2-4 g IV or isoproterenol. Do not use procainamide or quinidine
9. In cardiovascular collapse, administer dopamine, phenylephrine, or norepinephrine

18.9   DIGOXIN

Digoxin is the most frequently used of the cardiac glycosides, and is prescribed most commonly for CHF or dysrhythmias. The mechanism of digitalis toxicity involves interruption of potassium and calcium efflux from myocardial cells by inhibition of sodium-potassium-ATPase. Intoxication may be the result of acute accidental or suicidal ingestion or chronic overdose. The clinical findings are different in these two settings.

Clinical effects

Acute intoxication

1. Nausea, vomiting, and hyperkalemia
2. Dysrhythmias
   a. Bradycardia with sinus and AV block
   b. Ventricular dysrhythmias are uncommon

Chronic intoxication

1. Weakness, visual disturbances, and hypomagnesemia. Potassium is normal or low
2. Dysrhythmias
   a. Ventricular tachycardia and fibrillation are common
   b. Accelerated junctional rhythm and paroxysmal atrial tachycardia with block is common, especially in patients with chronic atrial fibrillation

Diagnostic studies

1. Digoxin level is more useful in chronic intoxication; it may be falsely high in acute overdose
2. Follow serum potassium, magnesium, BUN, and creatinine

Management

1. Induce emesis or perform gastric lavage if there is a history of significant ingestion. These may exacerbate bradycardia
2. Administer activated charcoal and cathartic
3. Digitoxin elimination is enhanced by a repeat dose of activated charcoal
4. Monitor cardiac rhythm continuously
5. Hyperkalemia
   a. If >5.5 mEq/L, administer sodium bicarbonate 1 mEq/kg IV; glucose 0.5 g/kg and regular insulin 0.1 U/kg IV; or polystyrene sulfonate 0.5 g/kg PO
   b. Do not administer calcium
6. Bradycardia
   a. Atropine 0.5-2 mg IV as needed
   b. Cardiac pacing may be required
7. Ventricular dysrhythmias
   a. Lidocaine 1 mg/kg IV bolus followed by 1-4 mg/min infusion or
   b. Phenytoin 15-20 mg/kg IV no faster than 50 mg/min or
   c. Magnesium sulfate 10%, 2 g IV over 20 min, and continuous infusion of 1-2 g/hr

Antidote

Digoxin-specific antibody fragments (Digibind)

1. These have a high affinity for digoxin, a lower affinity for digitoxin and other cardiac glycosides
2. Administer for life-threatening dysrhythmias due to digitalis intoxication, especially if hyperkalemia is present

3. Dosage: each 40 mg vial of digoxin-specific antibodies absorbs 0.6 mg of digoxin. Dosage of antibodies to be administered is calculated as follows
   a. Calculate body load of digoxin: dose ingested/0.8 or serum drug concentration in mg/ml by mean volume of distribution of digoxin (5.6 L/kg × patient weight) or digitoxin (0.56 L/kg × patient weight) and divided by 1000 to obtain load in mg
   b. Number of vials required: body load (mg)/0.6 mg
4. Administer IV over 30 min
5. There are no known contraindications. In patients with preexisting heart disease, there is withdrawal of the inotropic effect by removal of digitalis from the circulation. Monitor for development of heart failure
6. Reversal of signs of digitalis intoxication occurs within 30-60 min of administration. Complete removal of digoxin occurs by 3 hr

| 18.10 | NARCOTICS

Narcotics include naturally occurring and synthetic derivatives of opiates. These are used both medically and as drugs of abuse. Commonly used narcotics are found in the Box below. Extremely potent synthetic "designer" opioids are derivatives of meperidine and fentanyl (i.e., "China white") and are also included in this group. Narcotics may be ingested, injected parenterally, or inhaled.

Clinical effects

1. Sedation; myosis; respiratory depression; decreased heart rate, respiratory rate, and BP; diminished bowel sounds; and signs of transcutaneous injection (i.e., "track marks") may be present. Urine toxicology may confirm diagnosis but a negative result does not exclude it
2. In significant overdose: coma, pinpoint pupils, severe respiratory depression, and apnea
3. Complications of overdose include rhabdomyolysis and noncardiogenic pulmonary edema
4. Death is typically due to respiratory failure

Commonly Used Narcotics and Related Agents

Butorphanol (Stadol)
Codeine
Fentanyl
Hydrocodone (Anexsia, Vicodin)
Hydromorphone (Dilaudid)
Meperidine (Demerol)
Methadone
Morphine
Nalbuphine (Nubain)
Oxycodone (Percocet, Percodan, Tylox)
Pentazocine (Talwin)
Propoxyphene (Darvon)

Management

1. Maintain and assist ventilation as necessary
2. For oral ingestion, perform gastric lavage and administer activated charcoal and cathartic
3. Antidote: Naloxone
   a. Opioid antagonist competitively blocks CNS opiate receptors
   b. Administer 0.4-2 mg IV (may also be given IM, subcutaneously, intratracheally). Repeat prn. No response to a total of 10 mg is evidence against narcotic overdose
   c. Duration of action is 1-4 hr. Repeated administration may be required or administer as infusion of 0.4-0.8 mg/hr in 5% dextrose
   d. Use in opiate-dependent patients may produce narcotic withdrawal syndrome
   e. Higher doses are frequently required with pentazocine and designer opioids: begin with an initial dose of 4 mg
4. If respiratory distress continues, monitor with chest radiograph and ABGs
5. If noncardiogenic pulmonary edema (which may also be produced by naloxone) is present, treat according to guidelines for ARDS (see Chapter 15)

18.11   PHENCYCLIDINE

Phencyclidine (PCP), formerly used as a legal anesthetic agent, is now an illicit drug.

Clinical effects

1. Produces hallucinations, alteration of mental status, and bizarre or violent behavior. Clinical status tends to wax and wane, and severe symptoms may persist for as long as 2 weeks
2. Level of consciousness ranges from fully alert to comatose
3. Most common physical findings are nystagmus and hypertension. Pupils may be dilated or miotic

Medical complications

1. May be due to direct effect of the drug or to injury sustained during intoxication
2. Major complications are indications for ICU admission: seizures, hyperthermia, rhabdomyolysis, and acute renal failure (ARF)

Diagnostic studies

1. Serum and urine PCP levels correlate poorly with clinical effects
2. Check urine for myoglobin, which may indicate rhabdomyolysis

Management

1. Management is largely supportive
2. PCP is frequently smoked, so gastric decontamination is not useful in these cases. However, gastric lavage and activated charcoal may be indicated if large amounts have been ingested. Do not induce emesis
3. Hemodialysis and charcoal hemoperfusion are not effective in eliminating PCP

4. Acid diuresis may speed elimination but is rarely indicated
5. Severe agitation or violence: utilize physical restraints. May administer haloperidol 10 mg IM or IV or benzodiazepines
6. Hypertension is usually mild and does not require treatment
7. Seizures: if persistent treat with IV benzodiazepines

18.12   PHENYTOIN

Toxicity may be due to acute overdose or chronic overingestion.

Clinical effects

1. Nausea, vomiting, lethargy, ataxia, agitation, irritability, hallucinations, and seizures
2. Horizontal nystagmus is characteristic of overdose
3. At high very levels: coma and respiratory arrest
4. Cardiac toxicity occurs only with iatrogenic IV overdose, not with oral ingestion

Diagnostic studies

1. Phenytoin levels
   a. Therapeutic: 10-20 mg/L
   b. Levels >20 mg/L: nystagmus
   c. Levels >30 mg/L: ataxia
   d. Levels >40 mg/L: lethargy is common
2. Serum glucose: hyperglycemia may occur

Management

1. Induce emesis or perform gastric lavage
2. Administer activated charcoal. Multiple doses of charcoal may enhance elimination
3. Some recommend the use of charcoal hemoperfusion for severe intoxication
4. Remainder of treatment is supportive
5. Monitor cardiac rhythm in IV overdose

18.13   SALICYLATES

Used for analgesic, antipyretic, and antiinflammatory properties, these are found in a variety of both prescription and over-the-counter preparations (e.g., Alka-Seltzer, Ascriptin, Bufferin, Excedrin Extra Strength). Poisoning may be result of acute ingestion or chronic overdose.

Clinical effects

1. Result from CNS respiratory stimulation, uncoupling of oxidative phosphorylation, interference with platelet function, and bleeding time
2. Cerebral and pulmonary edema occur by uncertain mechanisms
3. Acute overdose
   a. Tachypnea, tinnitus, vomiting, lethargy, respiratory alkalosis, and metabolic acidosis
   b. Severe: hypoglycemia, hyperthermia, seizures, coma, and pulmonary edema

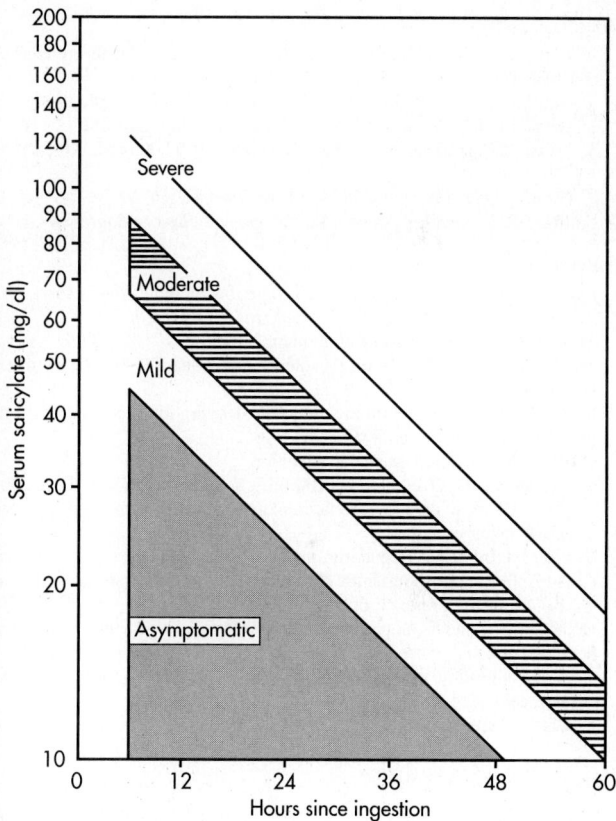

Figure 18-2
Done nomogram for salicylate poisoning. Note that this nomogram is not accurate for chronic ingestions. (From Done AK: Salicylate intoxication: significance of measurements of salicylate in blood in cases of acute ingestion. *Pediatrics* 1960; 26:800-7.)

4. Chronic overdose
    a. Confusion, dehydration, and metabolic acidosis. This presentation may mimic sepsis
    b. Pulmonary edema is more common in chronic overdose than in acute overdose

Diagnostic studies

1. In acute ingestion, obtain salicylate level and plot on Done nomogram (see Fig. 18-2 on p. 357)
    a. Multiple determinations may be necessary with sustained-release preparations. Obtain q 2-3 hr for 12 hr following ingestion
    b. Usual therapeutic levels in arthritis patients: 100-300 mg/L (10-30 mg/dl)
    c. Nomogram is not as useful in chronic intoxication
2. Follow ABGs, serum glucose, electrolytes, and chest radiographs

Management

1. Induce vomiting or perform gastric lavage if acute ingestion is suspected
2. Administer activated charcoal and cathartic
3. Monitor for development of pulmonary edema
4. Treat metabolic acidosis with IV sodium bicarbonate 1 mEq/kg to maintain pH at 7.40-7.50
5. Rehydrate with IV crystalloid solution if dehydration has resulted from vomiting or hyperventilation
6. Urinary alkalinization enhances excretion
    a. Administer D_5W containing 100 mEq sodium bicarbonate/L at 200-300 ml/hr. Use care in chronic intoxication; observe for development of pulmonary edema
    b. Check urinary pH frequently; maintain at 6.0-7.0
    c. Add 30-40 mEq potassium chloride (KCl) to each L of IV solution (except in the presence of renal failure)
7. Hemodialysis and hemoperfusion are effective in removing salicylates; hemodialysis also corrects fluid and acid-base disturbance. Indications
    a. Acute ingestion with serum levels >1200 mg/L (120 mg/dl) or severe acidosis
    b. Chronic intoxication with serum level >600 mg/L (60 mg/dl)

18.14 | SEDATIVES/HYPNOTICS

There are a large number of sedatives in medical use. The most common are barbiturates, nonbarbiturate sedatives/hypnotics (e.g., chloral hydrate, meprobamate, paraldehyde) and benzodiazepines (see the Box on p.359). The toxic:therapeutic ratio is very high for most benzodiazepines. Oral overdose with 20 times the therapeutic dose of diazepam may occur without significant CNS depression.

Clinical effects

1. The most prominent effect is CNS depression: lethargy, ataxia, slurred speech, and progression to coma and respiratory depression
2. Severe hypothermia, hypotension, and bradycardia may accompany deep coma due to barbiturates

Commonly Used Sedative/Hypnotic Agents

Barbiturates

Short-acting
   Secobarbital (Seconal)
   Pentobarbital (Nembutal)
Intermediate-acting
   Amobarbital (Amytal)
   Aprobarbital (Alurate)
   Butabarbital (Butisol)
Long-acting
   Phenobarbital

Nonbarbiturates

Chloral hydrate
Ethchlorvynol (Placidyl)
Meprobamate (Equagesic, Equanil, Miltown)
Paraldehyde

Benzodiazepines

Ultrashort-acting
   Midazolam (Versed)
   Temazepam (Restoril)
   Triazolam (Halcion)
Short-acting
   Alprazolam (Xanax)
   Lorazepam (Ativan)
   Oxazepam (Serax)
Long-acting
   Chlordiazepoxide (Librium)
   Clorazepate (Tranxene)
   Diazepam (Valium)
   Flurazepam (Dalmane)
   Prazepam (Centrax)

3. Chloral hydrate may have cardiac effects including dysrhythmias, hypotension, and myocardial depression

Diagnostic studies

Barbiturates

Serum levels >60-80 mg/L usually produce coma (>20-30 mg/L in short-acting barbiturates)

Benzodiazepines and others

Serum drug levels are of limited value

Management

1. Airway protection and ventilatory support are paramount
2. Induce emesis (if awake) or perform gastric lavage. Lavage is preferred for very short-acting agents such as triazolam
3. Administer activated charcoal and cathartic. A repeat dose of activated charcoal decreases the half-life of phenobarbital and meprobamate
4. Urinary alkalinization increases the elimination of phenobarbital (but not other barbiturates) and meprobamate
5. Charcoal hemoperfusion may be indicated for severe barbiturate overdose

Benzodiazepine antidote

1. Flumazenil (Romazicon [formerly called Mazicon]) is a selective benzodiazepine CNS receptor-competitive inhibitor; use it to reverse benzodiazepine-induced coma
2. Initial recommended dose is 0.2 mg IV over 30 seconds. Repeat 0.3 mg after 30 seconds, then 0.5 mg at 1-min intervals
3. Most patients respond to cumulative doses of 1-2 mg. Reversal of CNS depression is unlikely if a dose of 5 mg has been given without effect
4. Adverse effects
   a. Nausea and vomiting are most common
   b. May induce withdrawal syndrome (agitation, tachycardia, seizures) in patients dependent on benzodiazepines
5. Duration of action of a single dose is 1-2 hr. If there is prolonged reversal need, give repeated doses or administer as IV infusion of 0.1-0.5 mg/hr
6. Do not administer to patients suspected of taking cyclic antidepressants

18.15   THEOPHYLLINE

The mechanism of toxicity is via the release of endogenous catecholamines, stimulation of beta$_2$ receptors, and inhibition of adenosine receptors. Clinical effects may be delayed for several hours following acute ingestion if a sustained release formulation is involved. Toxicity may be acute or chronic.

Clinical effects

1. Common toxic effects include nausea, vomiting, tremor, tachycardia, and hypotension
2. Hypokalemia, hyperglycemia, and metabolic acidosis may occur (only in acute intoxication)
3. Seizures and ventricular dysrhythmias may occur, especially with very high serum levels and chronic intoxication

Diagnostic studies

1. Serum theophylline level
   a. Therapeutic: 15-20 mg/L
   b. In acute overdose with a level >100 mg/L: seizures, hypotension, and ventricular dysrhythmias are common
   c. Seizures may occur at levels of 40-60 mg/L in chronic overdose
   d. Repeat levels q 2-4 hr during treatment and monitor for 12-16 hr
2. Monitor serum pH, glucose, and potassium levels

Management

1. Perform gastric lavage
2. Administer activated charcoal 100 g and readminister 20-30 g q 2-3 hr. Continuous infusion of activated charcoal has been recommended. Dilute charcoal in normal saline and infuse at 0.25-0.5 g/kg/hr up to a maximum rate of 50 g/hr
3. Whole bowel irrigation has been recommended if there are undissolved sustained release tablets that cannot be removed with gastric lavage
4. Treat seizures and ventricular dysrhythmias in standard fashion as required. Magnesium has been successful in some cases
5. For supraventricular tachycardia or rapid sinus tachycardia, ventricular dysrhythmias, or hypotension administer esmolol 0.05 mg/kg/min or propranolol 0.01-0.03 mg/kg IV. Use with caution if wheezing is present
6. If the theophylline level >100 mg/L, or seizures or dysrhythmias do not respond to treatment, institute charcoal hemoperfusion
7. Hypokalemia usually resolves spontaneously

Selected readings

Albertson TE, Derlet RW, Foulke GE, et al: Superiority of activated charcoal alone compared with ipecac and activated charcoal in the treatment of acute toxic ingestion. *Ann Intern Med* 1989; 18:56-9.

Antman EM, Wenger TL, Butler VP, et al: Treatment of 150 cases of life-threatening digitalis intoxication with digoxin-specific Fab antibody fragments. *Circulation* 1991; 81:1744-52.

Bertino JS, Reed MD: Barbiturate and nonbarbiturate sedative hypnotic intoxication in children. *Pediatr Clin North Am* 1986; 33:703-22.

Bradberry JC, Roebel MA: Continuous infusion of naloxone in the treatment of narcotic overdose. *Drug Intell Clin Pharm* 1981; 15:945-50.

Chern TL, Hu SC, Lee CH, et al: Diagnostic and therapeutic utility of flumazenil in comatose patients with drug overdose. *Am J Emerg Med* 1993; 11:122-4.

Cregler LI, Mark H: Medical complications of cocaine abuse. *N Engl J Med* 1986; 315:1495-1500.

Cupit GC, Temple AR: Gastrointestinal decontamination in the management of the poisoned patient. *Emerg Med Clin North Am* 1984; 2:827-36.

Curry SC, Arnold-Capell P: Nitroprusside, nitroglycerin, and angiotensin converting enzyme inhibitors. *Crit Care Clin* 1991; 7:555-81.

Curtis RA, Barone J, Giacona N: Efficacy of ipecac and activated charcoal/cathartic. *Arch Intern Med* 1984; 144:48-52.

Durbin CG Jr: Neuromuscular blocking agents and sedative drugs: clinical uses and toxic effects in the critical care unit. *Crit Care Clin* 1991; 7:489-506.

Fine JS, Goldfrank LR: Update in medical toxicology. *Pediatr Clin North Am* 1992; 39:1031-51.

Frommer DA, Kulig KW, Marx JA, et al: Tricyclic antidepressant overdose. *JAMA* 1987; 257:521-6.

Henry J, Volans G: ABC of poisoning: diagnosis. *Br Med J* 1984; 289:172-4.

Karavokiros KAT, Tsipis GB: Flumazenil: a benzodiazepine antagonist. *DICP Ann Pharmacother* 1990; 24:976-81.

Kumar S, Rex DK: Failure of physicians to recognize acetaminophen hepatotoxicity in chronic alcoholics. *Arch Intern Med* 1991; 151:1189-91.

Leatherman JW, Schmitz PG: Fever, hyperdynamic shock, and multiple organ-system failure. *Chest* 1991; 100:1391-6.

Levy G: Gastrointestinal clearance of drugs with activated charcoal. *N Engl J Med* 1982; 307:676-8.

Miller PD, Heinig RE, Waterhouse C: Treatment of alcoholic ketoacidosis. *Arch Intern Med* 1978; 138:67-72.

Ohning BL, Reed MD, Blumer JL: Continuous nasogastric administration of activated charcoal for the treatment of theophylline intoxication. *Pediatr Pharmacol* 1986; 5:241-5.

Olson KR: *Poisoning and drug overdose,* Norwalk, Conn, 1990, Appleton & Lange.

Rolband GC, Marcuard SP: Cimetidine in the treatment of acetaminophen overdose. *J Clin Gastroenterol* 1991; 13:79-82.

Sanders LD, Pigott SE, Okell IR, et al: Reversal of benzodiazepine sedation with the antagonist flumazenil. *Brit J Anaesth* 1991; 66:445-53.

Sternbach GL, Varon J: Designer drugs: recognizing and managing their toxic effects. *Postgrad Med* 1992:91:169-76.

Tenenbein MD, Cohen S, Sitar DS: Whole bowel irrigation as a decontamination procedure after acute drug overdose. *Arch Intern Med* 1987; 147:905-7.

Varon J, Duncan SR: Naloxone reversal of hypotension due to captopril overdose. *Ann Emerg Med* 1991; 20:1125-7.

Weinstein RS: Recognition and management of poisoning with beta-adrenergic blocking agents. *Ann Emerg Med* 1984; 13:1123-31.

Trauma

19

George L. Sternbach and Joseph Varon

Trauma is the leading cause of death in persons between the ages of 1 and 44, and the fourth leading cause of death overall. About 140,000 traumatic deaths occur annually. Sepsis, adult respiratory distress syndrome, and multiorgan system failure are the leading causes of death in trauma patients who survive initial resuscitation and surgical repair of their injuries.

19.1 MULTISYSTEM TRAUMA

Establishment of priorities

1. The highest priorities in initial evaluation are:
   a. Airway maintenance
   b. Breathing and ventilation
   c. Circulation and shock management
2. Secondary evaluation includes vital signs and a complete physical (including rectal) examination. Nasogastric and urinary catheters (unless contraindicated) should generally be inserted to diagnose gastric or urinary tract hemorrhage and to allow for monitoring of urinary output
3. Rapid normalization of vital signs is one of the goals in trauma management

Severity of injury scoring systems

1. Glasgow coma scale (see Table 19-1) is used for assessing neurologic status in head injury
2. The trauma score (see Table 19-2) estimates the physiologic severity of injury and combines the Glasgow coma scale with other clinical indices of cardiovascular and pulmonary function

Airway management

1. Clear the airway of debris or secretions
2. Avoid chin-lift and neck-lift/tilt if cervical spine injury is considered. Obtain cervical spine radiographs as soon as possible

Table 19-1   Glasgow coma scale

	Score
Eye Opening	
Spontaneous	4
To verbal command	3
To pain	2
None	1
Best Motor Response	
Obeys verbal command	6
Localizes painful stimuli	5
Flexion withdrawal from painful stimuli	4
Decorticate (flexion) response to painful stimuli	3
Decerebrate (extension) response to painful stimuli	2
None	1
Best Verbal Response	
Oriented conversation	5
Disoriented conversation	4
Inappropriate words	3
Incomprehensible sounds	2
None	1

TOTAL SCORE: 3-15

From Teasdale G, Jennett B: Assessment of coma and impaired consciousness: a practical scale. *Lancet* 1974; 2:81-3.

Oxygenation and ventilation

1. If adequate respirations appear to be present, obtain baseline blood gases as soon as possible. Apply 100% O_2 by mask. If there are no spontaneous respirations, assist with bag and mask
2. Endotracheal intubation
   a. When necessary, intubation should usually be done by oral route with manual in-line stabilization
   b. Rapid sequence induction is often indicated in patients with major trauma, head or facial injury, diminished level of consciousness, and respiratory impairment. Preoxygenation, application of cricoid pressure, and administration of induction agents: vecuronium 0.2 mg/kg IV, followed 3 min later by succinylcholine 1-1.5 mg/kg (succinylcholine is contraindicated in penetrating eye injuries and massive crush injury), followed by intubation
3. Cricothyrotomy is the preferred procedure when a surgical airway is necessary

Table 19-2   Trauma score

	Points
Respiratory rate/min	
10-24	4
25-35	3
>35	2
<10	1
0	0
Respiratory effort	
Normal	1
Shallow or retractive	0
Systolic blood pressure	
>90 mm Hg	4
70-90 mm Hg	3
50-69 mm Hg	2
<50 mm Hg	1
0	0
Capillary refill	
Normal	2
Delayed	1
None	0
Glasgow coma score	
14-15	5
11-13	4
8-10	3
5-7	2
3-4	1
TOTAL	

From Champion HR, Sacco WJ, Carnazzo AJ, et al: Trauma score. *Crit Care Med* 1981; 9:672-6.

4. The most common causes for respiratory compromise are tension pneumothorax, open pneumothorax, and flail chest with pulmonary contusion

Circulation and shock management

1. Evaluation incudes assessment of vital signs, level of consciousness, skin color, character of pulse, and capillary refill
2. Shock in trauma is most commonly due to hypovolemia
   a. Likely sites for occult hemorrhage are the thorax, abdomen, pelvis, retroperitoneum, and thigh
   b. In addition, conditions producing shock that should be considered include tension pneumothorax, cardiac tamponade, myocardial contusion, and spinal trauma
3. Classification of hemorrhagic shock: see Table 19-3
4. Treatment
   a. Class I hemorrhage: replacement of primary fluid loss with electrolyte solution

Table 19-3   Classification of hemorrhage

	Blood Volume Lost	Clinical Signs
Class I	Up to 15%	Increased heart rate
Class II	15%-30%	Increased heart rate, decreased pulse pressure, minor delay in capillary refill, and anxiety
Class III	30%-40%	Increased heart rate, decreased blood pressure, delayed capillary refill, clouded sensorium
Class IV	>40%	Markedly increased heart rate; decreased blood pressure; negligible urine output; markedly depressed mental status; and cold, pale skin

From American College of Surgeons: *Advanced trauma life support instructor's manual,* Chicago, 1989, American College of Surgeons.

    b. Class II hemorrhage: initial stabilization with IV fluids; may require blood transfusion

    c. Class III hemorrhage: almost always requires transfusion

5. Establish at least two large-caliber (14- to 16-gauge or larger) IV lines. Initial fluid administration should be with isotonic electrolyte solution

    a. Administration rate should be commensurate with clinical condition and vital signs. Avoid fluid overload but achieve adequate intravascular volume, hematocrit (hct), and tissue perfusion

    b. In the hypovolemic patient at least 2 L (20 ml/kg in a child) can be rapidly infused and the patient then reassessed

6. If shock persists despite resuscitation with IV fluids, blood replacement is indicated

    a. Maintain hct of at least 30%

    b. Crossmatched blood is preferable if the patient's condition permits

    c. If there is insufficient time for a full crossmatch to be performed, administer type specific blood (ABO and Rh compatible)

    d. For patients in severe, life-threatening shock for whom type-specific blood is not available, administer type O blood (Rh-negative in women of child-bearing age), however, subsequent crossmatching may be more difficult

    e. Employ autotransfusion when feasible (especially administration of autologous blood from chest tube drainage)

7. Monitor for possible complications of transfusion

    a. Hemolytic transfusion reaction: fever; chills; chest, back and joint pain. Terminate transfusion, administer IV fluids and furosemide. Monitor urine output

b. Hypothermia may follow massive transfusion with refrigerated blood. Give blood through a warmer if possible. Monitor body temperature with core probe

c. Coagulopathy may result following massive transfusion, probably on the basis of quantity and function of platelets, as well as consumption of coagulation factors. Administration of platelets is advised following rapid transfusion of each 10 U of blood. If evidence of coagulopathy exists, consider administration of fresh frozen plasma (FFP) and cryoprecipitate

d. Banked blood is acidemic and high in potassium (K^+) preservative anticoagulant binds calcium [C_a^{2+}]. Monitor serum pH, K^+, magnesium, and Ca^{2+} levels

8. Monitor urine output; volume replacement should produce urine output of at least 1-1.5 ml/kg/hr.

Complications of hemorrhagic shock and volume resuscitation

Peripheral edema, hypothermia, cerebral edema, cardiac dysfunction (usually right ventricular failure), pneumonia, acute respiratory distress syndrome (ARDS), and multiorgan system failure

Cardiac arrest

1. Perform immediate thoracotomy in patients in extremis, especially with penetrating chest trauma
2. Therapeutic objectives include relief of cardiac tamponade, open cardiac massage, control of cardiac injuries, vascular control of major vessel or hilar injuries, and aortic occlusion for treatment of shock

19.2   HEAD TRAUMA

Head injury is a major entity often encountered in acute care. The head is the most frequently injured part of the body in trauma patients—over 80,000 persons sustain permanent disabling injuries of the head or spinal cord every year.

Assessment

History

1. Important components are the mechanism of injury and loss of consciousness. High-speed trauma (e.g, with ejection from a vehicle, impact with a windshield) produces a greater chance of significant injury
2. Incomplete recollection by the patient of details of the injury may imply a transient loss of consciousness. This is not as useful if the patient is intoxicated

Physical examination

1. Examine the scalp and face for signs of trauma such as lacerations, ecchymoses, hemotympanum, and bleeding or clear fluid from the nostrils or ears

2. Palpate the spine for tenderness or deformity. Always consider the possibility of concomitant spinal cord injury
3. Focus on other injuries that affect the airway or produce respiratory or circulatory impairment

Neurologic examination

1. This is the best tool for identifying the presence of significant intracranial injury
   a. Assess the mental status; this is the most important aspect of the neurologic examination
   b. Determine the focal neurologic deficit, abnormal posturing, and pathologic reflexes. Evaluate brain stem reflexes (light, corneal, gag) and ventilatory drive
   c. Absence of brain stem function usually indicates the need for urgent airway intervention
2. Frequent repetition of neurologic examination is necessary, especially within first 48 hr of injury

Glasgow coma scale

1. Determine the Glasgow coma scale score (see Table 19-1)
   a. Score of 13-15: mild injury
   b. Score of 9-12: moderate injury
   c. Score of 8 or less: severe injury
2. The Glasgow coma scale is of limited use in children <3 years of age

Management

Position

When associated injuries permit, elevate the head of the bed 30%- to 45°; this reduces intracranial pressure (ICP)

Airway and ventilation

1. The highest initial priority is prevention or reduction of secondary injury due to swelling or compression of cerebral tissue by cerebral edema and raised ICP
2. Proper airway management reduces increased ICP. Diminished mental status (particularly a Glasgow coma scale score of <9) is an indication for early endotracheal intubation
3. Chin-lift and neck-lift maneuvers are inappropriate if the patient with a head injury is suspected of having cervical spine injury
4. Initial management of increased ICP includes hyperventilation
   a. It is often recommended to maintain arterial carbon dioxide tension (Pco_2) of 25-30 torr, but there is no uniform agreement on this
   b. Many recommend not to hyperventilate below Pco_2 of 20 torr or pH >7.60 (see Chapter 11)
5. Endotracheal intubation
   a. Nasal intubation is relatively contraindicated; use orotracheal intubation with manual in-line stabilization

b. Precede intubation with bag-valve-mask ventilation, cricoid pressure, and pharmacologic induction: lidocaine 1.5 mg/kg and succinylcholine 1-1.5 mg/kg or vecuronium 0.1-0.2 mg/kg IV
6. When mechanical ventilation is instituted, avoid high levels (>10 cm) of positive end-expiratory pressure (PEEP) as this may increase ICP. Chest PT may also increase ICP

Osmotic therapy and diuresis

1. Reduces increased ICP by reducing intracranial volume
2. Mannitol: osmotic diuretic of choice. It is generally administered in the rapidly deteriorating patient and often for arresting neurologic deterioration when the patient is being prepared for urgent craniotomy
   a. Give as a 20% solution, 0.25-1 g/kg via rapid IV infusion
   b. ICP reduction usually occurs within 10-20 min
   c. Duration is limited to 2-6 hr following initial bolus. Continuous infusion may be required
   d. Monitor blood pressure (BP), serum electrolytes, and osmolarity
3. Diuretics may be used alone or in combination with osmotic diuretics to reduce intracerebral fluid volume
   a. Furosemide is the loop diuretic of choice. Administer IV bolus of 1 mg/kg. The onset of action is slower than mannitol, but concomitant use enhances the duration of ICP reduction by mannitol and decreases the risk of rebound ICP elevation. Repeated doses may be required
   b. Acetazolamide is a carbonic anhydrase inhibitor that decreases cerebrospinal fluid (CSF) production. Administer 250 mg qid. Monitor for production of acidosis
4. Corticosteroids are frequently administered, but whether they diminish ICP in head trauma is controversial

Cardiovascular support

1. Cerebral injury does not generally produce hypotension (except in the agonal state)
2. Look for an extracranial source if hypotension is present
3. Avoid fluid overload but provide adequate intravascular volume and hct. A pulmonary artery catheter may be required for monitoring

Monitoring

1. ICP
   a. Indicated in patients with severe head injury with computed tomography (CT) evidence of raised ICP. Monitoring ICP, however, has not been proven to affect survival
   b. Monitor by intraventricular catheter, subarachnoid bolt, or extradural pressure sensor
   c. It is generally advised to maintain ICP at ≤20 mm Hg
   d. Cerebral perfusion pressure (CPP): monitor this (CPP = mean arterial pressure [MAP] − ICP) and maintain at >60 mm Hg. If hypotension occurs, elevate arterial pressure to maintain CPP above this level, as ischemic damage may occur
2. Intravascular pressure: arterial catheterization to allow monitoring of MAP, as well as frequent blood gas determinations

3. Head trauma may produce the syndrome of inappropriate secretion of antidiuretic hormone (SIADH). This results in hyponatremia with a relatively concentrated urine (see also Chapters 6 and 16)

Diagnostic studies

Skull radiographs

1. Plain skull radiographs may demonstrate skull fracture but have poor sensitivity and specificity for identifying intracranial lesions
2. May be useful in children <2 years old, in whom skull fracture may identify the risk of hypovolemia due to extracranial bleeding, the formation of a leptomeningeal cyst, and child abuse

Computed tomography

1. Diagnostic procedure of choice in assessing acute head injury. Perform without contrast material. Indicated in the patient with a decreased level of consciousness (Glasgow coma scale score of ≤14), deteriorating mental status, focal neurologic deficit, seizures, or persistent vomiting
2. If the Glasgow coma scale score <9, obtain a CT immediately after endotracheal intubation when the patient is hemodynamically stable

Magnetic resonance imaging (MRI)

1. MRI is superior to CT in diffuse axonal injury
2. Limitations in acute injury are the duration of scanning and interference of monitoring and life-support equipment with its magnetic field

Ultrasound

May be an option in smaller children with suspected intraventricular hemorrhage

19.3 CRUSH INJURY

Traumatic asphyxia

1. Mechanism: direct massive thoracoabdominal compression
2. Clinical findings: blanching cyanosis of the upper chest, neck, and head; petechiae; edema; subconjunctival hemorrhage
3. Associated injuries: chest wall injury, pulmonary contusion, cardiac contusion, diaphragm rupture, and intraabdominal solid and hollow viscus injury
4. Sequelae: brachial plexus injury, spinal cord injury, and transient neurologic impairment

Abdominal and pelvic injury

1. Crush injury accounts for 5% of pelvic fractures. It may result in bladder laceration
2. Crush mechanism to abdomen results in a high proportion of hollow viscus injury

Skeletal muscle injury

1. Results in myonecrosis. May produce rhabomyolysis, hyperkalemia, hyperphosphatemia, hypocalcemia, and myoglobinuria

2. Sequelae include acute renal failure (ARF) and disseminated intravascular coagulation
3. Follow creatine kinase (CK), electrolytes, creatinine, and urine output
4. CK levels reach this maximum 24-36 hr after injury. The level should decline by 50% each 48 hr thereafter. If there is an increase in CK during this time, consider the recurrence of muscle necrosis
5. Treat ARF with fluid infusion, osmotic diuresis, and alkalinization (see Chapter 16)

19.4   CHEST TRAUMA

Chest trauma is the cause of death in up to 25% of cases of multiple-system trauma. Injury may occur to the chest wall, lung, great vessels, and mediastinal viscera

1. Most injuries can be initially managed with chest tube insertion and other nonoperative management
2. Indications for thoracotomy include cardiac tamponade and massive hemothorax (see below); pulmonary air leak >15-20 L/min; aortic arch, esophageal, tracheal, or major bronchial disruption; systemic air embolism; bullet embolism; and cardiac arrest

Chest wall trauma

1. Rib fracture is the most common chest wall injury. It is an important indicator of underlying injury
   a. First-third ribs: great vessel and bronchial injury. Diminished pulse or BP in arms and radiographic evidence of mediastinal hematoma (see below) are indications for arteriography
   b. Lower ribs: kidney, liver, or spleen laceration
2. Flail chest occurs when three or more ribs are fractured in two places or when there are multiple fractures associated with sternal fracture
   a. Clinical significance varies, depending on size and location of flail segment and the extent of underlying pulmonary contusion
   b. Obtain and follow arterial blood gases (ABGs)
   c. Splint thorax with weights, traction, or skeletal fixation
   d. Patients with severe hypoxemia require endotracheal intubation and positive pressure ventilation. Observe for late development of pneumothorax, especially tension pneumothorax in the mechanically ventilated patient
3. Sternal fracture is associated with myocardial contusion, cardiac rupture and tamponade, and pulmonary contusion. Early surgical fixation is often necessary; urgent surgery may be indicated when costosternal dislocations produce a compromise of the trachea or neurovascular structures at the thoracic inlet
4. Analgesic methods that may be required for treatment of major chest wall injuries include parenteral opiates, epidural analgesia, and intercostal nerve block

Pneumothorax

1. Usually results from a penetrating trauma or a blunt trauma with a rib fracture. It may be caused by positive pressure ventilation (barotrauma)

2. The presence of pneumothorax requires 28-40 Fr chest tube insertion. Smaller tubes may be utilized if pneumothorax is not accompanied by hemothorax
3. Open pneumothorax requires covering of the chest wall injury with air-tight dressing and insertion of a chest tube
4. Tension pneumothorax requires immediate needle decompression and chest tube insertion. Clinical findings include unilateral absence of breath sounds, severe dyspnea, tracheal shift, jugular venous distention, and cyanosis

Hemothorax

1. Initial treatment requires insertion of a chest tube to evacuate hemothorax, re-expand the lung, and monitor the rate of bleeding
2. Indications for thoracotomy include initial chest tube drainage of >1500 ml or continued bleeding of >300 ml/hr for >2-3 hr

Major vessel injury

1. Common cause of death in major trauma
2. In case of radiographic evidence of mediastinal hematoma, consider widened mediastinum, aortic knob obliteration, or tracheal or nasogastric tube deviation
3. Arteriography or CT is required for diagnosis

Cardiac tamponade

1. Most frequently occurs with penetrating injures. Suspect this in chest trauma with shock and jugular venous distention
2. Requires thoracotomy and pericardial decompression. Pericardiocentesis may be performed if diagnosis is uncertain or as a temporizing measure during preparation for thoracotomy

Pulmonary contusion

Management consists of supplemental oxygen administration and mechanical ventilation with the addition of PEEP (if indicated in patients with worsening hypoxemia)

Myocardial contusion

Management consists of cardiac monitoring, echocardiography, and treatment of dysrhythmias as necessary

19.5   ABDOMINAL TRAUMA

Evaluation

1. Physical findings may be unreliable if complicated by a head injury, other injury, or intoxication
2. Findings most consistently associated with internal abdominal injury are abdominal tenderness and guarding
3. Examine the thorax for rib fractures; palpate flanks and pelvis; and perform a rectal and pelvic examination
4. Obtain baseline hemogram, blood coagulation screen, and urinalysis (U/A)

Diagnostic peritoneal lavage

1. The use of this modality varies considerably from institution to institution
2. Indications may include equivocal abdominal findings. Abdominal injury may be obscured by diminished sensation due to head injury, spinal injury, or alcohol intoxication
3. The major advantage of diagnostic peritoneal lavage is the ability to obtain rapid indication of intraperitoneal hemorrhage
4. Relative contraindications are previous abdominal surgery, significant obesity, pregnancy, and preexisting coagulopathy
5. Positive lavage consists of aspiration of >10 ml of blood, aspiration of enteric contents, or lavage fluid that contains >100,000 red blood cells/mm^3, >500 white blood cells/mm^3, amylase ≥20 IU/L, or bile

Abdominal CT

1. Indicated in stable patients with possible intraabdominal injury and when diagnostic peritoneal lavage is being considered but is contraindicated
2. Advantages include the ability to visualize the urinary tract and retroperitoneum

Penetrating injury

1. Antibiotics
   a. Second- or third-generation cephalosporins (e.g., cefoxitin 2 g IV q6h or ceftazidime 1-2 g IV q8h)
   b. Alternatively, a combination of gentamicin (1.5-2 mg/kg IV loading and 3 mg/kg/day in 3 doses maintenance) or tobramycin (1 mg/kg q8h IV) and clindamycin 600-900 mg q8h IV

Indications for laparotomy

1. Gunshot wounds
2. Stab wounds that produce shock, signs of peritoneal irritation, gastrointestinal (GI) bleeding or evisceration of the bowel
3. Blunt trauma that produces unstable vital signs, GI bleeding, peritoneal irritation, pneumoperitoneum, or evidence of diaphragmatic injury
4. There may be a role for laparoscopy in the stable patient with a penetrating injury, but this method has not been used extensively in this setting

Postoperative complications

1. Intraabdominal hemorrhage
   a. May be due to recurrent bleeding from sites that were not identified during surgery due to hypotension
   b. Identify hemostasis deficiencies (thrombocytopenia, clotting dysfunction), especially if the patient has had massive transfusions
   c. If prothrombin time (PT) and partial thromboplastin time (PTT) are prolonged, administer FFP
2. Fever: consider wound infection, necrotizing fasciitis, peritonitis, and intraabdominal abscess
3. Missed intraabdominal injury: consider the diaphragm, biliary tree, duodenum, pancreas, ureter, colon, and rectum

Nonoperative management

1. May be suitable in the patient who remains hemodynamically stable following initial resuscitation with 1-2 L of IV fluids. Laparoscopic repair may be another option
   a. Normal vital signs, urine output >1-1.5 ml/hr, and no blood requirement
   b. Patient must be alert
   c. No coagulation defects
2. CT should establish the extent of the injury
3. Suitable injuries include
   a. Isolated splenic trauma with minor capsular tear or parenchymal injury
   b. Stab wounds without shock, peritoneal irritation, or GI bleeding
4. Monitoring
   a. Repeat abdominal examination for signs of peritoneal irritation at least q 4-6 hr
   b. Monitor vital signs q 1-2 hr during the first 24 hours
   c. Monitor serial hct q4hr. Also monitor amylase
   d. Repeat abdominal CT after 12 hr of observation and thereafter as indicated by clinical signs

Urinary tract injury

1. Evaluate with an intravenous pyelogram (IVP) or abdominal CT if there is gross hematuria; flank hematoma; or mass, penetrating trauma with suspected urinary injury
2. Bladder and urethra injury: see the following section on pelvic fractures

19.6   MULTIPLE FRACTURES

1. Identify fractures and dislocations; assess distal neurocirculatory function
2. Complications of fractures include arterial and neural injury, hemorrhage, compartment syndrome, ARDS, fat embolization, infection, and thromboembolism
3. Fractures of the pelvis and femur are particularly significant because of the potential for hemorrhage
4. Dislocations of the hip and knee require prompt reduction to avoid neurovascular complications

Initial management

1. Immobilize any injured extremity
2. Stabilize femur fracture in a Hare or comparable traction device

Arterial injury

1. Arterial injury may be due to transection, arterial spasm, occlusion by hematoma, external compression, or arteriovenous fistula formation
2. Acute loss of vascular function requires emergent surgical exploration or angiography

Compartment syndrome

1. Circulatory supply can be lost due to increased muscular compartment pressure. This is most common in the leg but also occurs in the forearm

2. The earliest sign is pain with passive stretching of the extremity. Suspect compartment syndrome if there is severe, constant pain despite reduction and immobilization
3. Measure compartment pressure by inserting a needle connected to a manometric pressure measurement system into the soft tissue of the extremity involved; the result should be <30 mm Hg in the normotensive pressure
4. Treatment is fasciotomy

Infection in open injuries

1. Give tetanus prophylaxis, especially for wounds with deep tissue penetration, devitalized tissue, and burns
2. IV antibiotics
   a. IV first-generation cephalosporins (e.g., cefazolin 1 g IV q6hr)
   b. If the wound is large or heavily contaminated, add gentamicin (1.5-2 mg/kg IV loading and 3 mg/kg/day in 3 doses maintenance) or tobramycin (1 mg/kg q8hr IV) if the patient has normal renal function
3. Observe for the appearance of gas gangrene (appearance of subcutaneous crepitation or soft tissue gas on radiographs)
   a. Occurs within 12-72 hr of injury and requires broad-spectrum antibiotics and aggressive wound debridement
   b. Most often occurs in grossly contaminated open fractures with soft tissue damage

Fat embolism

1. Occurs most commonly in multiple fractures, especially involving the femur, tibia, and pelvis
2. Onset of symptoms occurs 1-5 days following injury: tachypnea, hemoptysis, fever, petechiae, and mental status change
3. Hypoxemia (partial pressure of O_2 in arterial blood [Pao_2] <60 mm Hg on room air) is the most consistent finding
4. Treatment includes correction of hypoxemia and ventilatory support with PEEP (if arterial oxygenation cannot be maintained). Management is similar to that of ARDS (see Chapter 15). Maintain a negative fluid balance. A pulmonary artery catheter may be required to optimize management

Pelvic fracture

Pelvic fractures caused by high-energy forces have a significant mortality rate. Hemorrhage is a major cause, as are associated injuries, sepsis, multiorgan failure, and ARDS. Infection of pelvic hematoma may occur even in closed injuries due to hematogenous spread of bacteria.

Evaluation

1. Physical examination
   a. Palpate the pelvis to determine tenderness and instability
   b. Perform pelvic and rectal examination to ascertain open injury and sphincter tone
   c. Blood at urethral meatus or high-riding prostate on rectal examination indicates urethral tear

2. Radiographs
   a. Obtain pelvic radiographs in patients suspected of sustaining a pelvic fracture and in patients with multiple trauma
   b. CT is superior in demonstrating certain aspects of pelvic injury and should be utilized in the stable patient

Hemorrhage

1. Usually retroperitoneal, the result of venous injury to the pelvic venous plexus. Hemorrhage may be massive, exceeding several liters
2. Signs of persistent bleeding are an indication for external fixation of unstable pelvic fractures
3. Application of pneumatic antishock trousers may be helpful in temporarily controlling hemorrhage (although there is considerable controversy about their efficacy). Once antishock trousers are in place, do not remove them until vascular access is established and BP is stabilized
4. Consider arteriography and selective embolization for the patient with continued severe hemorrhage

Associated injuries

1. Injuries to consider are urinary bladder perforation, vaginal or rectal laceration, and posterior urethral tear
2. If signs of urethral injury are present, retrograde urethrogram should ascertain the integrity of the urethra before urinary catheter insertion

19.7	SPINAL CORD INJURY

Consider spinal injury in any patient with multiple-system injury, head or facial injury, and those who are unconscious. Maintain spinal immobilization until radiographs exclude spinal injury.

Evaluation

1. Perform a neurologic examination to determine the extent and level of the injury
   a. Examine and document motor function and sensory level
   b. Determine if there is sacral sensory sparing or anal sphincter contraction—these are signs that cord injury is incomplete
   c. Sacral reflexes (anal wink, bulbocavernosus reflex) are the first reflexes to return after spinal shock, usually within 24 hr following injury

Management

Endotracheal intubation

1. Patients may require endotracheal intubation because of paralysis of respiratory muscles
2. If intubation is necessary, it should be done with in-line cervical immobilization
3. The orotracheal approach is preferred, preceded by 100% oxygenation by mask and application of gentle cricoid pressure
4. Administer thiopental 25-200 mg and vecuronium 0.1-0.2 mg/kg IV or ethomidate 0.3-0.6 mcg/kg prior to intubation

Respiratory care

1. Monitor breathing with frequent vital capacity measurement. Vital capacity <10 ml/kg is an indication for ventilatory assistance
2. Monitor ABGs for hypoxemia and hypercapnia

Corticosteroids

1. It is generally accepted that high-dose steroid therapy reduces secondary injury if started within 8 hr of injury
2. Administer methylprednisolone initial IV bolus 30 mg/kg followed by 5.4 mg/kg/hr for next 23 hr
3. Naloxone (5.4 mg/kg IV followed by infusion of 4 mg/kg/hr for following 23 hr) is frequently used in addition to corticosteroids, though its effectiveness has not been proven

Neurogenic shock

1. Results from an injury to the descending sympathetic pathways (usually in cervical and thoracic cord injuries) with loss of vasomotor tone and sympathetic cardiac enervation
2. Injury produces neurogenic shock, that is characterized by bradycardia and hypotension, either of which can persist for days to weeks.
3. Administer IV fluids for initial treatment of hypotension. Administer phenylephrine or dopamine if hypotension persists
4. Atropine (0.5 mg) or isoproterenol may be given if the heart rate <45bpm

Abdominal

1. Insert nasogastric tube for ileus and acute gastric dilatation
2. Consider diagnostic testing (diagnostic peritoneal lavage or CT) to determine intraabdominal injury for patients with abdominal trauma

Urologic

1. A bladder catheter should be in place for at least 4 days following injury or until other injuries are stabilized and urine output is no longer being followed. After this, intermittent catheterization may be started
2. Tape the catheter over the pubis to prevent urethral traction injury

Traction immobilization

1. Traction with Gardner-Wells tongs may be required to immobilize and align cervical injuries
   a. Weight required varies with injury
   b. Perform a neurologic examination and take radiographs frequently to determine that alignment is correct and overdistraction does not occur

Autonomic hyperreflexia

1. Result of increased autonomic nervous system (primarily sympathetic) activity caused by noxious stimulus from below the level of the cord lesion
2. Produces paroxysmal hypertension, headache, sweating, bradycardia or tachycardia, and anisocoria

3. The most common cause is bladder distention. Other causes are fecal impaction, urinary tract infection, and ureterolithiasis
4. Treatment is for the underlying cause (e.g., catheterize bladder). Anticholinergic drugs may be used

Selected Readings

Baxa MD: Cardiac rupture secondary to blunt trauma: a rapidly diagnosable entity with two-dimensional echocardiography. *Ann Emerg Med* 1991; 20:902-4.

Borel C, Hanley D, Diringer MN et al: Intensive management of severe head injury. *Chest* 1990; 98:180-9.

Boyd CR, Merriman SJ: Airway management in trauma. *Adv Trauma* 1990; 5:49-71.

Bracken MB, Shepard MJ, Collins WF, et al: A randomized, controlled trial of methylprednisolone or naloxone in the treatment of acute spinal-cord injury. *N Engl J Med* 1990; 322:1405-11.

Canizaro PC, Pessa ME: Management of massive hemorrhage associated with abdominal trauma. *Surg Clin North Am* 1990; 70:621-34.

Capan LM, Miller SM, Turndorf H, editors: *Trauma anesthesia and intensive care*, Philadelphia, 1991, JB Lippincott.

Champion HR, Sacco WJ, Carnazzo, AJ, et al: Trauma score. *Crit Care Med* 1981; 9:672-6.

Cohen M: Initial resuscitation of the patient with spinal cord injury. *Trauma Quarterly* 1993; 9:38-43.

Dearden NM, Gibson JS, McDowal DG, et al: Effect of high-dose dexamethasone on outcome from severe head injury. *J Neurosurg* 1986; 64:81-88.

Falk JL, O'Brien JF, Kerr R: Fluid resuscitation in traumatic hemorrhagic shock. *Crit Care Clin* 1992; 8:323-40.

Honigman B, Lowenstein SR, Moore EE, et al: The role of the pneumatic antishock garment in penetrating cardiac wounds. *JAMA* 1990; 266:2398-2401.

Mattox KL: Indications for thoracotomy: deciding to operate. *Surg Clin North Am* 1989; 69:47-58.

Teasdale G, Jennett B: Assessment of coma and impaired consciousness. A practical scale. *Lancet* 1974; 2:81-83.

Other Emergencies

20

Joseph Varon

ANAPHYLAXIS

1. Definition
Anaphylaxis is an immediate, generalized, life-threatening reaction to the release of bioactive substances from mast cells and basophils.
2. Etiology
The most common causes of anaphylaxis are depicted in the Box on p. 380.
3. Clinical manifestations
   a. The onset may vary from individual to individual depending on the sensitivity of the person, as well as the route, quantity, and rate of administration of the "allergen."
   b. Early signs and symptoms that require a high index of suspicion include
      (1) Agitation
      (2) Dizziness
      (3) Headache
      (4) Nausea and vomiting
   c. Cutaneous involvement
      (1) Generalized pruritus
      (2) Flushing
      (3) Urticaria
   d. Upper-airway obstruction as a consequence of edema of the larynx, and swelling of the tongue and lips (angioedema). This may result in stridor and suffocation
   e. Respiratory failure (manifestations range from tachypnea to apnea) that may be related to the factors mentioned above and to broncho-constriction of the lower airways manifested by wheezing. These patients may also develop acute respiratory distress syndrome (ARDS)
   f. Cardiovascular collapse: pathophysiology is thought to be related to enhanced vascular permeability, peripheral vasodilation, and intravascular volume depletion. A heart rate increase >20 bpm from the baseline and a decrease of mean arterial pressure (MAP) >20 torr are characteristic
   g. Dysrhythmias: Both supraventricular and ventricular rhythm disorders have been described in patients with anaphylaxis

---

Common Causes of Systemic Anaphylactic Reactions

1. Drugs
   - Antibiotics (i.e, penicillins, cephalosporins, sulfonamides, vanco-mycin)
   - Local anesthetics (i.e., lidocaine, procaine)
   - Muscle relaxants
   - Others (i.e., insulin, protamine)
2. Foods
   - Nuts and seeds
   - Fish and shellfish
   - Milk and eggs
3. Food additives
   - Aspartame
   - Monosodium glutamate
4. Diagnostics
   - Iodinated radiographic materials
5. Insect and snakes (stings and bites)
6. Exercise
7. Other
   - Latex gloves
   - Heterologous serum (i.e., tetanus antitoxin)

---

4. Laboratory findings
   a. Do *not* wait for laboratory data to institute therapy!
   b. Patients with anaphylaxis may present with leukocytosis or leukopenia
   c. Thrombocytopenia may appear in severe cases
   d. IgE measurements may not be helpful as many patients may manifest non-IgE mediated anaphylaxis
5. Management
   a. Airway, breathing, and circulation (ABCs): secure the airway and assist with breathing and circulation as with all patients presenting with a potentially critical illness
   b. The drug of choice for patients with acute anaphylaxis is epinephrine. The dosage is 0.3-0.5 ml of 1:1000 dilution (0.3-0.5 mg) subcutaneously q 10-20 min, or IV as described below
   c. Antihistamines: traditionally H_1 receptor antihistamines have been used (e.g., diphenhydramine 25-50 mg IM, IV, or PO q 6-8 hr). In theory the combination of H_1 and H_2 receptor antihistamines might have a better chance of preventing further histamine-mediated reactions than H_1-blockers alone (e.g., cimetidine 300 mg IV or PO q6hr)
   d. Corticosteroids have an uncertain place in the management of acute reaction since there is a latent period of 4-6 hr before such agents are pharmacologically effective. The current recommended agents are hydrocortisone 250 mg IV q6hr or methylprednisolone 50 mg IV q6hr for 2-4 doses

> ## Preventive Measures for Patients at High Risk for Anaphylaxis
>
> 1. Avoid exposure
> 2. Slow administration of suspected agents under medical supervision in adequate facility (e.g., ICU)
> 3. Optimal management of underlying disorders
> 4. Short- and long-term desensitization (e.g., penicillin, aspirin)

   e. In cases of severe bronchospasm the following drugs can be used
     (1) Metaproterenol 0.3 ml (5% solution) in 2.5 ml of saline, inhaled through nebulizer
     (2) Aminophylline: loading dose 6 mg/kg IV over 30 min followed by 0.3-0.9 mg/kg/hr
   f. In patients with profound hypotension
     (1) Adequate IV fluid administration (up to 1 L q 20-30 min prn)
     (2) Epinephrine: 1 ml of 1:1000 dilution in 500 ml of D_5W at a rate of 0.5-5 mcg (0.25-2.5 ml)/min
     (3) Norepinephrine: 4 mg in 1 L of D_5W at a rate of 2-12 mcg (0.5-3 ml)/min
     (4) Glucagon may be particularly useful in patients taking beta-adrenergic blockers. The recommended dose is 1 mg in 1 L of D_5W at a rate of 5-15 mcg (5-15 ml)/min
6. Preventive measures for patients at high risk of anaphylaxis are depicted in the Box above.

20.2 STEVENS-JOHNSON SYNDROME (ERYTHEMA MULTIFORME)

1. Definition
Erythema multiforme (EM) is an erythematous maculopapular cutaneous eruption of variable form. When EM progresses to a more serious clinical state, the term *Stevens-Johnson syndrome* (SJS) is used.
2. Etiology
Common causes of EM and SJS are depicted in the Box on p. 382.
3. Clinical manifestations
   a. Prodromal symptoms may include
     (1) Malaise and headache
     (2) Pharyngitis and rhinorrhea
     (3) Diarrhea
     (4) Arthralgias
   b. The earliest lesions in EM are often red, edematous papules surrounded by blanching. They enlarge to form small plaques with concentric alterations in color and morphology
   c. The so-called target lesions are areas of central epidermal necrosis with or without bulla formation
   d. Patients admitted to the ICU with SJS usually present with extensive tissue necrosis and severe fluid depletion
4. Laboratory findings
   a. Usually nondiagnostic

Causes of Erythema Multiforme/Stevens-Johnson Syndrome

1. Infections
   - Viral (e.g., herpes simplex, measles, hepatitis B)
   - Bacterial (e.g., streptococcus, pseudomonas)
   - Mycobacterial (e.g., tuberculosis)
   - Spirochetal (e.g., syphilis)
   - Fungal (e.g., histoplasmosis)
2. Drugs
   - Analgesics (e.g., aspirin, NSAIDs)
   - Antibiotics (e.g., sulfonamides, penicillins, tetracycline)
   - Anticonvulsants (e.g., ethosuximide)
   - Antihypertensives (e.g., minoxidil)
   - Glucocorticoids
   - H_2-blockers (e.g., cimetidine)
3. Immunizations
   - Horse serum
   - Polio vaccine
   - Pertussis vaccine
4. Neoplasms (e.g., lymphomas)
5. Connective tissue disorders (e.g., lupus erythematosus)
6. Physical agents
   - Radiation therapy
   - Sunlight
7. Others
   - Inflammatory bowel disease
   - Sarcoidosis

---

    b. Skin biopsy reveals a perivascular lymphocytic infiltrate in the upper dermis, subepidermal bulla formation, and endothelial cell swelling

5. Management
   a. Immediately discontinue suspected drugs or agents as well as all *nonessential* drugs
   b. The usefulness of systemic corticosteroids in this setting is controversial. In the absence of controlled clinical trials, some authors recommend beginning therapy with prednisone 1 mg/kg/day (or IV equivalent)
   c. Fluid replacement as indicated by the severity of the disease
   d. Evaluate for infection and treat appropriately
   e. Obtain consultation depending on the degree and sites of involvement (e.g., ophthalmology, plastic surgery)

20.3   ANGIONEUROTIC LARYNGEAL EDEMA

1. Definition
   Angioneurotic laryngeal edema (ALE) is characterized by nonpruritic local swelling involving the face, larynx, and skin of the extremities

2. Etiology
   a. Allergic: related to foods (e.g., fish), drugs (e.g., angiotensin converting enzyme [ACE] inhibitors), inhaled substances, and insect stings (e.g., bees)
   b. Hereditary: caused by a deficiency in C_1 esterase inhibitor. It is autosomal-dominant. Precipitating events may include trauma and emotional stress
3. Clinical manifestations
   a. Swelling of the face, larynx, and skin of extremities
   b. Depending on the progression, stridor may be a prominent feature with ensuing respiratory distress
   c. Abdominal pain, nausea, and vomiting
4. Laboratory findings
   Nondiagnostic except in cases of hereditary ALE
5. Management
   a. Airway, breathing, and circulation (ABCs): Secure the airway and assist with breathing and circulation as with all patients presenting with a potentially critical illness
   b. Avoid precipitating allergens
   c. If ALE is thought to be allergic in origin, administer parenteral epinephrine and antihistamines (as noted above for anaphylaxis)
   d. Only rarely is intubation required for patients with allergic ALE; in patients with hereditary ALE, treatment of the acute episode may require urgent intubation or tracheostomy

Suggested readings

Araujo OE, Flowers FP: Stevens-Johnson syndrome. *J Emerg Med* 1984; 2:129-35.

Bochner BS, Lichtenstein LM: Anaphylaxis. *N Engl J Med* 1991; 324:1785-90.

Patterson R, Dykewicz MS, Gonzalzles A, et al: Erythema multiforme and the Stevens-Johnson syndrome—descriptive and therapeutic controversy. *Chest* 1990; 98:331-6.

Seiman MD, Lewandoswski CA, Potesta E, et al: Angioedema related to angiotensin converting enzyme inhibitors. *Otolaryngol Head Neck Surg* 1990; 102:727-31.

Slatter E, Merrill DD, Guess HA, et al: Clinical profile of angioedema associated with angiotensin converting enzyme inhibition. *JAMA* 1988; 260:967-70.

Sheffer AL, Austen KF: Exercise-induced anaphylaxis. *J Allergy Clin Immunol* 1980; 66:106-11.

Toogood JH: Risk of anaphylaxis in patients receiving beta-blocker drugs. *J Allergy Clin Immunol* 1988; 81:1-5.

Valentine MD: Anaphylaxis and stinging insect hypersensitivity. *JAMA* 1992; 268:2830-3.

Wong S, Dykewicz MS, Patterson R: Idiopathic anaphylaxis—a clinical summary of 175 patients. *Arch Intern Med* 1990; 150:1323-8.

Appendixes

APPENDIX I: USEFUL FORMULAS IN THE ICU

Anion gap (AG)

$$AG = (Na^+ + K^+) - (Cl^- + HCO_3^-)$$

Arterial-alveolar oxygen gradient ([A − a]DO$_2$)

$$(A - a)\, DO_2 = \left([BP - P_{H2O}] \times FIo_2 - \frac{Paco_2}{RQ} \right) - Pao_2$$

BP = Barometric pressure, P_{H_2O} = water vapor pressure, FIo_2 = fraction of inspired oxygen, RQ = respiratory quotient

Arteriovenous oxygen difference (DAVo$_2$)

$$DAVo_2 = (1.38 \times Hb) \times (Sao_2 - Svo_2)$$

Cardiac index (CI)

$$CI\ (L/min/m^2) = \frac{CO}{BSA}$$

Cardiac output (CO)

$$CO = HR \times SV$$

Colloid osmotic pressure (COP)

$$COP = (1.4 \times globulin) + (5.5 \times albumin)$$

Creatinine clearance (CCr)

$$CCr = \frac{(140 - age)\ (weight\ in\ kg)}{(72 \times Cr\ [mg/100\ ml])}$$

Ejection fraction (EF)

$$\text{EF (\%)} = \frac{\text{end-diastolic volume} - \text{end-systolic volume}}{\text{end-diastolic volume}}$$

Fractional excretion of sodium (FENa)

$$\text{FENa} = \frac{(\text{urine Na}^+ \times \text{serum Cr})}{(\text{serum Na}^+ \times \text{urine Cr})}$$

Mean arterial pressure (MAP)

$$\text{MAP} = \frac{(\text{SBP} + 2\text{DBP})}{3} = \text{mmHg}$$

Oxygen consumption (VO_2)

$$VO_2 = CO \times (CaO_2 - C\bar{v}o_2)$$

Oxygen content of arterial blood (CaO_2)

$$CaO_2 \text{ (ml } O_2/100 \text{ ml blood)} = (1.38 \times \text{Hb} \times \text{Sao}_2) + (\text{Pao}_2 \times 0.0031)$$

Oxygen delivery (DO_2)

$$DO_2 = CO \times CaO_2$$

Pulmonary capillary content (CcO_2)

$$CcO_2 = (\text{Hb} \times 1.39) + P_{A}o_2 \times 0.0031$$

Serum osmolarity (Osm)

$$\text{Osm} = 2(\text{serum Na}^+) + \frac{\text{BUN}}{2.8} + \frac{\text{glucose}}{18}$$

Shunt fraction (Q_S/Q_t)

$$Q_S/Q_t \text{ (\%)} = \frac{CcO_2 - CaO_2}{CcO_2 - C\bar{v}o_2}$$

Static compliance (Cst)

$$\text{Cst} = \frac{V_T}{(\text{Pplat} - \text{PEEP})}$$

Stroke volume (SV)

$$\text{SV (ml)} = \text{end-diastolic volume} - \text{end-systolic volume}$$

Stroke work (SW)

$$\text{SW} = \text{SV} \times (\text{BP-Pla})$$

Systemic vascular resistance (SVR)

$$SVR = \frac{MAP - CVP}{CO} \times 80$$

APPENDIX II: PHARMACOLOGIC AGENTS COMMONLY USED IN THE ICU

Acetaminophen (Tylenol)

Route: PO, PR
Dosage: 325-650 mg q 4-6 hr (adults); 60 mg/kg/24hr in divided doses q 4-6 hr (children)

Acetazolamide (Diamox)

Route: PO, IV
Dosage: for metabolic alkalosis
250 mg q 6-12 h

for altitude sickness
250 mg q 6-24 hr

Acetylcysteine (Mucomyst)

Route: PO, IV, nebulized
Dosage: for acetaminophen toxicity
PO: dilute to 5% with cola or other soft drink. Initial dose 140 mg/kg, then 70 mg/kg for 17 doses (do not give activated charcoal)
IV: load with 150 mg/kg in 200 ml D_5W over 15 min, then 50 mg/kg in 500 ml D_5W over 4 hr, followed by 100 mg/kg in 100 ml D_5W over 16 hr

Activated charcoal (Charcoaide)

Route: PO
Dosage: for poisoning
INITIAL: 30-100 g (1 g/kg) in 250 ml water
MAINTENANCE: 20-40 g q6hr until drug is removed from body

Adenosine (Adenocard)

Route: IV
Dosage: 3,6,9,12 mg (fast IV injection)

Ammonium chloride (generic)

Route: PO, IV
Dosage: for urine acidification
4-12 g/day PO in divided doses q 4-6 hr

Amrinone (Inocor)

Route: IV
Dosage: bolus 0.75-3 mg/kg over 2-3 min, followed by infusion of 5-20 mcg/kg/min

Atropine (generic)

Route: PO, IV, nebulized
Dosage: for bronchospasm
1.5-2 mg by nebulizer q6hr.
for bradycardia
0.5-1 mg IV push, repeat q5min to max 2 mg

Bretylium (Bretylol)

Route: IV, IM
Dosage: bolus 5-10 mg/kg over 10-20 min IV, followed by a continuous infusion 1-5 mg/min

Carbicarb (Carbicarb)

Route: IV
Dosage: for severe acidosis
initial dose is 1 mEq/kg, followed by 0.5 mEq/kg (adjust dose as indicated by clinical condition and blood pH)

Chlordiazepoxide (Librium)

Route: PO, IV, IM
Dosage: 15-100 mg/day in 3-4 divided doses

Chlorpromazine (Thorazine)

Route: PO, PR, IM
Dosage: for severe psychosis with agitation
25-100 mg IM q 1-4 hr until control is achieved

Clonidine (Catapres)

Route: PO, transdermal, ?PR
Dosage: in hypertensive emergencies: 0.2 mg PO, then 0.1 mg/hr to 0.8 mg or BP is controlled

Dantrolene (Dantrium)

Route: PO, IV
Dosage: for malignant hyperthermia
initial dose 1-2 mg/kg IV via rapid infusion. May repeat to total 10 mg/kg if needed

DDAVP (generic)

Route: intranasal, IV, SC
Dosage: hemostasis
0.3 mcg/kg in NS over 15-30 min.
for diabetes insipidus
0.5-1 ml IV/SC bid

Diazepam (Valium)

Route: PO, IV, IM
Dosage: for status epilepticus
5-10 mg IV (1-2 mg/min)

Diazoxide (Hyperstat)

Route: PO, IV
Dosage: for hypertensive crisis
 1-3 mg/kg IV (max 150 mg) q 5-15 min until BP is controlled

Digoxin (Lanoxin)

Route: PO, IV, IM
Dosage: for digitalization
 0.4-0.6 mg IV (may require up to 1.25 mg total)
 for maintenance
 0.125-0.25 mg/day PO or IV

Dobutamine (Dobutrex)

Route: IV
Dosage: 2.5-15 mcg/kg/min most commonly used

Dopamine (Intropin)

Route: IV
Dosage: for dopaminergic stimulation
 0.5-2 mcg/kg/min
 alpha, beta, dopaminergic effects
 >10 mcg/kg/min

Epinephrine (Epinephrine Injection)

Route: IV, SC
Dosage: for $beta_1$, $beta_2$ effects
 1-4 mcg/min
 for alpha effects
 4 mcg/min

Esmolol (Brevibloc)

Route: IV
Dosage: bolus 0.5-1 mg/kg followed by infusion at 50 mcg/kg/min
 MAINTENANCE: 50-200 mcg/kg/min

Fentanyl (Sublimaze)

Route: IV, IM
Dosage: for sedation/analgesia
 1 mcg/kg IV/IM

Flumazenil (Romazicon)

Route: IV
Dosage: 0.3 mg IV

Furosemide (Lasix)

Route: PO, IV, IM
Dosage: 10-120 mg IV/IM, adjusted as necessary until desired response
 obtained. May use continuous infusions

Glucagon (generic)

Route: SC, IM, IV
Dosage: for hypoglycemia
0.5-1 mg SC/IM/IV, may repeat in 15 min
for bradycardia
1-20 mg/hr

Haloperidol (Haldol)

Route: PO, IM, IV (not FDA-approved)
Dosage: for acute psychosis
2-5 mg IM q 1-2 hr until symptoms are controlled

Heparin (Liquaemin)

Route: IV, SC
Dosage: for DVT prophylaxis
5000 U SC q 8-12 hr.
for DVT/pulmonary emboli therapy
bolus with 100 U/kg followed by a continuous infusion of 800-1200 U/hr, titrated to maintain APTT 1½-2 × control

Hydralazine (Apresoline)

Route: PO, IV
Dosage: 5 mg IV bolus; 5-10 mg IV q6hr maintenance

Isoproterenol (Isuprel)

Route: IV, SC, PO, inhaled
Dosage: infusion 1-10 mcg/min

Ketorolac Tromethamine (Toradol)

Route: PO, IM
Dosage: initial dose 30-60 mg IM, then 15-30 mg q6hr

Labetalol (Normodyne)

Route: PO, IV
Dosage: for rapid BP control
IV bolus 5-20 mg (slowly), repeat after 5 min if needed. Continuous infusion of 1 mg/ml started at 1-2 mg/min and titrated to effect

Lidocaine (Xylocaine)

Route: IV, IM, SC
Dosage: bolus 1-1.5 mg/kg followed by 1-4 mg/min

Lorazepam (Ativan)

Route: PO, IV, IM
Dosage: 2-10 mg/day in divided doses PO/IV/IM (some patients may require continuous infusions)

Mannitol (Osmitrol)

Route: IV
Dosage: for cerebral edema
IV infusion 0.15-2 g/kg as 15%-25% solution over 30-60 min; max dose up to 6 g/kg/24hr

Meperidine (Demerol)

Route: PO, IM, IV, SC
Dosage: 50-150 mg q 3-4 hr

Midazolam (Versed)

Route: IV, IM
Dosage: 1-4 mg q 2-6 hr

Morphine (Duramorph)

Route: IM, IV, PO, PR
Dosage: 5-10 mg q 4-6 hr (some patients may require continuous infusions)

Naloxone (Narcan)

Route: IV, IM, SC
Dosage: 0.4-2 mg IV, may repeat up to 10 mg. Continuous IV infusion at 4-5 mcg/kg/min may be used

Nitroglycerin (Nitroglycerin)

Route: PO, IV, SL, topical
Dosage: 10-400 mcg/min IV

Norepinephrine (Levophed)

Route: IV
Dosage: 4-10 mcg/min

Phenobarbital (Barbita)

Route: PO, PR, IM, IV
Dosage: for status epilepticus
10 mg/kg IV at 50 mg/min; up to 20 mg/kg total (adults)

Phentolamine (Regitine)

Route: IV, IM
Dosage: ADULTS: 5 mg IV/IM prn, taper to effect
CHILDREN: 0.1 mg/kg IV prn

Phenylephrine (Neo-Synephrine)

Route: IV
Dosage: 15 mg dissolved in 250 ml D_5W (60 mcg/ml); start at 20-30 mcg/min, titrate to desired BP

Procainamide (Procainamide)

Route: PO, IV
Dosage: 100 mg/min IV to effect or to total dose of 1000 mg, followed
by infusion 2-6 mg/min

Prochlorperazine (Compazine)

Route: PO, IM, IV, PR
Dosage: 5-10 mg PO tid/qid; 5-10 mg IV q 3-4 hr; 25 mg PR bid

Propranolol (Inderal)

Route: PO, IV
Dosage: titrate 0.5-1 mg IV q5min to effect

Protamine (Protamine Sulfate)

Route: IV
Dosage: 1 mg for each 90 U of lung heparin or 1 mg for each 115 U
intestinal heparin by slow injection over 1-3 min; max dose 50
mg any 10 min

Sodium bicarbonate (Sodium Bicarbonate Injection)

Route: IV, PO
Dosage: for severe acidosis
initial dose 1 mEq/kg, followed by 0.5 mEq/kg; adjust dosage
as indicated by clinical condition and blood pH

Sodium nitroprusside (Nipride)

Route: IV
Dosage: mix 50 mg in 250 ml D_5W; start at 0.5 mcg/kg/min and titrate
to effect

Sodium polystyrene sulfonate (Kayexalate)

Route: PO, PR
Dosage: 15 g, PO q 6-24 hr

Succinylcholine (Anectine)

Route: IV, IM
Dosage: 1-1.5 mg/kg IV; 2-4 mg/kg IM (pediatric use only)

Thiopental (Pentothal sodium)

Route: IV, PR
Dosage: for general anesthetic
2-3 ml 2.5% solution (50-75 mg) IV q 20-40 sec until desired
effect reached
for seizures 75-125 mg IV

Trimethaphan (Arfonad)

Route: IV
Dosage: start at 0.3 mg/min and titrate to effect

APPENDIX III: ECG RHYTHM RECOGNITION

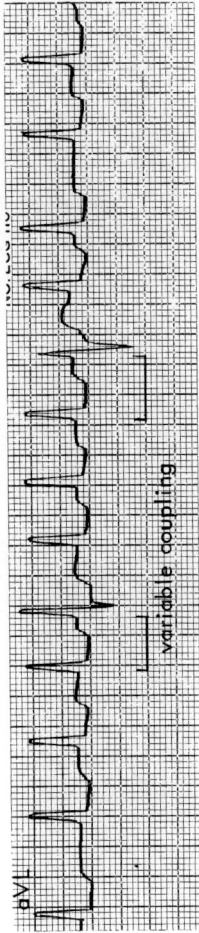

Figure 1
Atrial fibrillation

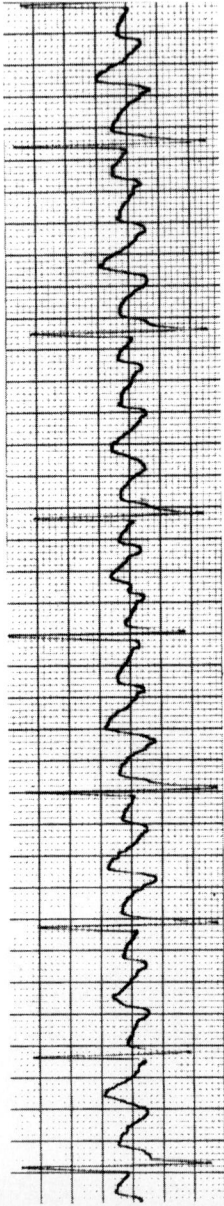

Figure 2
Atrial flutter

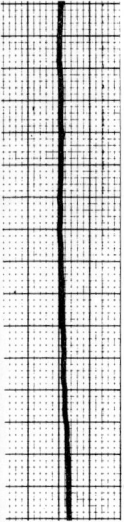

Figure 3
Asystole

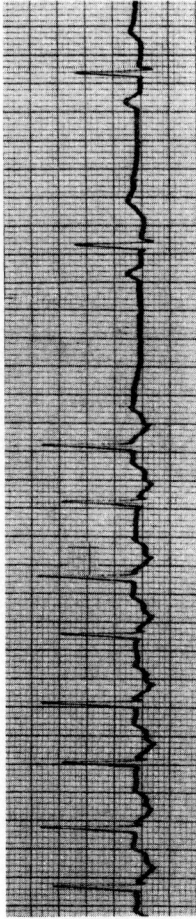

Figure 4
Supraventricular tachycardia

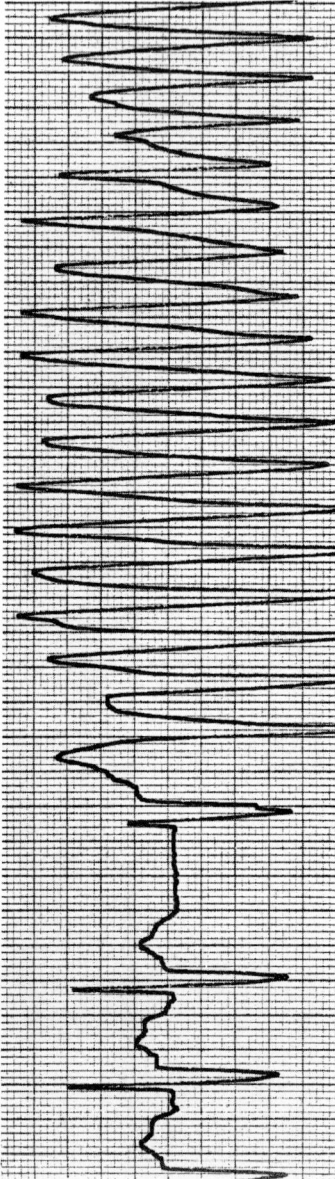

Figure 5
Torsades de pointes

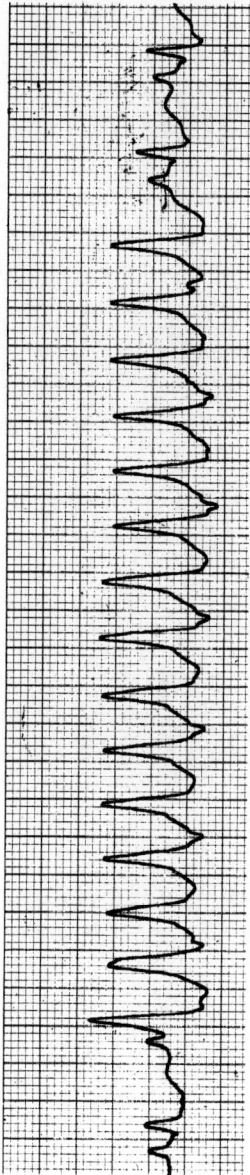

Figure 6
Ventricular tachycardia

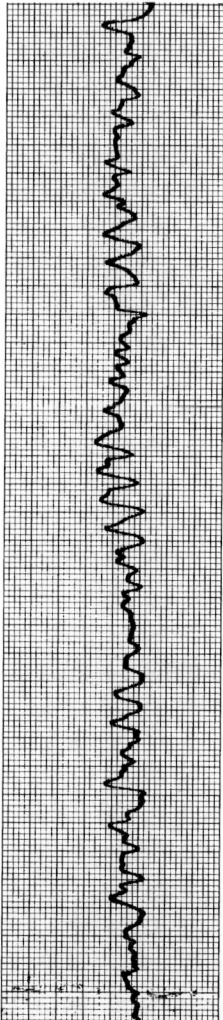

Figure 7
Ventricular fibrillation

Nomogram

| Height cm in | For children of normal height for weight | SA M² | Weight lb kg |

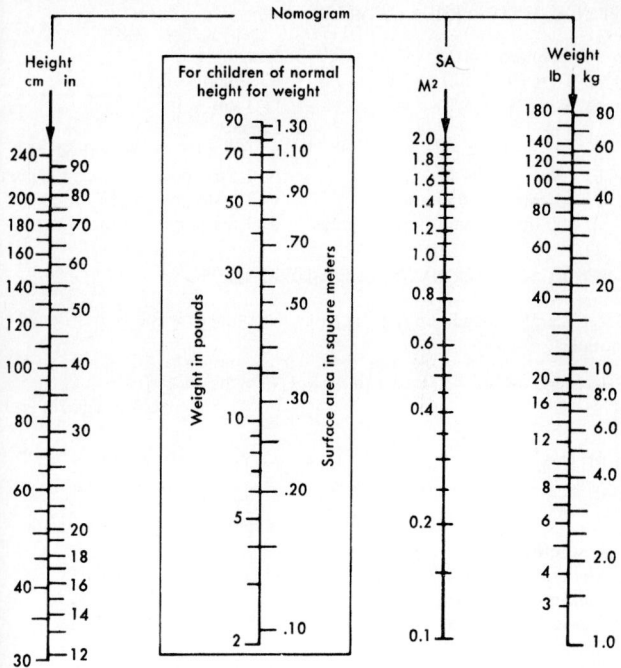

APPENDIX IV: NOMOGRAM FOR CALCULATION OF BODY SURFACE AREA

Place a straight edge from the patient's height in the left column to the weight in the right column. The point of intersection on the body surface area column indicates the body surface area (BSA). From Behrman RE, Vaughn VC (editors): *Nelson's textbook of pediatrics,* ed 12, Philadelphia, 1983, WB Saunders.

APPENDIX V: CONVERSION FORMULAS

1. Temperature
   a. °C = (°F − 32) × 5/9
   b. °F = (°C × 9/5) + 32
2. Weight
   a. 1 lb = 0.454 kg
   b. 1 kg = 2.204 lb
   c. 10 grains = 650 mg
   d. 400 micrograms = 1/150 grain
3. Length
   a. 1 inch = 2.54 cm
   b. 1 cm = 0.3937 inch
4. Liquid
   a. 100 ml = 3.38 fluid ounces
   b. 1 fluid ounce = 30 ml approx
   c. 1 tablespoon = 15 ml
   d. 1 teaspoon = 5 ml

APPENDIX VI: DETERMINATION OF CALORIC NEEDS

Basal energy expenditure (BEE) can be determined by the Harris-Benedict formulas*

BEE (male: 66 + (13.7 × wt [in kg]) + (5 × ht [in cm])
$$− (6.8 × age [in yrs])$$

[2]BEE (female: 65.5 + (9.6 × wt [in kg]) + (1.7 × ht [in cm])
$$−(4.7 × age [in yrs])$$

For states other than basal, the BEE is multiplied by a correction factor
   Low stress—1.3 × BEE
   Moderate stress—1.5 × BEE
   Cancer—1.6 × BEE
   Sepsis (normotensive)—1.7 × BEE
   Severe stress—2 × BEE
   Severe burn (>40% of body surface area, normotensive patient)—
      2.5 × BEE

APPENDIX VII: COMMON CAUSES OF ACIDOSIS

I. Non-anion gap acidosis
   A. Renal bicarbonate loss
      1. Renal tubular acidosis
      2. Interstitial renal disease
      3. Hypoaldosteronism
      4. Urinary tract obstruction
      5. Carbonic anhydrase inhibitors
   B. Gastrointestinal loss
      1. Diarrhea
      2. Ileal loop, ureterosigmoidostomy
      3. Enteric fistula
      4. Anion exchange resins

---

*From Rutten P, Blackburn GL, et al: Determination of optimal hyperalimentation infusion rate, *J Surg Res* 1975; 18:477.

B. Acidifying agents
1. Ammonium chloride
2. Arginine HCl
3. Lysine HCl
4. Hydrochloric acid
C. Miscellaneous
1. Dehydration
2. Hyperalimentation (with obsolete formulations)
3. Sulfur ingestion
II. Anion gap acidosis
A. Toxins
1. Methanol
2. Salicylates
3. Ethylene glycol
4. Paraldehyde
B. Diabetes
1. Diabetic ketoacidosis
2. Nonketotic hyperosmolar state
C. Nondiabetic ketoacidosis
1. Starvation
2. Ethanol intoxication
D. Renal failure
1. Uremic acidosis
E. Lactic acidosis
1. Shock (increased lactate production)
2. Excessive exercise (increased lactate production)
3. Liver failure (decreased metabolism)
F. Inborn errors of metabolism

APPENDIX VIII: COMMON CAUSES OF METABOLIC ALKALOSIS

Metabolic alkalosis results from conditions that cause base accumulation or net loss of hydrogen ions from the blood. It is usually characterized by an alkalemic pH (>7.45) and elevated serum bicarbonate (>27.0 mEq/L). Metabolic alkaloses often are classified according to whether they are responsive or unresponsive to sodium chloride administration. Responsiveness to sodium chloride administration implies that metabolic alkalosis is maintained as a consequence of intravascular volume depletion. A third, miscellaneous group is not well characterized.

I. Sodium chloride–responsive metabolic alkalosis
A. Gastrointestinal disorders
1. Vomiting
2. Villous adenoma

    3. Nasogastric suctioning
    4. Diarrhea
  B. Diuretic therapy
  C. Post-hypercapnia
  D. Cystic fibrosis
II. Sodium chloride–resistant metabolic alkalosis
  A. Excessive mineralocorticoid activity
    1. Hyperaldosteronism
    2. Licorice intoxication
    3. Cushing's syndrome
    4. Bartter's syndrome
  B. Profound potassium depletion
  C. Excessive use of chewing tobacco
III. Miscellaneous causes of metabolic alkalosis
  A. Administration of alkalinizing agents
  B. Milk-alkali syndrome
  C. Nonparathyroid hypercalcemia
  D. Massive doses of carbenicillin or penicillin
  E. Hypoparathyroidism
  F. Massive transfusion (secondary to citrate metabolism)
  G. Massive infusion of lactated IV solutions

APPENDIX IX: ANTIDOTES TO POISONING/OVERDOSE

I. General treatment
  A. Decrease absorption
    1. Emesis (apomorphine, ipecac)
    2. Lavage
    3. Activated charcoal
    4. Cathartics
  B. Increase elimination
    1. Diuresis (alkaline or acid)
    2. Activated charcoal
    3. Cathartics
    4. Dialysis
  C. Antidotes
II. Poison (overdose)/antidote
  A. Acetaminophen
    1. Acetylcysteine
      a. ADULT: Load with 140 mg/kg PO diluted with water, soft drink, or juice.
        (1) MAINTENANCE: 17 additional doses of 70 mg/kg q4hr; activated charcoal to absorb acetylcysteine
  B. Anticholinesterases, organophosphates, carbamate pesticides
    1. Atropine sulfate
      a. ADULT: 2-5 mg IV q 10-30 min prn
      b. PEDIATRIC: 0.05 mg/kg IV q 10-30 min prn
    2. Pralidoxime chloride:
      a. ADULT: 1 g IV over 2-30 min; repeat q8hr if muscle weakness persists

    b. PEDIATRIC: 25-50 mg/kg IV; repeat q8hr

C. Anticholinergics, tricyclics, antihistamines
   1. Physostigmine salicylate
     a. ADULT: 2 mg IV over 2-3 min; repeat with 1-2 mg dose in 20 min if symptoms persist
     b. PEDIATRIC: 0.5 mg IV over 2-3 min; repeat dose in 5-10 min if symptoms persist
   2. Sodium bicarbonate for tricyclics: raise pH >7.5
   3. Activated charcoal for tricyclics: increases elimination

D. Benzodiazepines
   1. Activated charcoal: increases elimination
   2. Flumazenil;—use contraindicated if other drugs were ingested

E. Calcium channel blockers
   1. Calcium for muscle contraction
   2. Glucagon, catecholamines, atropine for bradycardia

F. Carbon monoxide
   1. 100% oxygen or hyperbaric oxygen

G. Cyanide (nitroprusside)
   1. Amyl nitrite inhalant (step 1)
     a. ADULT: Inhale for 30 sec q 1-2 min
   2. Sodium nitrite (step 2)
     a. ADULT: 300 mg in 10 ml IV over 2-4 min; repeat if symptoms recur
   3. Sodium thiosulfate (step 3)
     a. ADULT: 12.5 g in 50 ml IV over 10 min
   4. Hydroxycobalamin IV, if available

H. Digoxin
   1. Digoxin immune fab (Digibind)
     a. ADULT: depends on amount to be neutralized (see package insert); if dose unknown, give 800 mg IV over 30 min

I. Ethanol
   1. Thiamine

J. Ethylene glycol
   1. Ethanol
     a. ADULT: 0.6 g/kg, then 110-130 mg/kg/hr
   2. Thiamine: 100 mg
   3. Pyridoxine: 100 mg q6hr × 4 doses
   4. Calcium for hypocalcemia
   5. Bicarbonate for acidosis
   6. Hemodialysis: level >50 mg/dl

K. Heavy metals
   IRON
   1. Deferoxamine mesylate
     a. ADULT/PEDIATRIC: 1000 mg IM/IV initially, then 500 mg q4hr × 2 doses. SUBSEQUENT DOSES: 500 mg q 4-12 hr may be given, to max 6 g/day (urine will turn pink)
   IRON, LEAD, MERCURY, COPPER, NICKEL, ZINC, CADMIUM, COBALT
   1. Calcium disodium edetate (EDTA)
     a. ADULT: 75 mg/kg/day deep IM or slow IV infusion given in 3-6 divided doses for up to 5 days

MERCURY, ARSENIC, GOLD
  1. Dimercaprol (BAL)
     a. ADULT: 3-5 mg/kg deep IM q4hr × 2 days; q 4-6 hr × 2 more days; then q 4-12 hr for up to 12 more days
     b. Requires adequate renal and hepatic function to excrete toxins
     c. Do not use for iron toxicity

LEAD, IRON, MERCURY, COPPER
  1. D-Penicillamine
     a. ADULT: 250 mg PO q6hr × 5 days (do not exceed 40 mg/kg/day)
     b. PEDIATRIC: 24-50 mg/kg PO q6hr

L. Heparin
   1. Protamine sulfate
      a. ADULT: 5 ml 1% solution slowly IV over 10 min (give 1-1.25 mg protamine for each 100 U heparin); max 50 mg as single dose

M. Hyperkalemia
   1. Calcium chloride: 5-10 ml 10% over 5 min
   2. Insulin and glucose: 5-10 U regular insulin with 1 amp $D_{50}W$
   3. Sodium bicarbonate: 44 mEq over 5 min
   4. Sodium polystyrene sulfonate (Kayexalate): 1 g binds 1 mEq K^+
      a. Give 20-50 g PO in 100 ml 20% sorbitol q 3-4 hr as indicated by clinical response
      b. RETENTION ENEMA: 50 g Kayexalate plus 50 g sorbitol in 200 ml water; retain 30-60 min; repeat hourly as indicated by clinical response
   5. Diuresis: furosemide
   6. Dialysis

N. Hypermagnesemia
   1. Calcium chloride: 5-10 ml 10% over 5-10 min
   2. Diuresis: furosemide
   3. Dialysis

O. Hyperphosphatemia
   1. Phosphate-binding antacids
      a. Aluminum containing (Amphojel)
   2. Diuresis
   3. Dialysis

P. Isopropyl alcohol
   1. Lavage
   2. Activated charcoal
   3. Nasogastric suction (secreted in saliva and gastric juice)
   4. Hemodialysis

Q. Methanol
   1. Ethanol
      a. ADULT: 0.6 g/kg; then 60-150 mg/kg/hr
   2. Folate: 1 mg/kg q4hr
   3. Bicarbonate for acidosis
   4. Hemodialysis: level >50 mg/dL

R. Opiates
   1. Naloxone hydrochloride
      a. ADULT: 0.4-0.8 mg IV bolus; may need to repeat q 20-60 min to maintain effect
      b. PEDIATRIC: 0.01 mg/kg IV bolus (naloxone action is shorter than narcotic action)
S. Salicylates
   1. Alkaline diuresis
   2. Activated charcoal
   3. Hemodialysis if severe
   4. Bicarbonate for metabolic acidosis
   5. Glucose for hypoglycemia
   6. Vitamin K for hypoprothrombinemia
T. Theophylline
   1. Activated charcoal: 50-100 g initially, then 30-50 g q 2-4 hr (mix in 100 ml 70% sorbitol)
   2. Charcoal hemoperfusion
U. Warfarin
   1. Fresh blood, coagulation factors
   2. Vitamin K analogs
      a. ADULT: 10 mg IM for large ingestion (can be given PO)
      b. PEDIATRIC: 1-5 mg IM

APPENDIX X: SELECTED SERUM/PLASMA DRUG LEVELS

Drug	Sample	Conventional Level	SI Units
Acetaminophen	Plasma	Toxic >5 mg/dl	>300 μmol/L
Amikacin	Serum	Peak/trough = 15-25/<10 μg/ml	
Carbamazepine	Plasma	4-10 mg/L	17-42 μmol/L
Chlorpromazine	Plasma	50-300 g/ml	150-950 mol/L
Chlorpropamide	Plasma	75-250 mg/L	270-900 μmol/L
Cyclosporine	Serum	125-300 μg/L	
Digoxin	Plasma	0.5-2.0 g/mL	0.6-2.6 mol/L
Disopyramide	Plasma	2-6 g/L	6-18 μmol/L
Ethanol	Plasma	Legal <80 mg/dl	<17 mmol/L
		Toxic >100 mg/dl	>22 mmol/L
Ethosuximide	Plasma	40-110 mg/L	280-780 μmol/L
Gentamicin	Serum	Peak/trough = 5-8/<2 μg/ml	
Gold	Serum	300-800 μg/dL	15-40 μmol/L
Lidocaine	Plasma	1-5 mg/L	4.5-21.5 μmol/L
Lithium	Serum	0.5-1.5 mEq/L	0.5-1.5 mmol/L
Meprobamate	Plasma	Therapeutic <20 mg/L	<90 μmol/L
		Toxic >40 mg/L	>180 μmol/L
Nitroprusside thiocyanate	Plasma	Toxic >10 mg/dl	>1.7 mmol/L

Continued.

Drug	Sample	Conventional Level	SI Units
Nortriptyline	Plasma	25-200 g/mL	90-760 mol/L
NAPA	Plasma	6-20 mg/L	
Pentobarbital	Plasma	20-40 mg/L	90-170 μmol/L
Phenobarbital	Plasma	2-5 mg/dl	85-215 μmol/L
Phenytoin	Plasma	10-20 mg/L	40-80 μmol/L
Primidone	Plasma	6-10 mg/L	25-46 μmol/L
Procainamide	Plasma	4-8 mg/L	17-34 μmol/L
Propoxyphene	Plasma	Toxic >2 mg/L	>5.9 μmol/L
Quinidine	Plasma	1.5-5 mg/L	4.6-15.4 μmol/L
Salicylate	Serum	Toxic >20 mg/dl	>1.45 mmol/L
Theophylline	Plasma	10-20 mg/L	55-110 μmol/L
Tobramycin	Serum	Peak/trough = 5-8/<2 μg/ml	
Vancomycin	Serum	Peak/trough = 30-40/5-10 μg/ml	

APPENDIX XI: COMPARISON OF MUSCLE RELAXANTS

	Advantages	Disadvantages
Tubocurarine	1. Inexpensive 2. Long-acting	1. Potential for histamine release 2. Long-acting
Metocurine	1. Inexpensive 2. Long-acting 3. Low potential for hemodynamic instability	1. Long-acting 2. Predominantly renally excreted, of concern in patients with renal failure
Pancuronium	1. Preserves hemodynamic function	1. Potential for tachycardia
Vecuronium	1. No hemodynamic effects 2. Predominantly biliary excretion (80%), good in patients with renal failure	1. Relatively short-acting
Atracurium	1. Minor, if any, hemodynamic alterations 2. Unique metabolism not requiring renal or hepatic function	1. Prolonged infusions in renal failure patients may produce significant serum laudanosine levels

	Advantages	Disadvantages
Succinylcholine	1. Short-acting (<5 min) 2. Does not require renal or hepatic metabolism	1. Potential for profound hyperkalemia (see text) 2. Prolonged action in patients with pseudo-cholinesterase deficiency 3. Potential for myalgias and myoglobinemia and myoglobinuria 4. Implicated as causative factor in malignant hyperthermia 5. Potential for dysrhythmias

Index